A Guide to Physiological Breech Birth
by Rixa Freeze, PhD, David Hayes, MD, and Kristine Lauria, CPM

Table of Contents

We want to thank Cynthia Caillagh, CPM, Betty-Anne Daviss, RM, and many other breech practitioners and parents for their input.

Introduction

A Guide to Physiological Breech Birth initially came about while Breech Without Borders was training Amish midwives, many of whom do not use electricity or internet. While some of them could watch our online content at "English" friends' houses, others were unable to do so. We wanted to create a printed version of our online breech training course to enable everyone to have the same learning opportunities.

With that audience in mind, the guide came into being. We kept the tone engaging and conversational, wanting it to sound less like a textbook and more like sitting in a room with us, learning about breech birth. We hope you enjoy it—wherever in the world you are and whatever language you speak.

Rixa Freeze, PhD
David Hayes, MD
Kristine Lauria, CPM

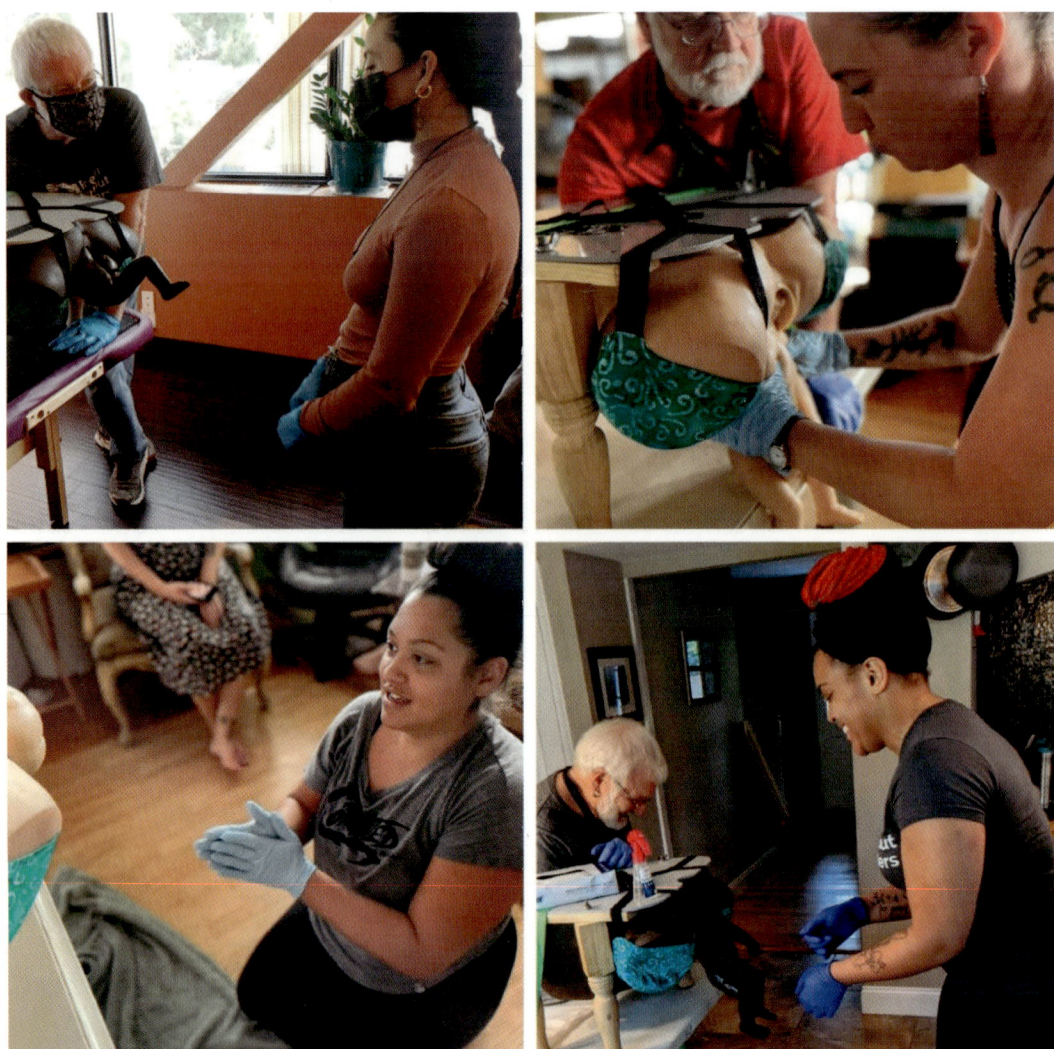

1st edition
ISBN: 979-8-9868301-0-0

10 steps of physiological breech

	Normal	Deviation	Possible Cause
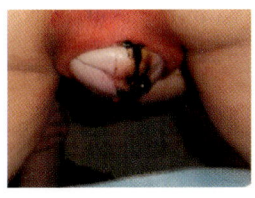	1. Baby rumps sacrum transverse	not ST when rumping	
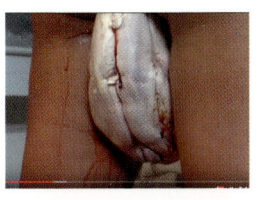	2. Baby turns SA as hips/torso emerge	Remains ST . . . . Turns SP . . . . Turns SA w/out descent . . . Turns SA w/ asymmetry . . .	Nuchal arm(s) Leg/knee/arm obstruction Head extended in inlet Raised arm
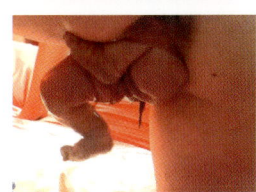	3. Legs release spontaneously	Legs do not release	Leg/knee obstruction (nonfrank) Head extended in inlet causing arrest of descent
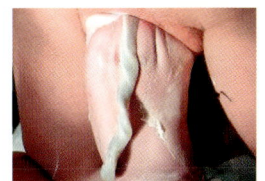	4. Chest crease ("cleavage") = arms NOT trapped	No chest crease; chest pulled tight on 1 or both sides	Nuchal arm(s)
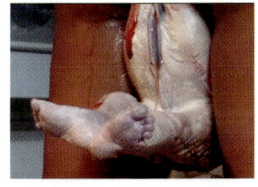	5. Tummy crunches flex head & bring arms down	No tummy crunches	Poor fetal condition
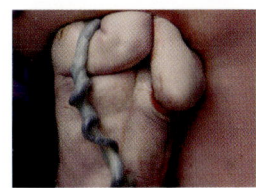	6. Arms release spontaneously. Arm lifts help flex head	Arms do not release spontaneously	Poor fetal condition Soft tissue dystocia
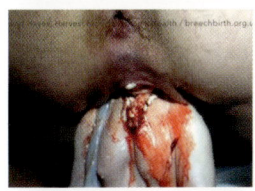	7. Full perineum = flexed head	Perineum appears hollow/deflated	Deflexed head
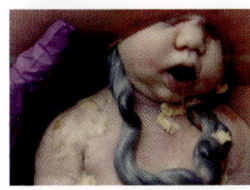	8. Head releases spontaneously	Head does not release spontaneously	Soft tissue dystocia
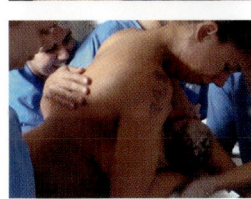	9. Baby passed to mother 10. Cord intact, incl. during resuscitation	Baby separated from mother Cord cut/clamped	Provider

Vaginal breech decision tree

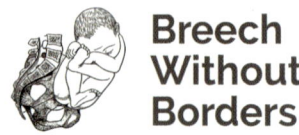

Breech Without Borders

1. Is there a deviation?

Yes   No ⟶ . . . .

2. What's causing the deviation?
legs/arms/head/maternal soft tissues

3. Is the deviation interfering with the birth?

Yes   No ⟶ . . . .

Unsure ⟶ . . . . . .

4. Do I need to intervene? Consider:
fetal condition (color/tone/FHR)
time elapsed
morbidity from intervention vs. risk of doing nothing

Yes   No ⟶ . . . .

> **Do nothing**
>
> **"Sit on your hands if you must" (Mary Cronk)**
>
> **Carefully observe progress (descent & rotation)**
>
> **Encourage maternal movement & position changes**

Continue encouraging maternal movement/position changes

release arms/shoulders

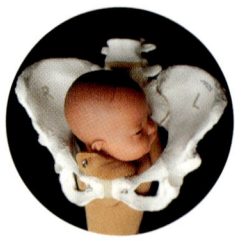

flex/disimpact head

Side to Side maneuver
- shoulder grip
- disimpact; rotate 180° through SA to the other side (baby "follows the rainbow")
- rotate 90° back to face you (SA)

Front to Back maneuver
- prayer hands or shoulder grip
- disimpact; rotate 90° to sacrum posterior
- sweep anterior arm
- rotate 180° back to face you (SA)

Head in midpelvis/outlet
- shoulder press
  - if ineffective, try rock & roll
- gluteal lift / perineal lift

Then try other flexion techniques:
- Ritgen
- Crowning Touch
- upright MSV

Head in pelvic inlet (rare)
- Elevate baby against counterpressure until the head **flexes** and **flops** to the side, then **drop** head into oblique with fundal pressure

Posterior deflexed head (rare)
- Chin tuck or disimpaction & 180° rotation

Weigh potential morbidity of intervention vs. risk of waiting

Problems

Solutions

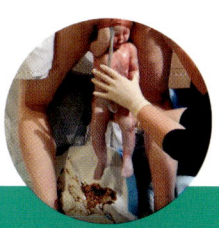

Upright

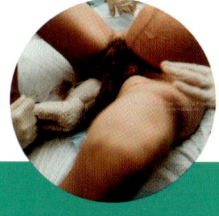

Supine

Fundal pressure

- Maternal exhaustion
- Poor contraction pattern
- Poor fetal condition
- Diagnosing an obstruction

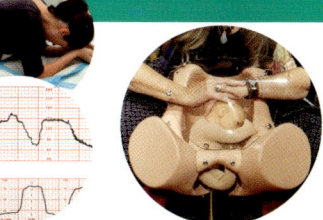

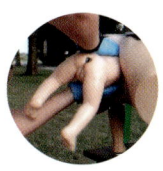

- Can augment a contraction or replace a missing/delayed contraction
- Done only after buttocks are on the perineum

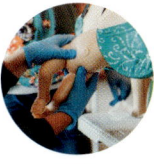

Release arms/shoulders (between contractions)

Baby stuck in a side-facing position with no progress

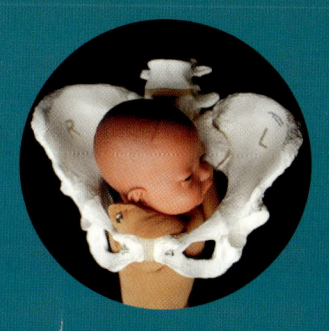

Side to Side (Louwen) maneuver
"face to thigh, then spine"

- Disimpact, rotate 180° through SA to the other side
- Rotate 90° back to SA

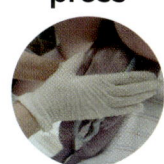

Front to Back maneuver
"face to pubes, then spine"

- Disimpact, rotate 90° to SP (face to pubes)
- Sweep anterior arm
- Rotate 180° back to SA

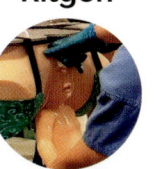

Løvset maneuver
- Lateral flexion towards pubic bone
- 180° rotation w/ traction
- 1st shoulder delivers under pubic arch
- Repeat flexion & rotation for other shoulder
- Rotate baby 90° to SA

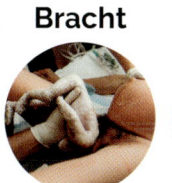

Upright Løvset
- Same as supine Løvset, but thumbs on front of baby's pelvis

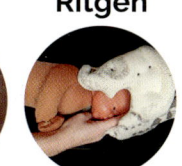

Flex/disimpact head (between or during contractions)

Extended head in the pelvic outlet

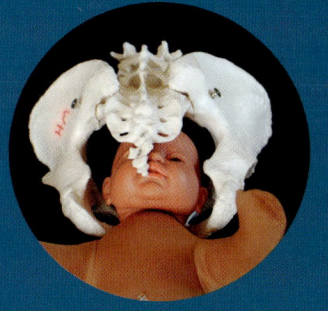

Shoulder press

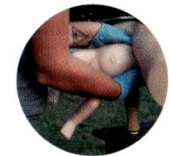

Rock & Roll

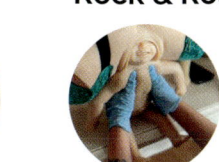

Ritgen

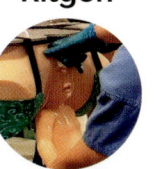

Crowning Touch

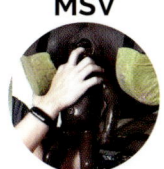

Upright MSV

Bracht

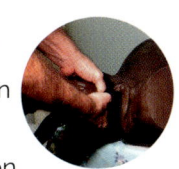

Burns-Marshall

Ritgen

MSV

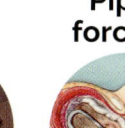

Piper forceps

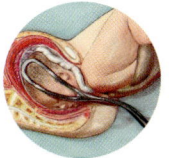

Flex, flop, & drop

Hyperextended head in pelvic inlet (rare)

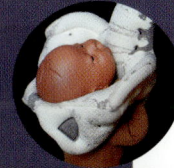

Elevate head against counterpressure until it **flexes** and **flops** to the side, then **drop** head into oblique with fundal pressure

Tuck chin under pubic bone - or -
Disimpact & rotate 180° back to SA

SP chin stuck on pubic bone (rare)

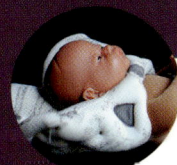

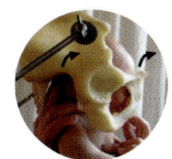

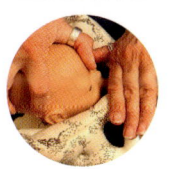

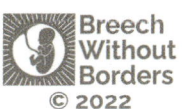

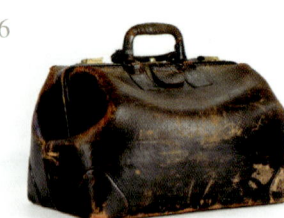

6 essential breech birth tools

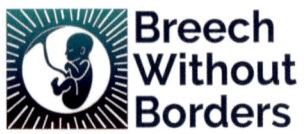

**Breech
Without
Borders**

Head flexion

Disimpaction, rotation, &/or extraction

1. Shoulder press

- Shoulder grip or flat hand
- Press directly towards pubic bone
- Rock & roll if head doesn't release

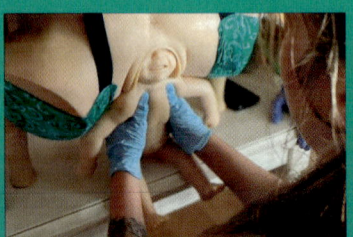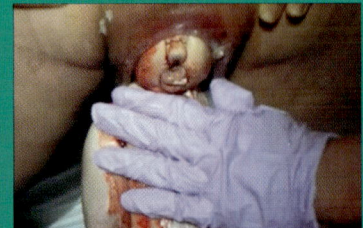

2. Crowning touch

- 2 fingers along cheekbone until you touch the ear
- Angle fingers down behind neck & occiput
- Tilt wrist forward, using your other 2 fingers as a fulcrum

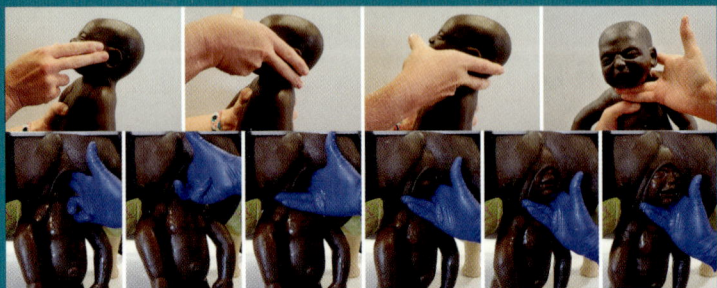

3. Ritgen

- Insert 1-2 lubricated fingers into the rectum
- Reach as far back as you can and flex the top of the baby's head forward
- Can be done upright or supine

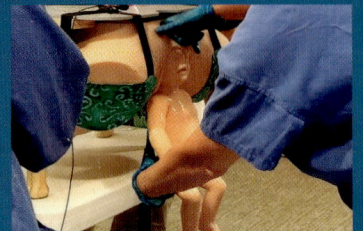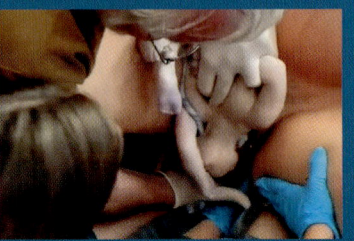

4. Side to Side

- Baby stuck sacrum transverse
- Shoulder grip or scissor grip
- Upright = thumbs anterior
- Disimpact & rotate 180° to the other side, then 90° back to SA

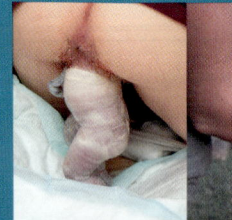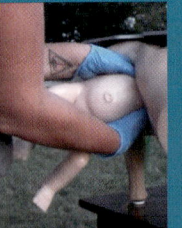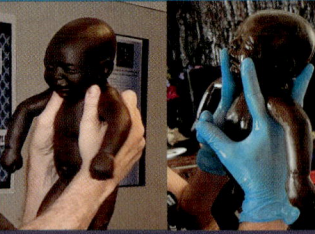

5. Fundal pressure

Indications:
- Maternal exhaustion or poor contraction pattern
- Poor fetal condition or to expedite the birth
- To diagnose an obstruction

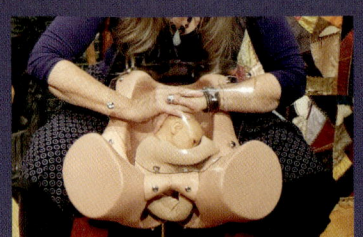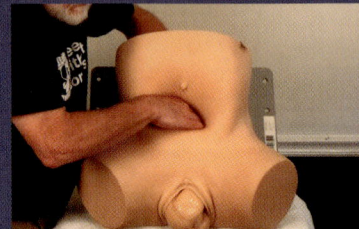

6. Flex, flop, & drop

- For a hyperextended head in the pelvic inlet
- Grasp femurs, disimpact against counterpressure
- Head will **flex** and **flop** to one side
- **Drop** head into pelvis with fundal pressure
- Løvset to extract the baby, if necessary

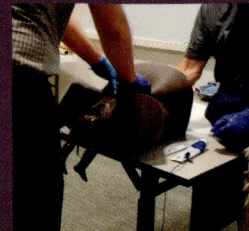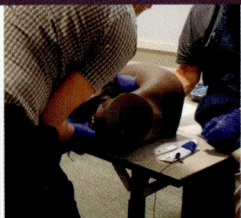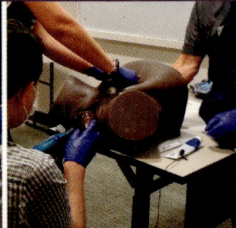

Lesson 1: Core Values

Breech Without Borders upholds the following core values, which should guide all decision-making and counseling.

#1: Autonomy

A pregnant woman has an absolute right to decide what does or does not happen to her body and to the baby she is carrying. This includes freedom from coercion, bullying, or scare tactics. Legally and ethically, she has the right to informed consent, which includes the right to refuse any recommended treatment.

A care provider's role is to provide her with unbiased information, including the full range of risks, benefits, and alternatives of any proposed procedure or treatment; to give her the time and space to make a decision; and to support her once she has made the decision.

When a woman's decision diverges from a provider's recommendations, institutional policies, protocols, or governmental regulations, the care provider has a duty of non-abandonment. The provider should provide the best possible care without eroding the mother's legal and ethical right to refuse any proposed treatment. A care provider should be protected from censure or punishment for upholding maternal autonomy.

From a care provider's perspective, maternal autonomy can be communicated to the pregnant woman with one short statement: "You lead, we follow."

#2: Trauma-Informed Care for All Women

Assume all women have a background of trauma and treat them accordingly. How can a provider demonstrate trauma-informed care?

- Whenever a provider enters the room, they should ask the woman's permission to approach and enter her space.
- They should ask permission prior to any touch or intervention, giving the woman the time and space to agree or decline.
- They should repeatedly assure the woman that she can say no, that she can ask for more time, that she can withdraw her consent at any time–and most importantly, that she can do any of these things without fear of reprisal.

#3: Culturally Relevant and Responsive Care

A care provider should know and respect the cultural/religious traditions of the populations they are serving and adjust their care accordingly. Guidelines and protocols should never override individual values and preferences.

#4: Burden of proof rests upon the intervention, not physiology

Childbirth is a complex physiological process, honed over hundreds of thousands of years of evolution. We still understand very little about the complex interplay of factors that determine the course of labor & birth. Interfering in these processes without fully understanding the short- and long-term consequences is inadvisable. For any proposed intervention into the normal physiological process–anything that may interrupt what would otherwise happen if the woman were left undisturbed–the burden of proof rests upon the intervention. When there is no evidence that the intervention improves outcomes without incurring undue risks, the inherent physiology should be supported.

A note about evidence-based medicine

Evidence-based medicine is a worthy goal. However, most interventions in childbirth are not well studied and do not take into account the complexity of the process. It is very hard to isolate the effectiveness of a single intervention or to randomize women into care paths, given how intricate labor and birth are. In addition, interventions that get studied require funding, and funding is often tied to the potential profitability of the intervention. This complicates our ability to fully understand the consequences, intended or unintended, of interfering with the birth process. No study is fool-proof and conflicting evidence is common.

With vaginal breech birth specifically, good studies are even scarcer. There has only ever been one relatively large randomized controlled trial studying planned vaginal breech birth (pVBB) vs planned C-section (pCS)—the 2000 Term Breech Trial—and that study was subsequently found to be flawed in both its design and implementation. No other RCTs since the Term Breech Trial have evaluated the effects of specific interventions during vaginal breech births. We are left with only a few options: looking at observational data, extrapolating data from cephalic births, following decades or centuries of traditions (which may or may not be harmful), or simply guessing.

Again, when the effect of an intervention is otherwise unknown or unstudied, we defer to physiology as the default and implement any interference with extreme caution.

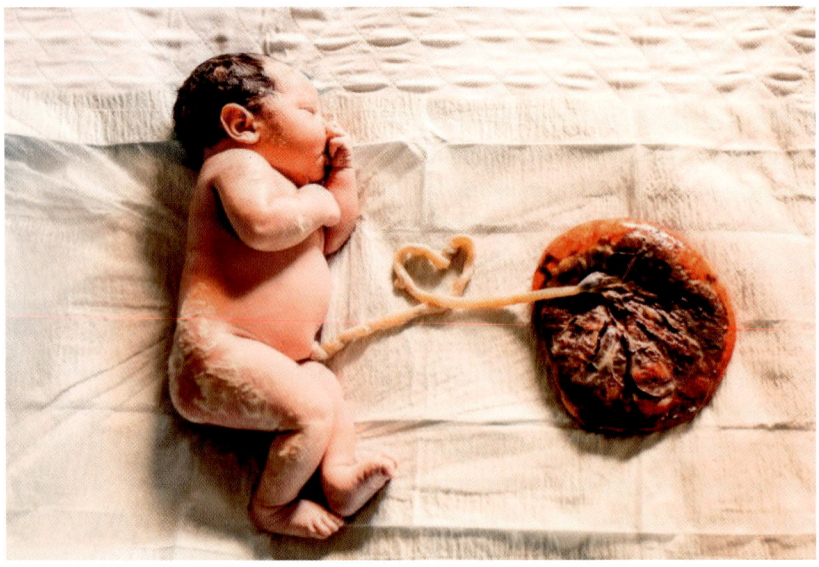

A note on terminology: we have adopted the NICE approach in using woman/women/mother: "In this guideline we use the terms 'woman' and 'women', based on the evidence used in its development. The recommendations will also apply to people who do not identify as women but are pregnant or have given birth." (nice.org.uk)

An undiagnosed breech baby born shortly after the provider had trained with BWB

Lesson 2: Care Providers' Responsibilities

#1: Respect autonomy

We have already outlined our position on maternal autonomy. Below is a sampling of other statements upholding maternal autonomy from various obstetric organizations:

- <u>2016 ACOG statement on Refusal of Medically Recommended Treatment During Pregnancy</u>: "Pregnancy is not an exception to the principle that a decisionally capable patient has the right to refuse treatment, even treatment needed to maintain life. Therefore, a decisionally capable pregnant woman's decision to refuse recommended medical or surgical interventions should be respected. The use of coercion is not only ethically impermissible but also medically inadvisable because of the realities of prognostic uncertainty and the limitations of medical knowledge. As such, it is never acceptable for obstetrician-gynecologists to attempt to influence patients toward a clinical decision using coercion. Obstetrician-gynecologists are discouraged in the strongest possible terms from the use of duress, manipulation, coercion, physical force, or threats, including threats to involve the courts or child protective services, to motivate women toward a specific clinical decision." (Committee opinion n. 664, June 2016)
- <u>2019 SOGC breech guidelines (Canada)</u>: "A woman's choice of delivery mode should be respected….Women with a contraindication to a trial of labour should be advised to have a Caesarean section. Women choosing to labour despite this recommendation have a right to do so and should be provided the best possible in-hospital care." (No. 384–Management of Breech Presentation at Term, August 2019)
- <u>ALARM guidelines</u>: "The woman's wishes, in collaboration with the attending health care providers' judgment, should determine which delivery method is the most appropriate course of action."
- <u>2020 French breech guidelines:</u> "The decision about the planned route of delivery should be shared by the woman and her healthcare provider, who must respect her right to autonomy." (Sentilles 2020)

#2: Disclose experience levels, training, and biases

Care providers should disclose their skill and experience level, including how many vaginal breech births they have attended and whether they were upright or supine, breech trainings they have completed, and how they ensure ongoing competency.

Care providers should give women information and recommendations that are as unbiased as possible, providing the full range of options and the associated risks, benefits, and alternatives. Providers should freely disclose any biases they may hold to ensure that parents can make decisions without undue influence.

The provider's skill and experience level may influence the range of situations they may or may not be comfortable with. The provider should disclose this to the woman and her family and have a frank discussion when their comfort levels are being surpassed. We recommend that less experienced providers consult with or invite an experienced breech provider to attend the birth alongside them, if that option is available.

#3: Acquire breech skills via training and/or mentorship

Because ¼ to ⅓ of all breech presentations are undiagnosed before labor, all maternity care providers should be proficient in attending vaginal breech births. Breech training should include both upright and supine techniques, which will allow the provider to attend the birth in whatever position the mother chooses.

Breech Without Borders offers an online breech training course, Breech Pro, as well as vaginal breech workshops (Breech Pro + in-person simulation training). We have translated Breech Pro into Spanish (Podálica Pro) and have other translations in process.

#4: Practice regularly

We recommend regular skills training. At a bare minimum, providers should practice all upright & supine maneuvers monthly and keep records that document this ongoing practice.

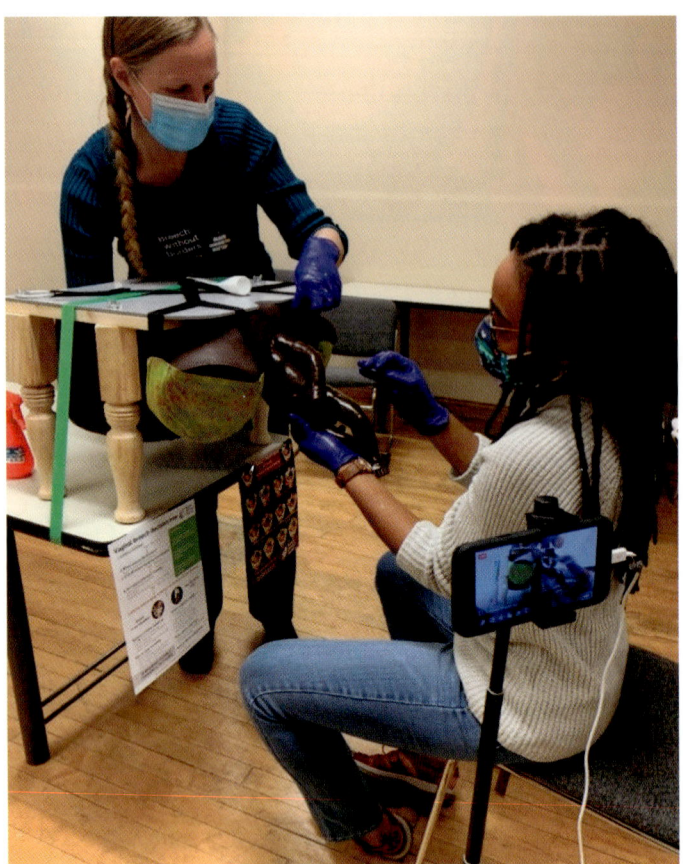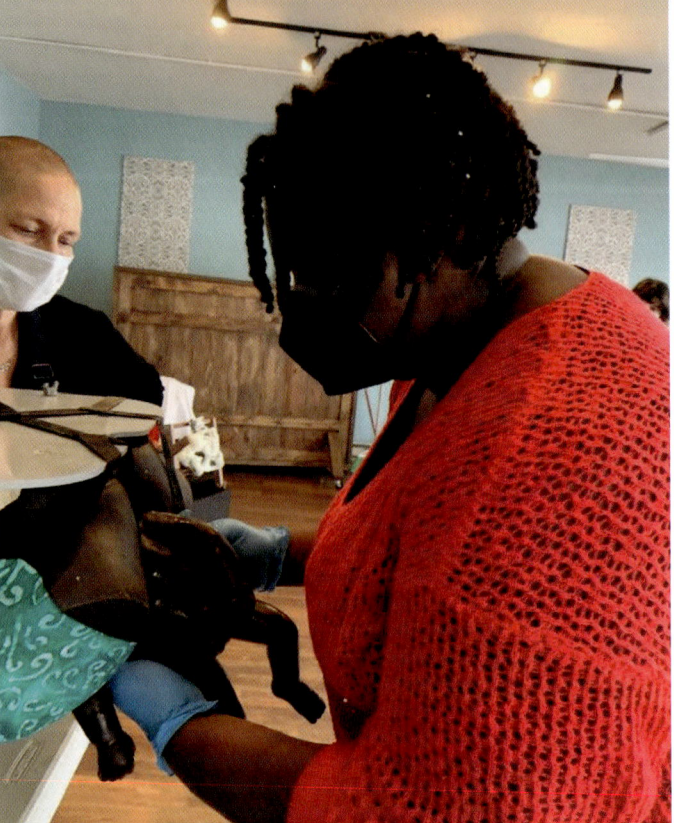

Breech training during the Covid-19 pandemic

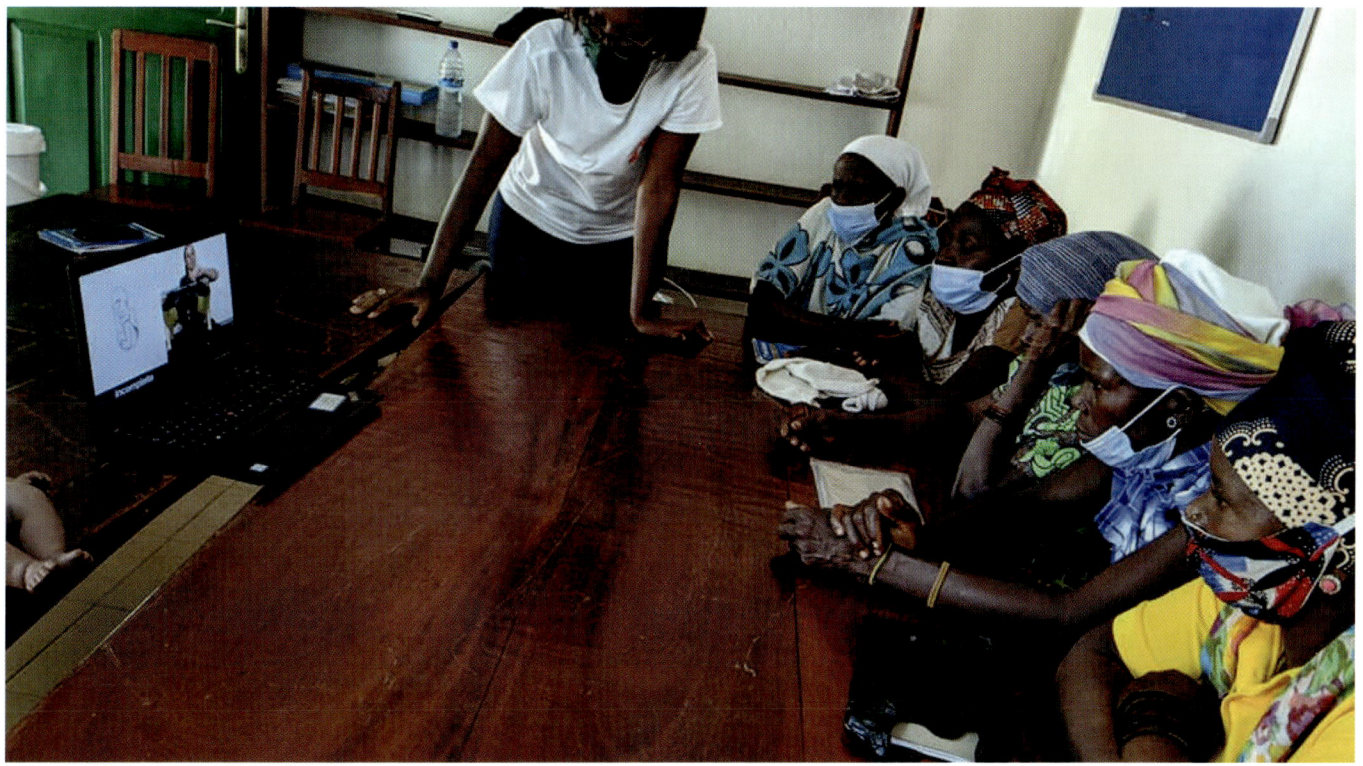

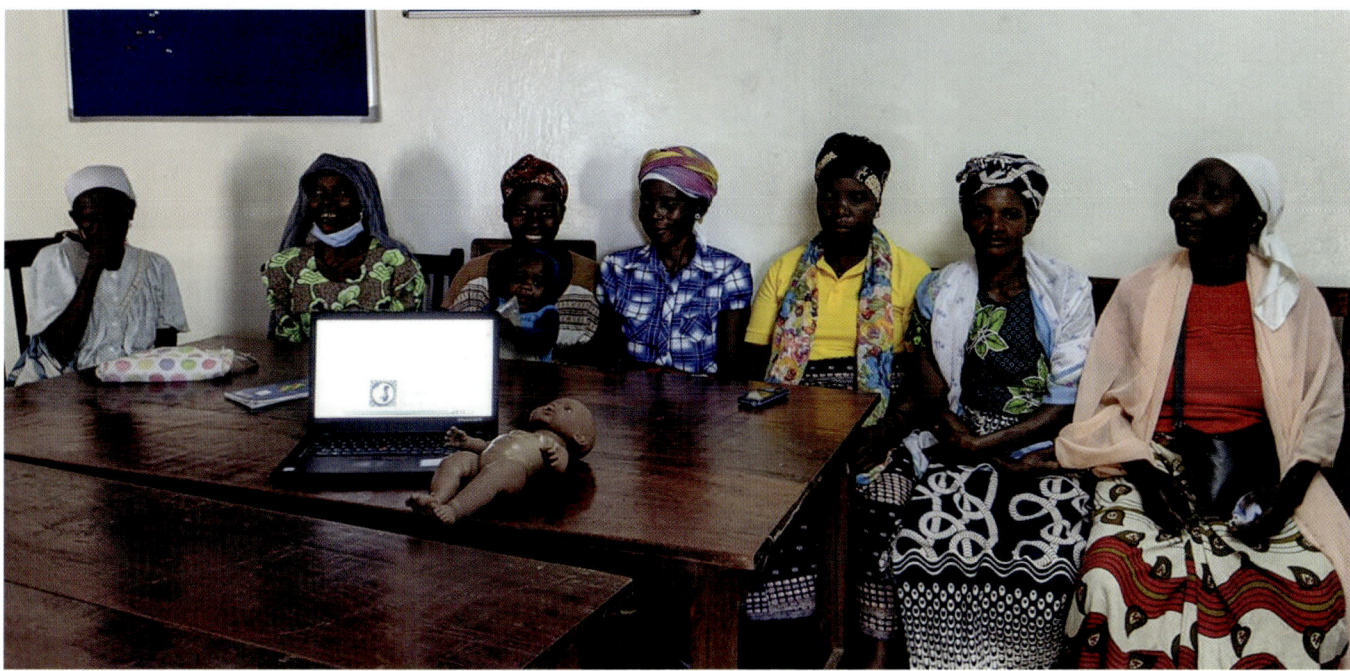

*Traditional Birth Attendants in Mozambique learning vaginal breech techniques
from Breech Without Borders materials*

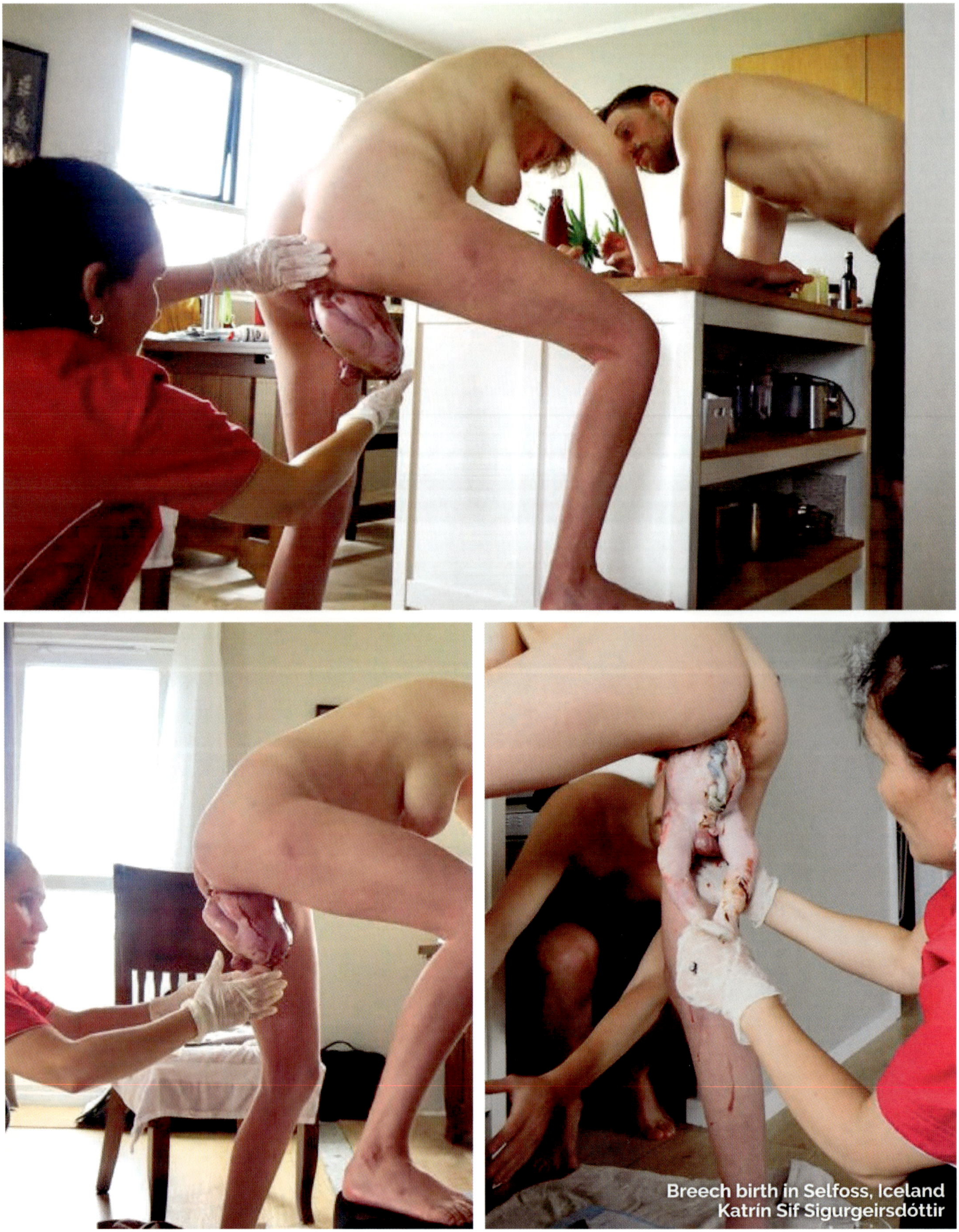

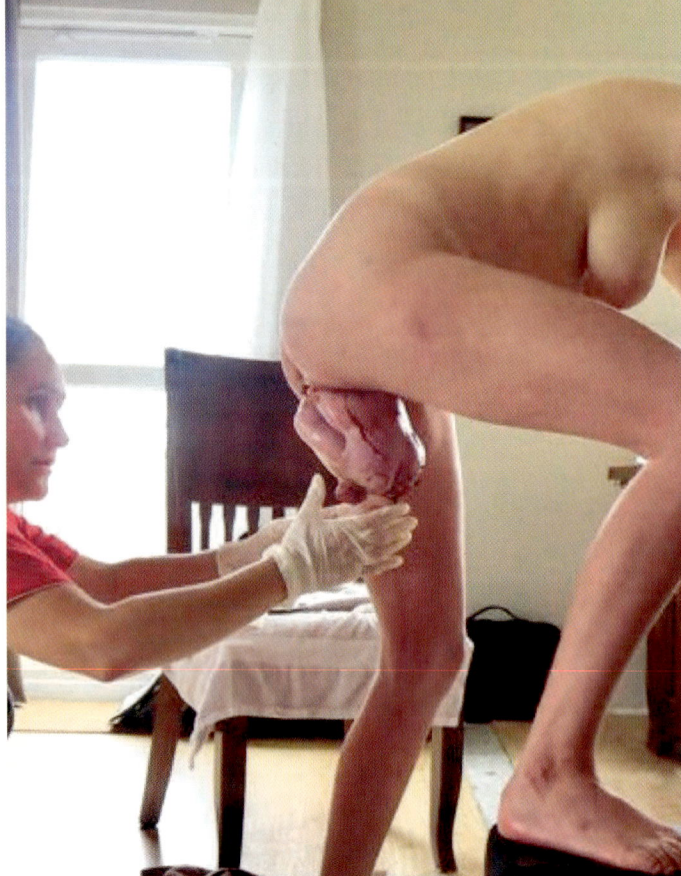

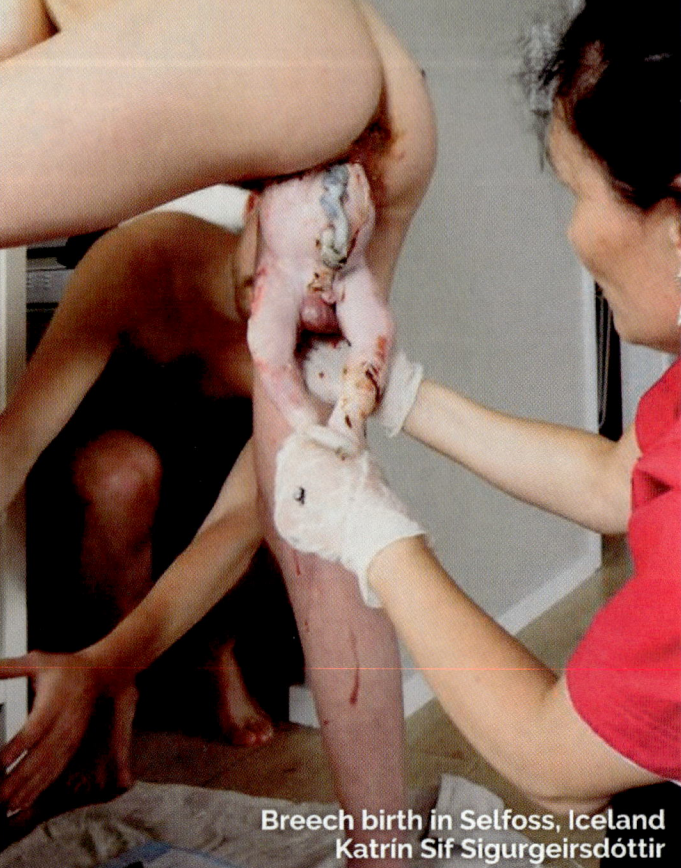

Breech birth in Selfoss, Iceland
Katrín Sif Sigurgeirsdóttir

Lesson 3: The Safety of Vaginal Breech Birth vs Cesarean Section

By Rixa Freeze, PhD

Instead of giving a long and complicated lesson about the medical evidence (something that normally takes over 2 hours when we teach in-person workshops), I am going to give you a short article in the next lesson, "The Bottom Line on Breech." This article summarizes the evidence on planned vaginal breech birth (pVBB) versus planned C-section (pCS) in both hospital and home settings.

After reviewing 20 years of evidence on term breech outcomes, I have identified six key takeaway points:

1. When we ask, "Is a vaginal breech birth safe?" we have to ask, "Safe for whom? Safe when?"

There are 5 main categories of safety to consider:
1. Short-term safety for the baby (during late pregnancy, labor, and in the first few weeks after the birth)
2. Long-term safety for the baby as it becomes a child and adolescent
3. Short-term safety for the mother (during labor and in the first few weeks after the birth)
4. Long-term safety for the mother (for the rest of her reproductive lifetime until she is finished having children, including any future pregnancies and births)
5. Safety for the mother's next child or children

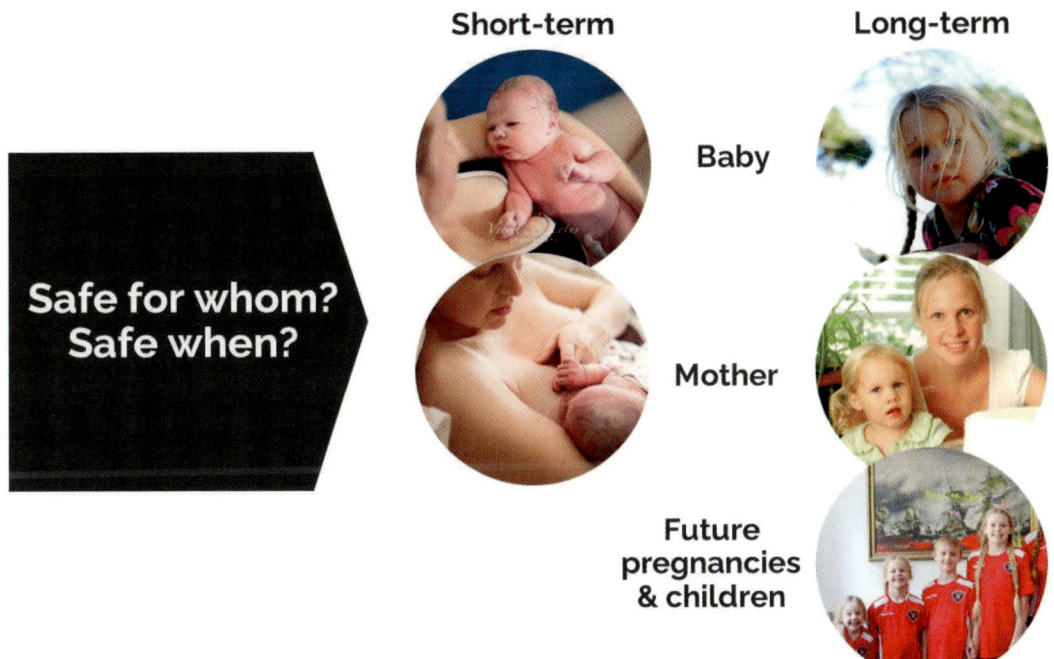

© 2022 Breech Without Borders

If we look at the global body of research, vaginal breech birth is slightly riskier for the baby in the short-term (see point #2 below). However, the more experienced the provider, the lower the risk. In centers or in countries that are highly experienced, vaginal breech birth seems to pose no additional short-term neonatal risk, either for morbidity (injury) or mortality. But for the other four categories, a vaginal birth is safer for mother, child, and any future babies.

2. Vaginal breech birth is not as dangerous as previously thought.

This next illustration shows current estimates for term breech **perinatal mortality** (risk of the baby dying during labor and in the first few weeks after birth). The red dots are planned CS, the green dots are planned VBB, and the purple dot is planned cephalic (head-down) vaginal birth. (These numbers are all per 1,000 births.)

The 2000 Term Breech Trial found a larger difference between pCS and pVBB and is one of the reasons that almost no hospitals "allow" vaginal breech birth anymore. However, over the past 2 decades, many large studies have found a much smaller difference in perinatal risk. Notice how much closer together the red and green dots are in the other studies.

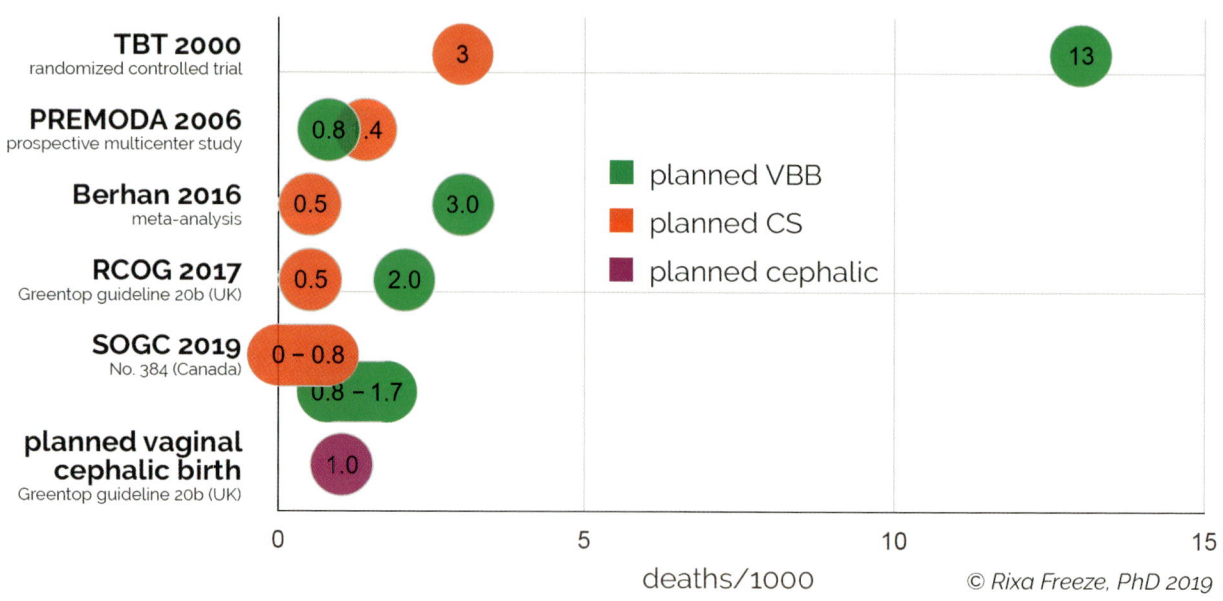

Perinatal/neonatal mortality for term breech: TBT versus recent evidence

In terms of neonatal morbidity (injuries), recent studies have also found much smaller differences than previously thought. For example, this illustration compares the findings of the 2000 Term Breech Trial against studies from countries or centers that are skilled in VBB. Note that there are no statistically significant differences in severe neonatal morbidity in the more recent studies (circled in red—things like seizures, serious birth trauma, extremely low 5-minute Apgar scores, intubation and ventilation for > 24 hours, and long NICU stays).

Comparison of severe neonatal morbidity

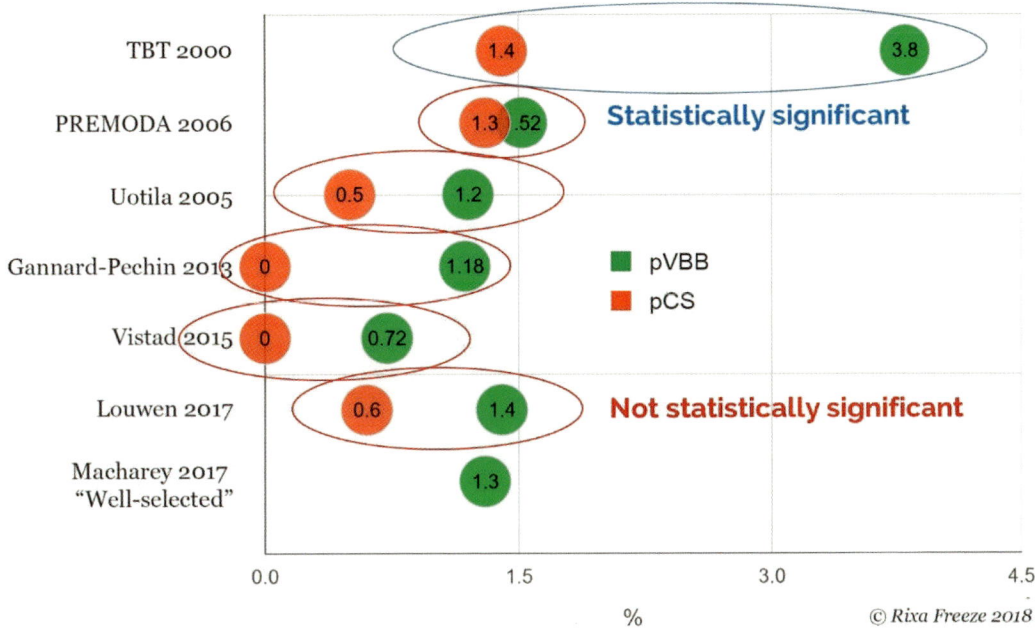

© Rixa Freeze 2018

3. Half of the perinatal mortality risk of breech birth comes just from being pregnant and having a vaginal birth; the other half comes from the breech part specifically.

The RCOG—the obstetrical society in the UK—has estimated the risk of perinatal death to be:
- **1/2000 (0.5/1000) for a planned C-section**
- **1/1000 for a planned cephalic (head-down) vaginal birth**
- **1/500 (2/1000) for a planned vaginal breech birth**

Note that a head-down vaginal birth adds extra "risk," about 1 death per every 2,000 births, compared to pCS at 39 weeks. This makes sense: if a woman is pregnant for a few additional weeks and then goes through labor, there will be a slightly higher chance of an adverse outcome. However, we still tend to see that higher risk as acceptable, since most women still plan vaginal births when they have head-down babies, given the risks that come with surgical births.

A baby being breech adds another 1/1,000 risk (1/1000 for having a baby vaginally + 1/1000 for the breech part = 1/500 total), but somehow that is seen as unacceptably high. But is it? That is a question that only the mother and family can answer.

4. Safety is more than about just the baby.

Our society tends to focus only on one of the 5 safety categories: short-term safety for the baby. The other four often get ignored or dismissed as less important.

5. Breech birth has a risk-benefit trade-off

A C-section has a small chance of preventing a neonatal death and possibly a neonatal injury, but it also adds risks to the baby as it grows up, risks to the mother, and risks to the mother's future pregnancies. There is a risk-benefit trade-off with breech. You can't get rid of risk; it just goes downstream for you to swim in later.

1. We should be giving women the time, information, and space to make the choice that is best for them.

To support the choice of a VBB, providers must be well-trained. They also need to be honest about their skill and experience levels and do everything they can to practice and to learn from more experienced midwives or doctors. I love this quote from a textbook written in the UK. It should serve as a guide for how providers support women with breech babies:

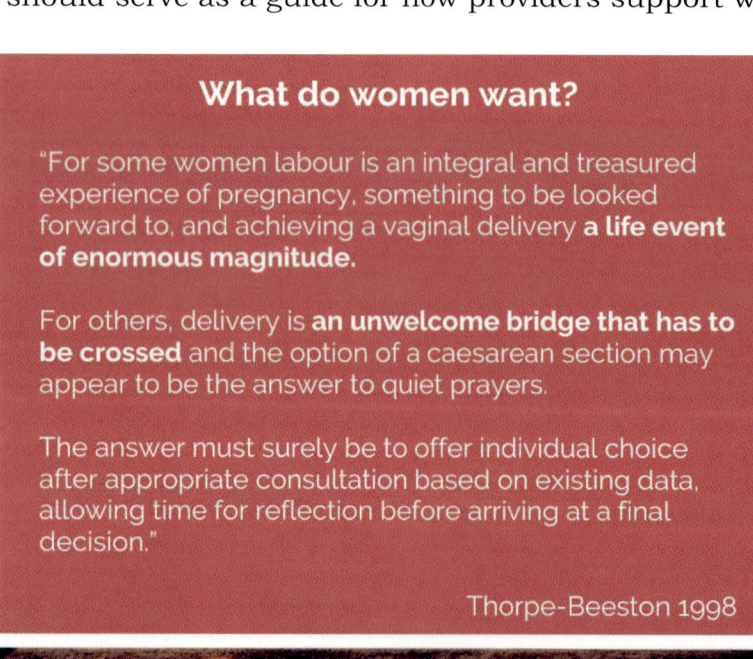

What do women want?

"For some women labour is an integral and treasured experience of pregnancy, something to be looked forward to, and achieving a vaginal delivery **a life event of enormous magnitude.**

For others, delivery is **an unwelcome bridge that has to be crossed** and the option of a caesarean section may appear to be the answer to quiet prayers.

The answer must surely be to offer individual choice after appropriate consultation based on existing data, allowing time for reflection before arriving at a final decision."

Thorpe-Beeston 1998

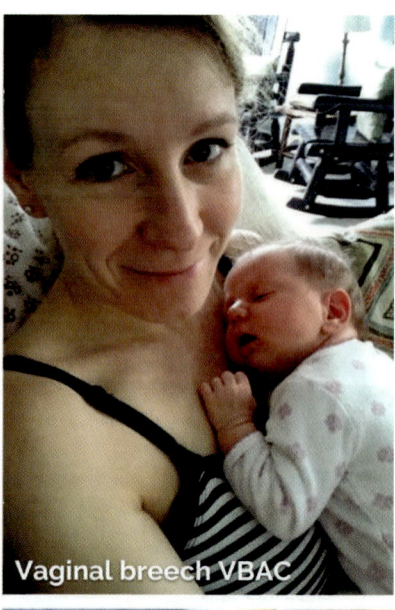

Vaginal breech VBAC

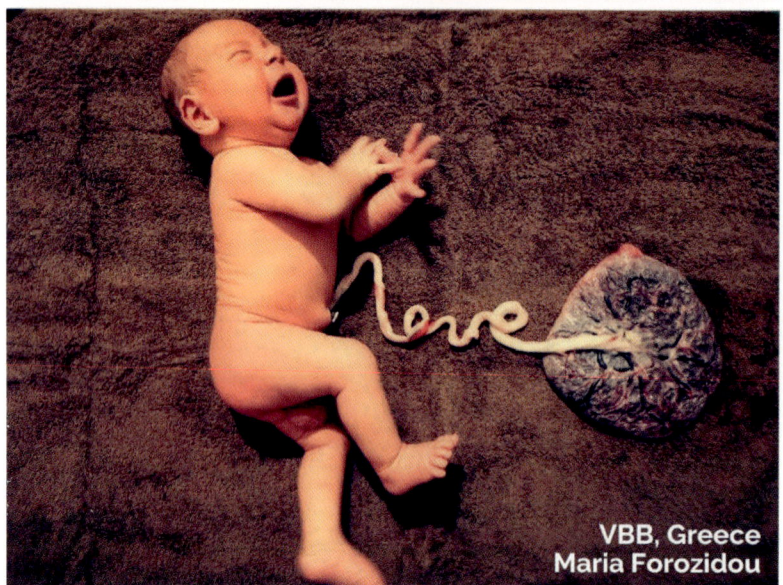

VBB, Greece
Maria Forozidou

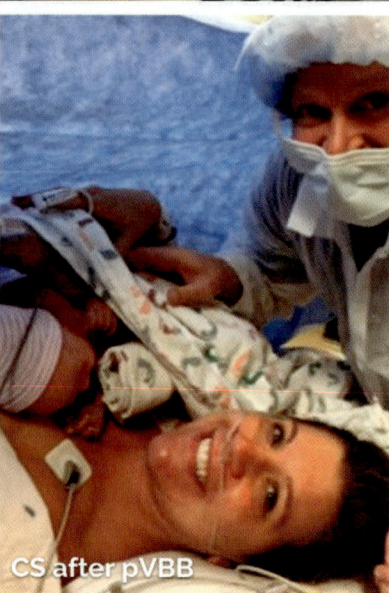

CS after pVBB

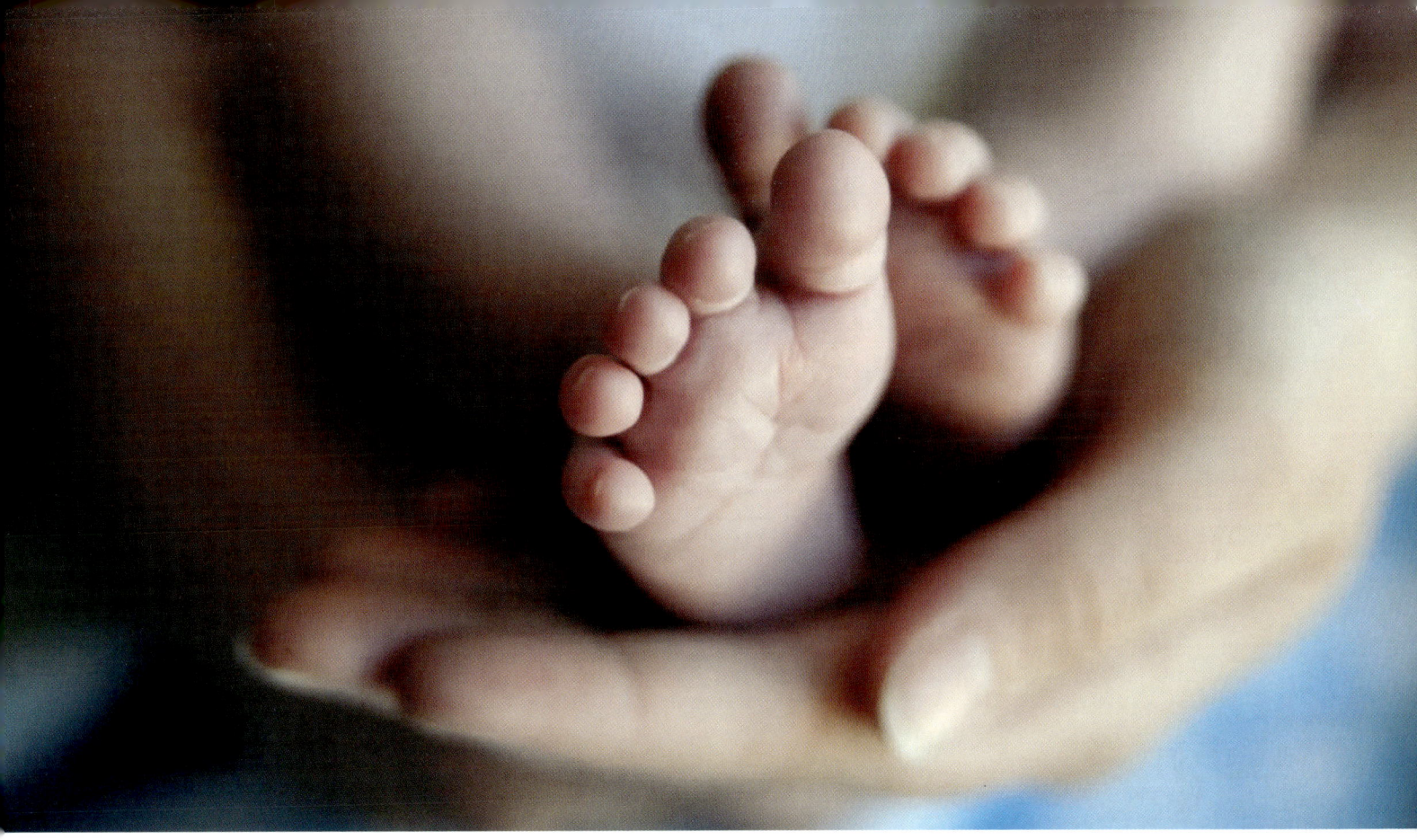

The Bottom Line on Breech

Home, Hospital, and Birth Center Outcomes and Suggestions for Birth Attendants

by Rixa Freeze

Since the 1960s, the cesarean rate for breech presentation has been rising. When a much-awaited randomized controlled trial on term breech was published in 2000 (the Term Breech Trial, or TBT), the cesarean rate for breech in the US was already over 83% (Hannah et al. 2000; Lee, El-Sayed, and Gould 2008). The TBT firmly cemented the practice of routine cesarean for breech. The study has since been critiqued for flaws in recruitment, randomization, implementation, and labor management protocols (Glezerman 2006; Kotaska 2004). In addition, a long-term analysis of children participating in the TBT found no significant differences in outcomes at ≥2 years of age (Whyte et al. 2004). Studies on term breech since the TBT have found either no difference in outcomes between planned cesarean section and planned vaginal breech birth (Goffinet et al. 2006, also called the PREMODA study) or a difference that is much less significant than in

the TBT (Berhan and Haileamlak 2016). However, the damage had already been done after the TBT. Hospitals and physicians around the world stopped allowing vaginal breech births, bringing the 2016 cesarean rate for breech (including twins and premature babies) in the US to 93.2% (1).

Despite the near-extinction of vaginal breech birth in a hospital setting, many women continue to value vaginal birth. When the only option offered is mandatory cesarean, some women will opt out of the hospital altogether. In many parts of the US, the only place a woman can have a vaginal breech birth is at home or in some birth centers (2). Breech educators report that their workshops are mostly attended by home or birth center midwives, and my own experience organizing and teaching breech workshops confirms that observation. The small number of hospital-based providers who continue to offer vaginal breech birth do so in isolation and often

face significant opposition and hostility from their colleagues (3).

For better or for worse, breech birth is occurring at home and in birth centers. What are the outcomes of breech birth in hospital settings and in home- and birth center births? What should midwives (and the rare homebirth physicians) and their clients know in order to make an informed decision?

Safety of Vaginal Breech Birth

To answer the question, "Is vaginal breech birth safe?" we must look at both short- and long-term risks and benefits to the baby, to the mother, and to the mother's future pregnancies and future babies. I reviewed all single-center, multi-center, and national registry/birth certificate studies in PubMed from 2000 onward to understand how planned vaginal breech birth (pVBB) compares to planned c-section (pCS) for term breeches.

Photograph | Brandee Noelee Photography

Perinatal/neonatal mortality and short-term neonatal morbidity. Vaginal breech birth does present some short-term risks to the baby. The RCOG updated its breech guidelines in 2017 and estimated the risk of perinatal mortality (PNM) during a planned vaginal breech birth at around 1/500, compared to 1/1000 for a planned cephalic birth and 1/2000 for a pCS (RCOG 2017). This number aligns with many large national registry studies and meta-analyses. However, in France and Belgium, which have retained a strong tradition of vaginal breech birth and continue to teach breech in residency programs, large high-quality prospective studies have found no difference in neonatal outcomes between pVBB and pCS (Goffinet et al. 2006; Vendittelli et al. 2002; Vendittelli et al. 2006). These findings are in stark contrast with the TBT, which found the risk of mortality from pCS at 3/1000 and pVBB at 13/1000. (See Figure 1.)

We can expect a slightly higher rate of short-term neonatal morbidity after a planned vaginal breech birth, although at a much lower rate than found in the TBT. Below is an illustration of rates of severe neonatal morbidity in the TBT compared with more recent studies using the same criteria. Again, some studies find no difference at all, while others find some advantage to pCS, although at a much lower rate than the TBT. (See Figure 2, page 14.)

The only point of consensus on short-term neonatal outcomes is to anticipate suppressed Apgar scores after a pVBB, especially in the first minute. This may occur because the cord is often compressed as the baby's head passes through the maternal bony pelvis.

Long-term childhood outcomes. Of the 18 studies since 2000 that investigate long-term childhood outcomes of breech birth, three find some disadvantage to pVBB: increased risk of neurodevelopmental delay (Molkenboer et al. 2006), increased risk of CP and cognitive impairment (Andersen et al. 2009), and lower school exam scores (Mackay et al. 2015). A fourth concluded that the long-term benefits of pCS were "modest" (Jensen and Wust 2015). On the other hand, 12 studies found no difference in long-term outcomes between pCS and pVBB (see the list below).

- Munstedt et al. 2001
- Giuliani et al. 2002
- Hellsten, Lindqvist, and Olofsson 2003
- Ulander et al. 2004
- Eide et al. 2005
- Pradhan, Mohajer, and Deshpande 2005
- Uotila, Tuimala, and Kirkinen 2005
- Andreasen, Nielsen, and Oian 2010
- Preis et al. 2012
- Vistad et al. 2015
- Abdessalami et al. 2017
- Macharey et al. 2017

Finally, while one study noted that childhood asthma was associated with breech extraction and/or low Apgars (Xu, Pekkanen, and Jarvelin 2000), another found that 75% of breech infants with low Apgars have no handicap or disability at long-term follow up (Krebs, Langhoff-Roos, and Thorngren-Jerneck 2001).

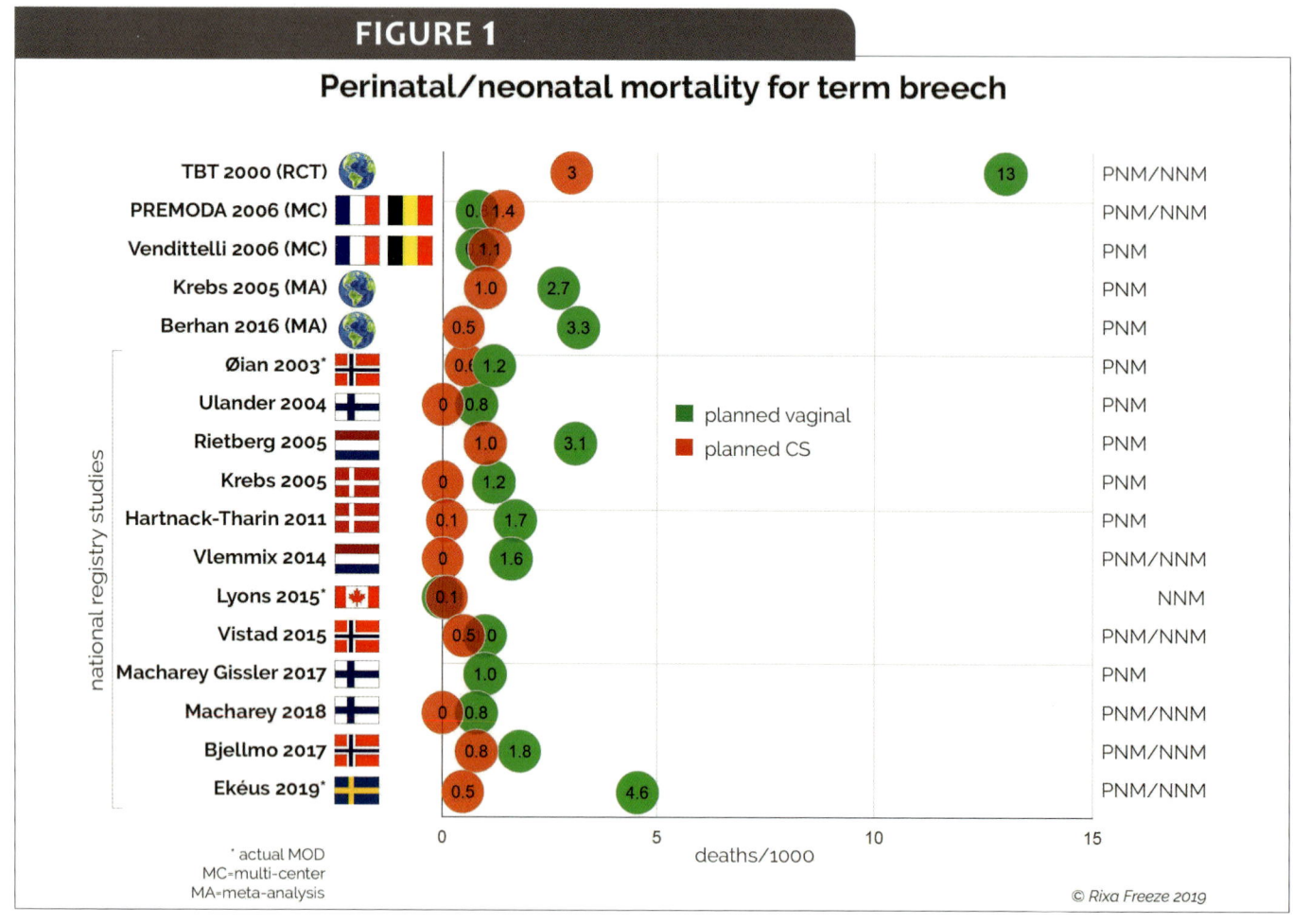

FIGURE 1

Perinatal/neonatal mortality for term breech

Study	planned CS	planned vaginal	measure
TBT 2000 (RCT)	3	13	PNM/NNM
PREMODA 2006 (MC)	0.?	1.4	PNM/NNM
Vendittelli 2006 (MC)	1.1		PNM
Krebs 2005 (MA)	1.0	2.7	PNM
Berhan 2016 (MA)	0.5	3.3	PNM
Øian 2003*	0.?	1.2	PNM
Ulander 2004	0	0.8	PNM
Rietberg 2005	1.0	3.1	PNM
Krebs 2005	0	1.2	PNM
Hartnack-Tharin 2011	0.1	1.7	PNM
Vlemmix 2014	0	1.6	PNM/NNM
Lyons 2015*	0.1		NNM
Vistad 2015	0.5	0	PNM/NNM
Macharey Gissler 2017	1.0		PNM
Macharey 2018	0	0.8	PNM/NNM
Bjellmo 2017	0.8	1.8	PNM/NNM
Ekéus 2019*	0.5	4.6	PNM/NNM

national registry studies

■ planned vaginal
■ planned CS

deaths/1000

* actual MOD
MC=multi-center
MA=meta-analysis

© Rixa Freeze 2019

FIGURE 2

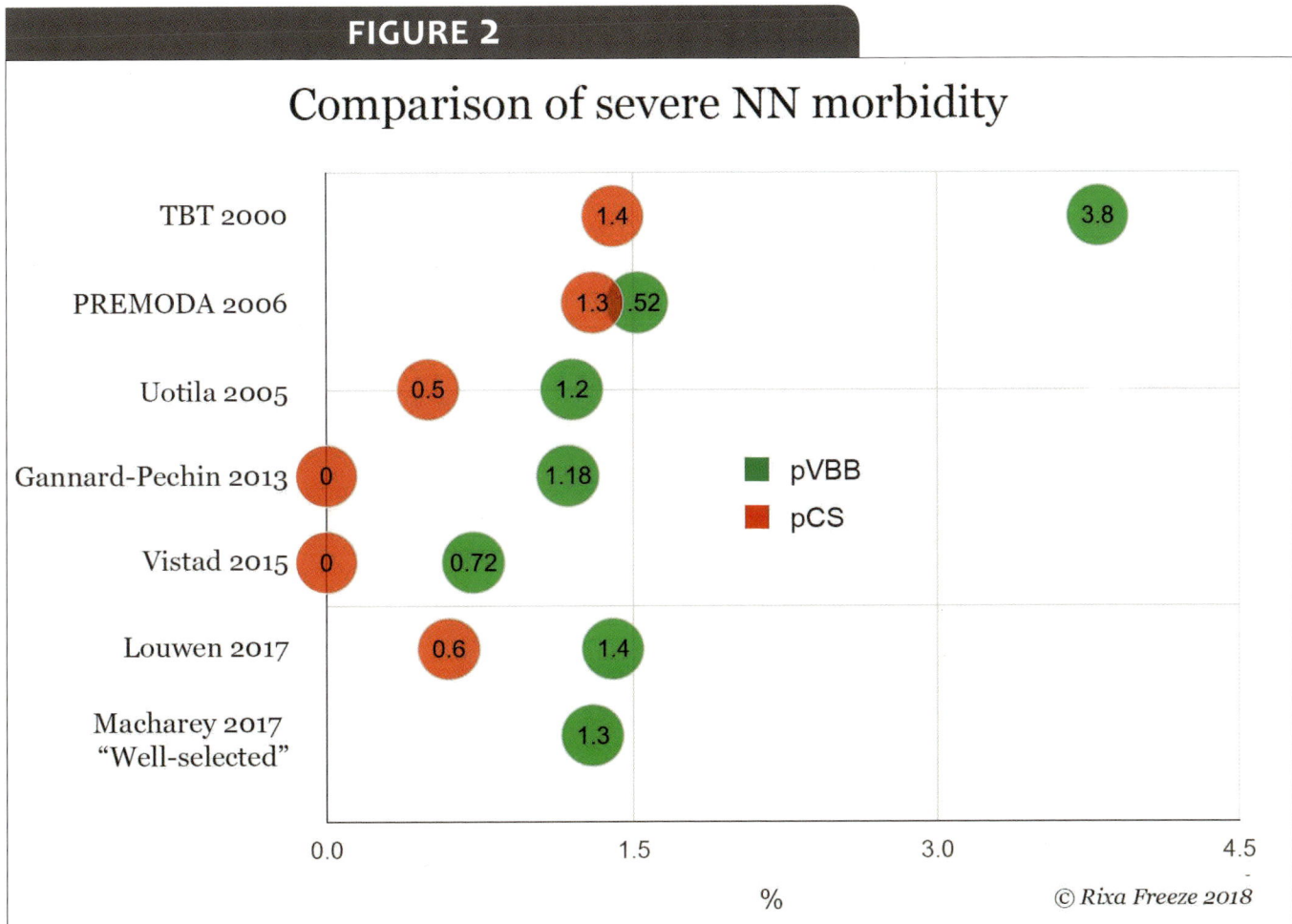

Comparison of severe NN morbidity

TBT 2000 — 1.4 (pCS), 3.8 (pVBB)
PREMODA 2006 — 1.3 (pCS), .52 (pVBB)
Uotila 2005 — 0.5 (pCS), 1.2 (pVBB)
Gannard-Pechin 2013 — 0 (pCS), 1.18 (pVBB)
Vistad 2015 — 0 (pCS), 0.72 (pVBB)
Louwen 2017 — 0.6 (pCS), 1.4 (pVBB)
Macharey 2017 "Well-selected" — 1.3 (pVBB)

■ pVBB
■ pCS

0.0   1.5   3.0   4.5

%

© Rixa Freeze 2018

We also have to consider the emerging research on the long-term risks of c-section in general, such as increased rates of childhood asthma (Thavagnanam et al. 2008), infant leukemia (Marcotte et al. 2018), type I diabetes (Cardwell et al. 2008), autoimmune and allergic diseases (Neu and Rushing 2011; Sandall et al. 2018), altered gut microbiome (Butel, Waligora-Dupriet, and Wydau-Dematteis 2018; Tun et al. 2018), and altered stem cell epigenetics (Almgren et al. 2014).

Short- and long-term maternal outcomes and subsequent births. Of 37 studies that compare the short-term maternal morbidity of breech births, planned vaginal breech birth is either superior or equivalent to pCS in 35 of the studies (4). Two studies found some disadvantage to pVBB in terms of urinary incontinence and perineal lacerations. Thus, in the short-term, a planned vaginal breech birth is better for the mother, even taking into account the higher morbidity of cesareans performed during labor.

Maternal mortality after breech birth is extremely rare. However, in the Netherlands four women died as a direct result of elective CS (eCS) for breech between 2000 and 2002, leading to a case fatality rate of 0.47/1000 (Schutte et al. 2007). Three other studies report maternal breech deaths:

- one pCS death in a Finnish hospital (out of 497 pCS), described as a "complicated cesarean" (Toivonen et al. 2012).
- two deaths in a Tanzanian hospital: one after CS (of 747 CS) due to anesthetic complications and one after a VBB (of 908 VBB) due to a ruptured uterus (Högberg et al. 2016).
- three deaths in a Danish registry study: two deaths 40 and 55 days after in-labor CS and one long-term death; the mother had a CS for breech and then a VBAC, after which she died (Krebs and Langhoff-Roos 2003).

In general, cesareans lead to a higher rate of severe acute maternal morbidity (SAMM) than planned vaginal births. SAMM is also called a *maternal near miss*, in which a pregnant woman nearly dies (Chhabra 2014). After a cesarean, SAMM persists into the next pregnancy. This means that women will have a higher rate of SAMM in the *next* birth after their cesarean, regardless of how their subsequent babies are born (van Dillen et al. 2010).

I have identified five studies that compare long-term maternal outcomes after breech birth, including complications after the current pregnancy and complications with subsequent pregnancies and future fertility:

- Krebs and Langhoff-Roos 2003
- Hannah et al. 2004
- Verhoeven, de Leeuw, and Bruinse 2005
- Molkenboer et al. 2007
- Su et al. 2007

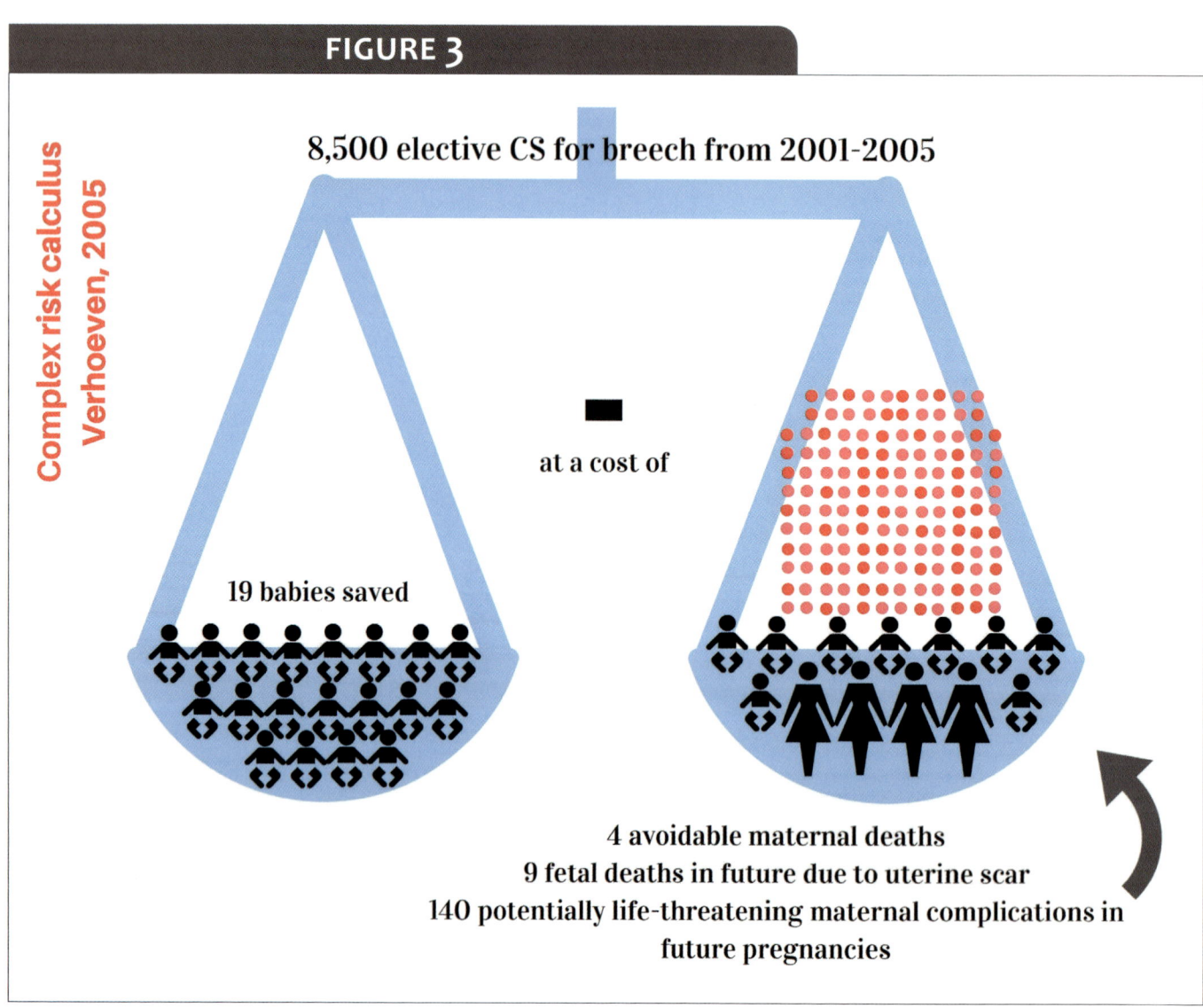

FIGURE 3

Complex risk calculus Verhoeven, 2005

8,500 elective CS for breech from 2001-2005

— at a cost of

19 babies saved

4 avoidable maternal deaths
9 fetal deaths in future due to uterine scar
140 potentially life-threatening maternal complications in future pregnancies

Unsurprisingly, a planned vaginal birth is equivalent or better for mothers in the long term as well as the short term, with a lower rate of long-term morbidity and fewer complications with future pregnancies, such as miscarriage, ectopic pregnancy, uterine rupture, placental complications, or adverse neonatal outcomes in subsequent births. In addition, researchers investigating cesarean scar pregnancies and morbidly adherent placentas found that the main indication for these previous CS in both groups was breech presentation (Pekar-Zlotin et al. 2017).

In studies that track the results of a woman's next pregnancy after a breech baby, we find a complex risk tradeoff. For example, let's look at what happened to Dutch women before and after the Term Breech Trial. A small number of breech babies were saved by doing more elective cesareans (an estimated 19 babies saved by performing 8500 elective cesareans). However, those cesareans came at a cost: four avoidable maternal deaths, nine additional fetal deaths in the next pregnancy due to the uterine scar, and 140 cases of SAMM in future pregnancies (Verhoeven, de Leeuw, and Bruinse 2005). (See Figure 3.)

Universal cesareans for term breech babies do not remove the risk entirely. Instead, they remove some short-term neonatal risk in exchange for transferring other risks downstream to the mother, to the mother's subsequent pregnancies, and to the mother's next babies.

Outcomes of Home Breech Birth

The studies mentioned above all came from hospital data, including individual centers, multi-center studies, and national registry or birth certificate data. What about home or birth center breech outcomes? We have some data, but most of those studies have several significant weaknesses: we usually do not know the providers' experience or skill level, the selection criteria, the type of breech presentation, whether there were congenital anomalies (diagnosed or undiagnosed), or whether the breech presentation was diagnosed before labor and, thus, whether it was truly a planned breech birth.

"High-risk" births. Four studies have examined the influence of breech presentation on homebirth perinatal outcomes, usually by comparing "high-" and "low-" risk births. Breech would often be included with several other "high-risk" situations, such as twins or postdates. None of these studies parse out the role of breech specifically. (See Table 1.)

Mehl-Madrona and Madrona (1997) matched 1000 midwife-attended homebirths with 1000 physician-attended homebirths. Although the PNM was significantly higher among the midwife-attended group, that difference disappeared when the authors removed "high-risk" homebirths from both groups (breech, twins, postdates, and lethal congenital anomalies). There were 31 breeches, 32 postdates, 9 twins, and 5 anomalies among the 2000 births studied.

Symon et al. (2009) compared outcomes between UK's independent midwives (majority planned homebirths) and National Health Service (NHS) maternity unit births (almost all hospital births). Each IM birth was matched with up to five NHS births for age, parity, year of birth, and socioeconomic status (but not other factors such as gestational age, presentation, or singleton/multiples). When "high-risk" births were excluded (premature, breech, twins, pre-existing obstetric or medical conditions), there was no significant difference in PNM between the 1462 IM and 7214 NHS births (0.5% vs 0.3%). Looking specifically at term single-ton breech births, the IM cohort had four perinatal deaths (three born vaginally, one by CS), compared with no PNDs in the NHS cohort.

Nove's 2011 PhD dissertation analyzed more than a half-million home- and hospital births in the UK's SMMIS registry from 1988 to 2000. She found that malpresentation (including but not limited to breech) was associated with a "slightly higher risk of negative maternal and infant outcomes if a homebirth is attempted." However, even with such a large number of births, the small number of perinatal deaths after a planned homebirth (n=12) "makes it impossible to estimate the magnitude of the increased risk of perinatal death in these three situations (cord prolapse, resuscitation, malpresentation) with any confidence."

Davies-Tuck et al. (2018) looked at births from the Victorian Perinatal Data Collection, which records all births in Victoria from 20 weeks gestation. This study examined births ≥37 weeks, excluding the newly established public homebirth programs, in order to compare planned homebirths attended by a private midwife with planned hospital births. Eighty-one percent of planned homebirths and 85%of planned hospital births were defined as low risk, according to the Australian College of Midwives (ACM) guidelines. Breech presentation was one of several factors defined as high risk. Comparing just the high-risk groups, planned homebirths had:

- lower rates of maternal morbidity and obstetric intervention (CS, forceps, vacuum, episiotomy, and anesthesia).
- lower rates of SCN (special care nursery) admission, birth trauma, intrauterine hypoxia, and composite perinatal morbidity.
- similar rates of stillbirth, 5-minute Apgar scores, hypoxic-ischemic encephalopathy, and other perinatal morbidity.
- higher rates of neonatal death (NND) and neonatal intensive care unit (NICU) admissions.

In other words, high-risk homebirth conferred significant advantages to the mother and some to the baby in terms of birth trauma and other morbidities, had equivalent outcomes for several other perinatal factors, but also came with a higher rate of NND and NICU admission.

Table 2 (see page 18) lists outcomes of home/birth center breech births from studies or reports with a range of infor-

Table 1: Role of Malpresentation and "High Risk" Births in Neonatal Outcomes

Lead author & year	Years	Country	Data set (cohort size)	Findings
Mehl-Madrona 1997	1969–1985	USA	MW & FP homebirths (2000)	Non-significant difference in PNM (0.3% vs 0.2%) after excluding "high risk" (incl. breech) cases. 31 total breech births.
Symon 2009	2002–2005	UK	IM & NHS (1462 IM, 7214 NHS)	Non-significant difference in PNM (0.5% vs 0.3%) after excluding "high risk" (incl. breech) cases. 4 term breech PNDs in IM cohort.
Nove 2011	1988–2000	UK	SMMIS (515,777)	Malpresentation (incl. breech) associated with slightly higher risk of negative maternal/fetal outcomes in planned homebirths
Davies-Tuck 2018	2000–2015	Australia	VPDC (3945 home, 829,286 hosp.)	Planned homebirth among high risk women (incl. 81 non-vertex) was associated with significantly higher rates of PNM but an overall significant decrease in composite perinatal and maternal morbidities.

mation and sample sizes. The first category is a group of five studies that reported breech fatalities in planned out-of-hospital (OOH) births, but without other context, including the overall number of breech births. Sullivan and Beeman (1983) and Koehler, Solomon, and Murphy (1984) looked at outcomes of homebirth practices in Arizona and in Sonoma County, California—each reporting one death. Doser (2012) reported on outcomes of home or birth center transports to an Oregon hospital over a five-year period, finding three fatalities among the 17 breech transports. Hargand and Stiefvater (2012) collated homebirth outcomes in Oregon in 2012, noting two deaths due to breech presentations. Cox et al. (2015) looked at VBACs in the MANA Stats 2.0 database, finding one breech death out of an unspecified number of breeches.

Smaller breech cohorts. Bastian, Keirse, and Lancaster (1998) analyzed Homebirth Australia, a consumer database that collected outcomes of homebirths from a number of sources. The breeches had a mortality rate of 1:14, or 7%. This means that there were *at least* four breech deaths among an unspecified number of breech births (although an exact number cannot be ascertained). The CPM 2000 study by Johnson and Daviss (2005) included two breech deaths; there were at least 80 identified breech presentations (including one urgent and three non-urgent transports) and likely more in the "malpresentation" group (Daviss, personal communication). We have no other additional details about the circumstances or outcomes in these two studies.

Larger breech cohorts. Only four studies include relatively large numbers of home breech births: the MANA Statistics Project (MANA Stats) 2.4/4.0 data analyzed by Cheyney et al. (2014) and Bovbjerg et al. (2017) and Centers for Disease Control and Prevention (CDC) birth certificate data analyzed by Grünebaum et al. (2017) and Bachilova, Czuzoj-Shulman, and Abenhaim (2018). However, we still know very little, other than whether the neonate survived, especially in the CDC data. In all four studies, we do not know if the breech presentation was diagnosed

before labor, the type of breech presentation, the selection criteria, or the skill level of the provider. Grünebaum and Bachilova's studies both examined neonatal deaths only, as intrapartum deaths are not recorded on birth certificates. Both also looked only at states using birth certificates that noted the *planned* location of birth. Grünebaum found seven NNDs in 553 home breech births between 2009 and 2013 (1.27%). In Bachilova's group, there were four early NNDs among the 652 non-vertex presentations (0.61%), compared to 50 (0.11%) among the 47,158 vertex presentations (roughly 1/3 of the birth certificates did not specify presentation).

Cheyney and Bovbjerg both analyzed MANA Stats data, a voluntary collection of OOH births by mainly North American providers. Cheyney looked at the 2.0 data (2004–2009), while Bovbjerg analyzed both 2.0 and 4.0 (2012–2014). Because these two datasets overlap, I will only discuss Bovbjerg's findings. Out of 539 breech births, nine neonates died (1.68%). Over half the breech cohort transferred to a hospital, mostly intrapartum, and 44.7% were born by CS. This suggests a high rate of undiagnosed breeches. Bovbjerg also analyzed several other maternal and neonatal outcomes. Interestingly, compared to cephalic birth, breech birth was protective of the maternal genital tract.

Only three studies looked at home or birth center breech outcomes with the breech diagnosed before labor, a known type of breech presentation, a skilled provider, and clear selection criteria. Deline et al. (2012) analyzed outcomes of an Amish birth center in SW Wisconsin that accepted frank breeches as well as other "high-risk" births. Births were attended by a family physician and a licensed midwife. Of the 22 breech presentations, two were frank breech but the parents chose eCS, three turned successfully during intrapartum ECV, and three remained non-frank and were transferred for CS. The remaining 14 women with frank breech presentations labored at the birth center; 8 gave birth vaginally and 6 were eventually transported for CS. There were no bad outcomes and the overall CS rate was 50%.

Fischbein (2015) and Fischbein and Freeze (2018) discuss outcomes of breech and cephalic births with a homebirth ob-

stetrician. The 2018 publication is an update of the 2015 data, so I will discuss only the newer article. The OB had several decades' experience attending vaginal breech births, mainly in hospital, before he began a homebirth practice. His selection criteria included frank or complete presentation, flexed or neutral head, EFW 5–9.9 lbs, adequate pelvimetry by history or exam, no gross anomalies, spontaneous labor, maternal/fetal tolerance to labor, and informed and motivated parents. Fifty women with breech presentations were still in the OB's care at the onset of labor. Overall, 84% gave birth vaginally, including 100% of multips. The rate of low Apgars was significantly lower at 1 minute but not statistically different at 5 minutes compared to the OB's cephalic births.

Ten women were transported for stalled labor (all primips), of whom eight had CS and two birthed vaginally with augmentation, vacuum, and/or forceps. In the breech group, there was one brachial plexus injury among the completed homebirths, ongoing at 6 months of age. There were three other serious neonatal morbidities (two short-term, one with ongoing mild developmental delay) and one mortality—all in the hospital transfer group. All three morbidities were associated with augmentation and attempted vaginal birth after hospital transfer to one of the few local physicians who attended vaginal breech births. Two of those births ended vaginally with augmentation and vacuum/forceps and one in urgent CS after bradycardia during placement of an IUPC. A fourth woman transferred in stable condition for stalled labor and prolonged ROM. She was admitted for a CS in a hospital that did not offer vaginal breech birth. The surgery took place over two hours after admission, and the baby died.

From these data, we can conclude that home breech birth seems to have poorer short-term neonatal outcomes compared to hospital breech birth—but the absolute risk is difficult to quantify. We do not know how much of the additional risk resulted from inexperienced providers, diagnosed or undiagnosed congenital anomalies, or delays or miscommunication during transfers, versus how much of the risk is inherent in a low-technology community setting and cannot be improved by better train-

Table 2: Breech Outcomes in Home or Birth Center Settings

Lead author & year	Date range & country	Data set	Skill level	Selection criteria	Type of BP	Dx before labor	# breech	CS rate	# deaths (NN/PN)	Mortality (%)
Sullivan 1983	1978–1981 USA	AZ LMs	-	-	-	-	-	-	1	-
Koehler 1984	1976–1982 USA	Sonoma county HBs	-	-	-	-	7[a]	-	1	-
Doser 2012	2004–2008 USA	OR OOH transfers	17 OOH breech transfers (IP/PP) out of 223 total. 14 born vaginally and 3 by CS. 3 fatalities.							
Hargand 2013	2012 USA	OR OOH births	-	-	-	-	-	-	2	-
Cox 2015	2004–2009 USA	MANAStats 2.0 VBACs	-	-	`	-	-	-	1	-
Bastian 1998	1985–1990 Australia	Homebirth Australia	-	-	-	-	-	-	≥4[b]	7.0%
Johnson 2005	2000 USA	NARM	-	-	-	-	≥80	-	2	-
Cheyney 2014	2004–2009 USA	MANAStats 2.0	-	-	-	-	222	42.8%	5/222	2.3%
Bovbjerg 2017	2004–2009, 2012–2014 USA	MANAStats 2.0 & 4.0	-	-	-	-	539	44.7%	9/539	1.7%
Grunebaum 2017	2009–2013 USA	CDC birth certificates	-	-	-	-	553	-	7/553	1.3%
Bachilova 2018	2011–2013 USA	CDC birth certificates	-	-	-	-	652[c]	-	4/652	0.61%
Deline 2012	1993–2010 USA	Amish birth center	Y	Y	Y	Y	22	50%	0/22	0
Fischbein 2015	2010–2015 USA	single OB practice	Y	Y	Y	Y	27	18.5%	0/27	0
Fischbein 2018	2010–2017 USA	single OB practice	Y	Y	Y	Y	50	16%	1/50[d]	2%

a: total # unclear; breech stillbirth d/t double footling breech w/cord prolapse
b: at least four breech deaths
c: "non-vertex"
d: mother transferred for stalled labor and prolonged ROM at 7 cm; CS performed >2 hrs after admission
   for cesarean

ing. In her analysis of over a half-million births in the UK, Nove stated that the slightly poorer outcomes for malpresentation could lead to two different proposed solutions: 1) recommend hospital birth or 2) improve midwife training. She makes the case for considering the second solution:

"[I]t could be argued that there should be more midwives who specialise in delivering malpresented foetuses vaginally in low-technology settings. If all midwives had the requisite skills/experience to cope with vaginal deliveries of malpresented foetuses, we could speculate that the risk of adverse outcomes with a planned homebirth would not be higher than with a planned hospital birth. Until this option has been fully explored, it is premature to state that homebirth is intrinsically less safe than hospital birth in cases of malpresentation" (2011).

In most of these studies, we do not know whether the baby had a congenital anomaly and, if so, whether it was diagnosed prenatally. This is significant, as breech presentation is associated with a higher rate of congenital anomalies. Women in homebirth populations often choose not to undergo prenatal testing or ultrasound examinations, and after the birth they often forego autopsy when a perinatal death occurs. For example, Cheyney et al. commented:

[S]ome of the intrapartum fetal deaths, as well as some additional neonatal deaths, reported in MANA Stats may have been congenital anomaly-related. There were several incidences when the midwife or receiving physician suspected congenital defect based on visual assessment, but an autopsy or other testing was declined and no official cause of death was assigned. The number of unknown causes of death in our sample is also at least partially attributable to parents declining autopsies (49); of the 35 intrapartum and neonatal deaths not attributed to congenital anomaly, only six received an autopsy (2014).

Thus, congenital anomalies or other underlying conditions may play a role in some or many of these breech deaths.

Context is important, too, because most American women with a breech presentation have *no* hospital option for a vaginal birth. Women in some northern European and Scandinavian countries may have more options, but they have no guarantee of vaginal breech birth in every maternity unit. Even in countries such as Canada, where the SOGC's 2009 breech guidelines strongly support vaginal breech and skill retraining, the vaginal birth rate has only risen minutely from 2.7% in 2003 to 3.9% in 2011 (Lyons et al. 2015). In today's context, outlawing breech birth at home or in a birth center is, essentially, equivalent to forcing women to have cesareans, unless they are lucky enough to live near a hospital breech provider or desperate enough to have an unassisted birth. Mandating c-sections goes against state and federal rulings that protect a person's right to refuse surgery, as well as moral and ethical mandates to respect bodily autonomy (ACOG Committee on Ethics 2016; Standler 2012).

Let me share some suggestions for midwives planning to attend breech births at home or in birth centers. Although I do not have hands-on experience attending breech births, I have been immersed in breech for several years as an academic, researcher, educator, and advocate.

1. **Share all of the available information.** Women with breech presentations need accurate information about the risks and benefits of a vaginal birth versus a planned cesarean, including short-and long-term outcomes. If we only share information from hospital studies, however, we are not providing a fully honest picture. We should also share information on home breech outcomes, noting that mortality rates seem to be higher. However, we also do not know the true risks of a planned home vaginal breech birth with a skilled provider, a known breech presentation, and clear selection criteria.

2. **Be honest about your skills and experience level.** Let clients know how many breeches you have attended and in what roles (primary, assistant, etc.). How many breech simulations have you done? What workshops or conferences have you attended?

What situations would you feel comfortable with, and in what situations would make you want a more skilled provider to assist you?

3. **Invite other experienced providers to assist.** If there are experienced breech providers in your area, invite them to attend the birth with you. Have someone present who is an expert in neonatal resuscitation, including intubation.

4. **Resuscitate with the cord intact.** Given the higher rate of low Apgar scores after a vaginal breech birth, birth attendants must keep their NRP skills current and be prepared to resuscitate. Keeping the cord intact is a key step in physiological breech birth and allows the baby to receive its full blood volume, which is especially important for a "shocky" breech newborn. Home and birth center providers typically resuscitate with the cord intact—an evidence-based practice that ought to be adopted in all birth settings. Resuscitation equipment and surfaces must be portable and easily accessible no matter where the mother ends up giving birth.

5. **Avoid simplistic catch-phrases.** I often hear the sayings "Breech is just a variation of normal" and "Trust birth." These sound lovely, but what do they really mean? Might they instill false confidence in a situation that may require life-saving skills and experience? Instead of relying on slogans or sayings, let's focus on studying the literature, learning the mechanisms and maneuvers, and improving our skills as much as possible.

Another catch-phrase to avoid is "Hands off the breech." Yes, that is often true. However, sometimes a breech needs hands on in order to be born quickly and safely. I have seen videos of birth attendants keeping hands off during a breech birth when the baby clearly needed assistance! The essential skill is *knowing* when to be hands-off and when to be hands-on and not hesitating to assist when the baby shows signs that it needs help.

A breech birth, especially with the mother in an upright position, will follow predictable mechanisms. My non-profit organization, Breech Without Borders (breechwithoutborders.org), has produced a series of educational videos illustrating the normal mechanisms of an upright breech birth. We can, essentially, "read" the baby as it wiggles its way down and out. The baby will tell us whether it is managing to birth itself or whether it needs your help. *Listen to the baby and respect what it is telling you.*

6. **Create an optimal environment for undisturbed, physiological birth.** Midwives generally excel at this. But Dr. Michel Odent reminds midwives to be mindful of their fear level as well as their skill level while attending a breech. With experience attending around 300 vaginal breech births, Dr. Odent recommends treating the first stage of labor as a trial: "If it is straightforward, easy, and fast, the vaginal route is possible. If the first stage is long and difficult, a caesarean should be decided upon without delay, before a point of no return is reached" (Culpin and Odent 2003). On the other hand, other highly experienced breech attendants treat breech labors no differently than cephalic and accept a wide range of labor patterns (Caillagh 2019; Hayes 2019; Louwen et al. 2017).

7. **Counsel women about non-medical risks.** Besides the health risks and benefits, women also need to think about the non-medical risks of a vaginal breech birth at home or in a birth center. If something goes wrong, they (and their midwives) will likely face blame from family, friends, and strangers, and possible legal/criminal charges. This is an unfortunate reality in our litigious, fearful culture that believes that a cesarean equals absolute safety and that does not accept uncertainty in birth.

8. **Collect and share your data.** Those who plan to attend breech births in their homebirth or birth center practice need to keep good records. Vaginal breech birth at home with a skilled attendant might be safer than we thought, but we will never know unless we have the data to support it! Even if you never publish your out-comes, analyze them periodically and share the results with your birth team and your clients.

I know of at least two midwives who have consented to have their breech outcomes analyzed; both of these midwives have done hundreds of breech births and are likely some of the most experienced breech providers in the US. When these results are published, we might have more data points on home breech outcomes than MANA Stats and the CDC combined. I am also aware of researchers planning to collect prospective data on vaginal breech births; please consult Breech Without Borders for updates.

9. **Demand breech options at your local hospitals.** I am an ardent supporter of homebirth—head-first or bum-first. However, I also want women to have good options in their local hospitals so they are not forced into choosing homebirth because that is the only way to avoid a cesarean. If hospitals disapprove of breech births occurring at home, they ought to change their own policies rather than persecute providers who are willing to support women's wishes.

10. **Don't sell breech down the river (5).** As more states regulate direct entry midwifery, breech, twins, and VBAC often get traded away in order to pass legislation. As much as I understand why this happens, I find it a great travesty. Midwives, advocates, and legislators: Don't give away a woman's fundamental right to bodily autonomy in exchange for midwifery licensure. Insist on keeping a woman's right to choose how her baby is born—and on a midwife's right to not abandon her client.

11. **Work with local hospitals to ensure seamless transfers.** Whether a transfer is urgent or not, women deserve a smooth, nonjudgmental transition from home or birth center to hospital. I recommend using the transfer guidelines created by the Home Birth Summit Collaboration Task Force (Vedam et al. 2014).

Notes:

1. This number comes from personal correspondence on September 13, 2017, between Evidence Based Birth and Anne Driscoll, PhD, at the Centers for Disease Control and Prevention. "The Evidence on: Breech Version." Updated February 2, 2018. evidencebasedbirth.com/what-is-the-evidence-for-using-an-external-cephalic-version-to-turn-a-breech-baby.
2. In the US, breech birth is not allowed in CABC-accredited birth centers.
3. Ongoing research project, IRB #1610303, interviewing US providers, hospital administrators, and allied health professionals who provide or support VBB in hospital settings.
4. I am happy to share a reference list; please contact me at breechwithoutborders@gmail.com.
5. This expression signified ultimate betrayal in the slave-owning era. "What does sold down the river really mean?" Last modified 27 January 2014. Accessed March 21, 2019. npr.org/sections/codeswitch/2014/01/27/265421504/what-does-sold-down-the-river-really-mean-the-answer-isnt-pretty?t=1552399357316.

References:

Abdessalami, S, et al. 2017. "The Influence of Counseling on the Mode of Breech Birth: A single-center observational prospective study in the Netherlands." *Midwifery* 55: 96–102.

ACOG Committee on Ethics. 2016. "Committee Opinion No. 664 Summary: Refusal of Medically Recommended Treatment during Pregnancy." *Obstet Gynecol* 127(6): 1189–90.

Almgren, M, et al. 2014. "Cesarean Delivery and Hematopoietic Stem Cell Epigenetics in the Newborn Infant: Implications for Future Health?" *Am J Obstet Gynecol* 211(5): 502.e1–e8.

Andersen, GL, et al. 2009. "Is Breech Presentation a Risk Factor for Cerebral Palsy? A Norwegian Birth Cohort Study." *Dev Med Child Neurol* 51(11): 860–65.

Andreasen, S, EW Nielsen, and P Oian. 2010. "Delivery of a Breech Presentation." *Tidsskr Nor Laegeforen* 130(6): 605–08.

Bachilova, S, N Czuzoj-Shulman, and HA Abenhaim. 2018. "Effect of Maternal and Pregnancy Risk Factors on Early Neonatal Death in Planned Home Births Delivering at Home." *J Obstet Gynaecol Can* 40(5): 540–46.

Bastian, H, MJ Keirse, and PA Lancaster. 1998. "Perinatal Death Associated with Planned Home Birth in Australia: Population Based study." *BMJ* 317(7155): 384–88.

Berhan, Y, and A Haileamlak. 2016. "The Risks of Planned Vaginal Breech Delivery versus Planned Caesarean Section for Term Breech Birth: A Meta-analysis including Observational Studies." *BJOG* 123(1): 49–57.

Bjellmo, S, et al. 2017. "Is Vaginal Breech Delivery Associated with Higher Risk for Perinatal Death and Cerebral Palsy Compared with Vaginal Cephalic Birth? Registry-based cohort study in Norway." *BMJ Open* 7(4): e014979.

Bovbjerg, ML, et al. 2017. "Perspectives on Risk: Assessment of Risk Profiles and Outcomes among Women Planning Community Birth in the United States." *Birth* 44(3): 209–21.

Butel, MJ, AJ Waligora-Dupriet, and S Wydau-Dematteis. 2018. "The Developing Gut Microbiota and Its Consequences for Health." *J Dev Orig Health Dis* 9(6): 590–97.

Caillagh, Cynthia. 22 March 2019. Personal communication.

Cardwell, CR, et al. 2008. "Caesarean Section is Associated with an Increased Risk of Childhood-onset Type 1 Diabetes Mellitus: A Meta-analysis of Observational Studies." *Diabetologia* 51(5): 726–35.

Cheyney, M, et al. 2014. "Outcomes of Care for 16,924 Planned Home Births in the United States: The Midwives Alliance of North America Statistics Project, 2004 to 2009." *J Midwifery Womens Health* 59(1): 17–27.

Chhabra, P. 2014. "Maternal Near Miss: An Indicator for Maternal Health and Maternal Care." *Indian J Community Med* 39(3): 132–37.

Cox, KJ, et al. 2015. "Planned Home VBAC in the United States, 2004–2009: Outcomes, Maternity Care Practices, and Implications for Shared Decision Making." *Birth* 42(4): 299–308.

Culpin, E, and M Odent. 2003. "Home Breech Birth." *Pract Midwife* 6(1): 10–11.

Davies-Tuck, ML, et al. 2018. "Planned Private Home-birth in Victoria 2000–2015: A Retrospective Cohort Study of Victorian Perinatal Data." *BMC Pregnancy Childbirth* 18(1): 357.

Daviss, Betty-Anne. 16 March 2019. Personal communication.

Deline, J, et al. 2012. "Low Primary Cesarean Rate and High VBAC Rate with Good Outcomes in an Amish Birthing Center." *Ann Fam Med* 10(6): 530–37.

Doser, L. 2012. "Perinatal Mortality of Planned Out-of-hospital Births Transferred to an Oregon Hospital." DNP diss, Oregon Health & Science University School of Nursing.

Eide, MG, et al. 2005. "Breech Delivery and Intelligence: A Population-based Study of 8738 Breech Infants." *Obstet Gynecol* 105(1): 4–11.

Fischbein, SJ. 2015. "'Home Birth with an Obstetrician: A Series of 135 Out of Hospital Births." *Obstet Gynecol Int* 2(4): 00046.

Fischbein, SJ, and R Freeze. 2018. "Breech Birth at Home: Outcomes of 60 Breech and 109 Cephalic Planned Home and Birth Center Births." *BMC Pregnancy Childbirth* 18(1): 397.

Gannard-Pechin, E, et al. 2013. "Term Breech Presentations in Singleton Pregnancies: A Continuous Series of 418 Cases." *J Gynecol Obstet Biol Reprod (Paris)* 42(7): 685–92.

Giuliani, A, et al. 2002. "Mode of Delivery and Outcome of 699 Term Singleton Breech Deliveries at a Single Center." *Am J Obstet Gynecol* 187(6): 1694–98.

Glezerman, M. 2006. "Five Years to the Term Breech Trial: The Rise and Fall of a Randomized Controlled Trial." *Am J Obstet Gynecol* 194(1): 20–25.

Goffinet, F, et al. 2006. "Is Planned Vaginal Delivery for Breech Presentation at Term Still an Option? Results of an observational prospective survey in France and Belgium." *Am J Obstet Gynecol* 194(4): 1002–11.

Grünebaum, A, et al. 2017. "Planned Home Births: The Need for Additional Contraindications." *Am J Obstet Gynecol* 216(4): 401.e1–e8.

Hannah, ME, et al. 2000. "Planned Caesarean Section versus Planned Vaginal Birth for Breech Presentation at Term: A Randomised Multicentre Trial. Term Breech Trial Collaborative Group." *Lancet* 356(9239): 1375–83.

——— 2004. "Maternal Outcomes at 2 Years after Planned Cesarean Section versus Planned Vaginal Birth for Breech Presentation at Term: The International Randomized Term Breech Trial." *Am J Obstet Gynecol* 191(3): 917–27.

Hargand, S, and A Stiefvater. 2012. "Out-of-hospital Births in Oregon." Presentation, Oregon Public Health Association, Portland, OR.

Hartnack-Tharin, JE, S Rasmussen, and L Krebs. 2011. "Consequences of the Term Breech Trial in Denmark." *Acta Obstet Gynecol Scand* 90(7): 767–71.

Hayes, David. 22 March 2019. Personal communication.

Hellsten, C, PG Lindqvist, and P Olofsson. 2003. "Vaginal Breech Delivery: Is It Still an Option?" *Eur J Obstet Gynecol Reprod Biol* 111(2): 122–28.

Högberg, U, et al. 2016. "Breech Delivery at a University Hospital in Tanzania." *BMC Pregnancy Childbirth* 16(1): 342.

Jensen, VM, and M Wust. 2015. "Can Caesarean Section Improve Child and Maternal Health? The Case of Breech Babies." *J Health Econ* 39: 289–302.

Johnson, KC, and BA Daviss. 2005. "Outcomes of Planned Home Births with Certified Professional Midwives: Large Prospective Study in North America." *BMJ* 330(7505): 1416.

Koehler, NU, DA Solomon, and M Murphy. 1984. "Outcomes of a Rural Sonoma County Home Birth Practice: 1976–1982." *Birth* 11(3): 165–70.

Kotaska, A. 2004. "Inappropriate Use of Randomised Trials to Evaluate Complex Phenomena: Case Study of Vaginal Breech Delivery." *BMJ* 329(7473): 1039–42.

Krebs, L. 2005. "Breech at Term. Early and Late Consequences of Mode of Delivery." *Dan Med Bull* 52(4): 234–52.

Krebs, L, and J Langhoff-Roos. 2003. "Elective Cesarean Delivery for Term Breech." *Obstet Gynecol* 101(4): 690–96.

Krebs, L, J Langhoff-Roos, and K Thorngren-Jerneck. 2001. "Long-term Outcome in Term Breech Infants with Low Apgar Score—a Population-based Follow-up." *Eur J Obstet Gynecol Reprod Biol* 100(1): 5–8.

Lee, HC, YY El-Sayed, and JB Gould. 2008. "Population Trends in Cesarean Delivery for Breech Presentation in the United States, 1997–2003." *Am J Obstet Gynecol* 199(1): 59.e1–e8.

Louwen, F, et al. 2017. "Does Breech Delivery in an Upright Position instead of On the Back Improve Outcomes and Avoid Cesareans?" *Int J Gynaecol Obstet* 136(2): 151–61.

Lyons, J, et al. 2015. "Delivery of Breech Presentation at Term Gestation in Canada, 2003–2011." *Obstet Gynecol* 125(5): 1153–61.

Macharey, G, et al. 2017. "Risk Factors and Outcomes in 'Well-selected' Vaginal Breech Deliveries: A Retrospective Observational Study." *J Perinat Med* 45(3): 291–97.

Macharey, G, M Gissler, et al. 2017. "Risk Factors Associated with Adverse Perinatal Outcome in Planned Vaginal Breech Labors at Term: A Retrospective Population-based Case-control Study." *BMC Pregnancy Childbirth* 17(1): 93.

Macharey, G, et al. 2018. "Neurodevelopmental Outcome at the Age of 4 Years According to the Planned Mode of Delivery in Term Breech Presentation: A Nationwide, Population-based Record Linkage Study." *J Perinat Med* 46(3): 323–31.

Mackay, DF, et al. 2015. "Educational Outcomes following Breech Delivery: A Record-linkage Study of 456,947 Children." *Int J Epidemiol* 44(1): 209–17.

Marcotte, EL, et al. 2018. "Cesarean Delivery and Risk of Infant Leukemia: A Report from the Children's Oncology Group." *Cancer Epidemiol Biomarkers Prev* 27(4): 473–78.

Mehl-Madrona, L, and MM Madrona. 1997. "Physician- and Midwife-attended Home Births. Effects of Breech, Twin, and Post-dates Outcome Data on Mortality Rates." *J Nurse Midwifery* 42(2): 91–98.

Molkenboer, JF, et al. 2006. "Birth Weight and Neurodevelopmental Outcome of Children at 2 Years of Age after Planned Vaginal Delivery for Breech Presentation at Term." *Am J Obstet Gynecol* 194(3): 624–29.

——— 2007. "Maternal Health Outcomes Two Years after Term Breech Delivery." *J Matern Fetal Neonatal Med* 20(4): 319–24.

Munstedt, K, et al. 2001. "Term Breech and Long-term Morbidity–Cesarean Section versus Vaginal Breech Delivery." *Eur J Obstet Gynecol Reprod Biol* 96(2): 163–37.

Neu, J, and J Rushing. 2011. "Cesarean versus Vaginal Delivery: Long-term Infant Outcomes and the Hygiene Hypothesis." *Clin Perinatol* 38(2): 321–31.

Nove, A. 2011. "Home Birth in the UK: A Safe Choice?" PhD diss., University of Southampton, School of Social Science.

Pekar-Zlotin, M, et al. 2017. "Cesarean Scar Pregnancy and Morbidly Adherent Placenta: Different or Similar?" *Isr Med Assoc J* 19(3): 168–71.

Pradhan, P, M Mohajer, and S Deshpande. 2005. "Outcome of Term Breech Births: 10-year Experience at a District General Hospital." *BJOG* 112(2): 218–22.

Preis, K, et al. 2012. "Long-term Follow-up for Organic Dysfunction in Breech-presenting Children." *Med Sci Monit* 18(12): CR741–46.

Royal College of Obstetricians and Gynaecologists. 2017. "Management of Breech Presentation: Greentop Guideline No. 20b." *BJOG* 124(7): e151–e177.

Sandall, J, et al. 2018. "Short-term and Long-term Effects of Caesarean Section on the Health of Women and Children." *Lancet* 392(10155): 1349–57.

Schutte, JM, et al. 2007. "Maternal Deaths after Elective Cesarean Section for Breech Presentation in the Netherlands." *Acta Obstet Gynecol Scand* 86(2): 240–43.

Standler, RB. "Legal Right to Refuse Medical Treatment in the USA." Last modified 29 July 2012. Accessed 21 March 2019. rbs2.com/rrmt.pdf.

Su, M, et al. 2007. "Factors Associated with Maternal Morbidity in the Term Breech Trial." *J Obstet Gynaecol Can* 29(4): 324–30.

Sullivan, DA, and R Beeman. 1983. "Four Years' Experience with Home Birth by Licensed Midwives in Arizona." *Am J Public Health* 73(6): 641–45.

Symon, A, et al. 2009. "Outcomes for Births Booked under an Independent Midwife and Births in NHS Maternity Units: Matched Comparison Study." *BMJ* 338: b2060.

Thavagnanam, S, et al. 2008. "A Meta-analysis of the Association between Caesarean Section and Childhood Asthma." *Clin Exp Allergy* 38(4): 629–33.

Toivonen, E, et al. 2012. "Selective Vaginal Breech Delivery at Term—Still an Option." *Acta Obstet Gynecol Scand* 91(10): 1177–83.

Tun, HM, et al. 2018. "Roles of Birth Mode and Infant Gut Microbiota in Intergenerational Transmission of Overweight and Obesity from Mother to Offspring." *JAMA Pediatr* 172(4): 368–77.

Ulander, VM, et al. 2004. "Are Health Expectations of Term Breech Infants Unrealistically High?" *Acta Obstet Gynecol Scand* 83(2): 180–86.

Uotila, J, R Tuimala, and P Kirkinen. 2005. "Good Perinatal Outcome in Selective Vaginal Breech Delivery at Term." *Acta Obstet Gynecol Scand* 84(6): 578–83.

van Dillen, J, et al. 2010. "Severe Acute Maternal Morbidity and Mode of Delivery in the Netherlands." *Acta Obstet Gynecol Scand* 89(11): 1460–65.

Vedam S, et al. 2014. "Transfer from Planned Home Birth to Hospital: Improving Interprofessional Collaboration." *J Midwifery Womens Health* 59(6): 624–34.

Venditelli, F, et al. 2002. "Breech Presentation at Term: Evolution of French Practices and an Analysis of Neonatal Results in Regards to Obstetrical Management of Breech Presentation, from AUDIPOG Database." *J Gynecol Obstet Biol Reprod (Paris)* 31(3): 261–72.

——— 2006. "The Term Breech Presentation: Neonatal Results and Obstetric Practices in France." *Eur J Obstet Gynecol Reprod Biol* 125(2): 176–84.

Verhoeven, AT, JP de Leeuw, and HW Bruinse. 2005. "Breech Presentation at Term: Elective Caesarean Section is the Wrong Choice as a Standard Treatment Because of Too High Risks for the Mother and Her Future Children." *Ned Tijdschr Geneeskd* 149(40): 2207–10.

Vistad, I, et al. 2015. "Neonatal Outcome of Singleton Term Breech Deliveries in Norway from 1991 to 2011." *Acta Obstet Gynecol Scand* 94(9): 997–1004.

Vlemmix, F, et al. 2014. "Term Breech Deliveries in the Netherlands: Did the Increased Cesarean Rate Affect Neonatal Outcome? A Population-based Cohort Study." *Acta Obstet Gynecol Scand* 93(9): 888–96.

Whyte, H, et al. 2004. "Outcomes of Children at 2 Years after Planned Cesarean Birth versus Planned Vaginal Birth for Breech Presentation at Term: The International Randomized Term Breech Trial." *Am J Obstet Gynecol* 191(3): 864–71.

Xu, B, J Pekkanen, and MR Jarvelin. 2000. "Obstetric Complications and Asthma in Childhood." *J Asthma* 37(7): 589–94.

Rixa Freeze is a professor, researcher, and mother of four children, all born at home. She is the founder of the nonprofit organization Breech Without Borders (breechwithoutborders.org). She also blogs at Stand and Deliver (rixarixa.blogspot.com).

Lesson 5: Physiological Breech Birth

By Rixa Freeze, PhD

In this lesson, we will learn about the normal physiological mechanisms of breech birth.

First, I'm going to walk you through some of the key principles of upright physiological breech birth. Then we're going to look at the mechanics and the cardinal movements of the breech as it comes through the maternal pelvis.

Why upright or physiological breech?

For as long as humans have been giving birth, midwives have been attending upright or physiological births, head-up or head-down. However, much of this knowledge has been lost over time, especially with the advent of Western male-dominated obstetrics and the associated supine (on-the-back) positioning.

Over the past few decades, there has been a Renaissance in physiological breech birth and a renewed convergence between hospital and community-based providers in sharing this knowledge. Midwives and physicians around the globe are researching and publishing about physiological breech birth, bringing it back into the mainstream.

What does the medical literature tell us about physiological breech birth? One of the earliest studies I have identified is a German study by **Burger & Safar in 1996**, in which they document outcomes of 82 breech births occurring on a birth stool out of 138 total breech presentations between 1990-1995. They note that all vaginal breech births were born using the birth stool since 1992 and "could not identify any disadvantages with this new technique." (I have not yet been able to translate the article into English, so I am limited to reading the abstract.)

In **2014**, **Borbolla-Foster** and colleagues (including Australian obstetrician **Andrew Bisits**) published a study on vaginal breech outcomes in a university hospital. Although the study itself does not mention positioning, the vast majority were on a birth stool and a minority on hands & knees or supine (personal correspondence with Andrew Bisits, 2022). In **2015**, **Bogner** and colleagues published a matched-pair analysis comparing upright (all fours) vs. supine births at their clinic in Austria, finding better outcomes with upright birth. Each of 41 upright breech births was matched with a supine breech birth during the same study period. The researchers found several advantages: only 30% of upright breeches required assistance and maternal injuries were fewer.

These findings and more were confirmed by a large study, published in **2017** by **Frank Louwen, Anke Reitter**, and other colleagues in Frankfurt Germany. They analyzed outcomes of all term breech presentations at their institution (750 total). They found no differences in perinatal mortality or morbidity between planned C-sections (315) and planned vaginal breech births (435). Looking at outcomes of upright vs. supine vaginal breech births, they found several significant advantages to upright positioning: shorter 2nd stage, fewer maternal and neonatal injuries, higher rate of vaginal birth, and fewer maneuvers required.

Louwen and colleagues have since published several sub-analyses of the Frankfurt data, which is called **FRABAT** (Frankfurt Breech At Term), including examinations of parity (Kielland-Kaisen et al. 2020), outcomes of labors occurring before or after the due date (Möllmann et al. 2020), VBAC (Paul et al. 2020), MRI as a predictor of a successful VBB (Klemt et al. 2019), role of MRI and fetal birth weight in predicting mode of birth (Zander et al. 2022), fetal leg position (Jennewein et al. 2019), and birth weight (Jennewein et al. 2018). They also published on the role of preexisting experience in learning upright breech techniques (Jennewein et al. 2021). The FRABAT dataset currently has well over 1,000 planned VBBs and continues to grow.

Besides studies on perinatal and maternal outcomes, there are many other scholarly articles on the topic of upright or physiological breech birth. Shawn Walker, a midwife/PhD in the UK, has published a large number of articles on physiological breech birth along with Emma Spillane and other colleagues and is coordinating the Opti-Breech Study, a multicenter study across the UK that will involve a RCT of various breech care pathways and that centers physiological breech in its design (see Selected References incl. Walker S, Spillane E, Mattiolo S, and Reitter 2020).

Midwives Maggie Banks (New Zealand) and Jane Evans (UK) have both published about upright breech birth in various birth and midwifery journals (see Selected References). Wildschut 2017 published a case study of an undiagnosed breech birth in the Netherlands. Stefanovic 2018 is another case study of an upright breech birth among a woman with a very high BMI. Fahy 2011 discusses whether the findings of the Term Brech Trial apply to spontaneous vaginal breech birth. In addition, French obstetrician Michel Odent addresses upright breech birth in his 1984 book Birth Reborn. American midwife Anne Frye has an extensive section on upright breech birth in her textbook *Holistic Midwifery*, vol II. Canadian midwife Betty-Anne Daviss, who trained extensively at Frank Louwen's clinic, has published a breech birth guide, *Rethinking the Physiology of Vaginal Breech Birth*.

Upright breech techniques have been introduced, shared, and refined in several international conferences: the 2006 International Breech Conference in Vancouver, BC, Canada; the 2nd International Breech Conference in 2009 in Ottawa, Ontario, Canada, the 3rd International Breech Conference in 2012 in Washington, DC, the 2016 Amsterdam Breech Conference, the 2017 North of England Breech Conference, the 2019 Madison Breech Conference, and more. Reports of most of these conference proceedings are available at breechwithoutborders.org/conferences.

Key principles of physiological breech

- Mother and baby are both active participants in the birth
- Mother in upright positions of her choice (kneeling, hands & knees, standing, squatting)

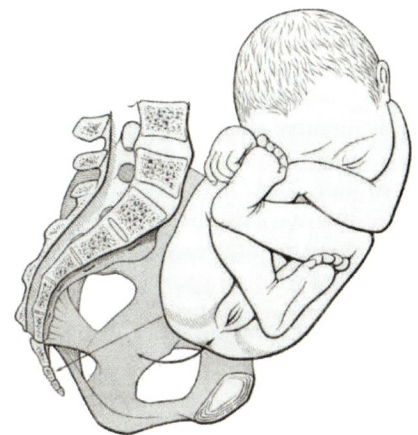

The first key principle is that the mother and the baby are both active participants in the birth, rather than passive participants. When the mother is in an upright position of her choice, she's able to be mobile. Her pelvis can flex and change diameters. MRI research on pelvises in both pregnant and non-pregnant women shows that being in an upright position, compared to on the back, results in significantly increased diameters in the mid-pelvis and pelvic outlet (Reitter 2014).

I want to illustrate that with this beautiful photograph, taken by taken by Melissa Espey-Mueller of North Dallas Doula Associates at Baylor University Medical Center in Dallas, TX, USA. The mother is in second stage, and the lighting allows you to see the sacrum (Rhombus of Michaelis) being moved up and out of the way as the head descends through the pelvis.

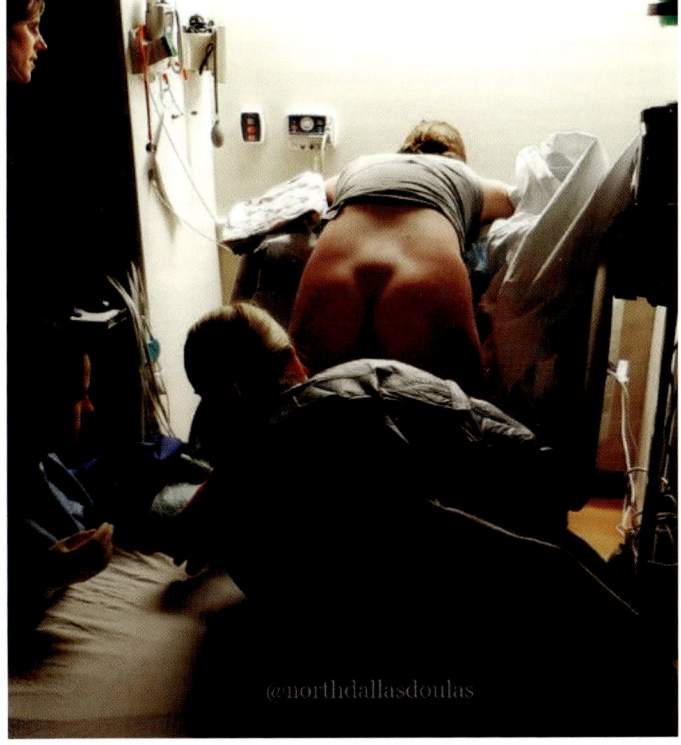

@northdallasdoulas

When the mother is in on her back and basically flipped 180°, all the weight of her body is on the sacrum. The sacrum cannot move up and out of the way, as it does with an upright breech birth. Anecdotally, when I've been attending births, I've had women say to me, "I can feel my back opening up." You can almost see the shift in the sacrum as the baby is emerging. This is the beauty of a mobile and a flexible pelvis.

1. Know the mechanisms

Respect the mechanisms when normal
Restore the mechanism when abnormal

Another key principle is that you need to know your mechanisms inside and out, backwards and forwards. They need to be so ingrained in you that you don't even have to stop and think about it. The way that we suggest approaching breech birth, whether it's normal or abnormal, is: "respect the mechanism when it's normal and restore the mechanism when it's abnormal."

This saying comes from Shawn Walker, a midwife in the UK. Instead of saying something like "Hands off the breech"—which isn't necessarily the best solution to breeches that get into trouble—we want you to really think about the mechanisms. If the mechanisms are normal and the baby's vital signs are otherwise fine, then you can trust that the birth is going as it should be, and you don't need to do anything. On the other hand, if the mechanisms are abnormal, the goal of an upright intervention is to help restore the baby to the normal mechanisms. We'll talk about that as we illustrate our mechanisms in the next part.

2. What you see on the outside tells you what's going on inside

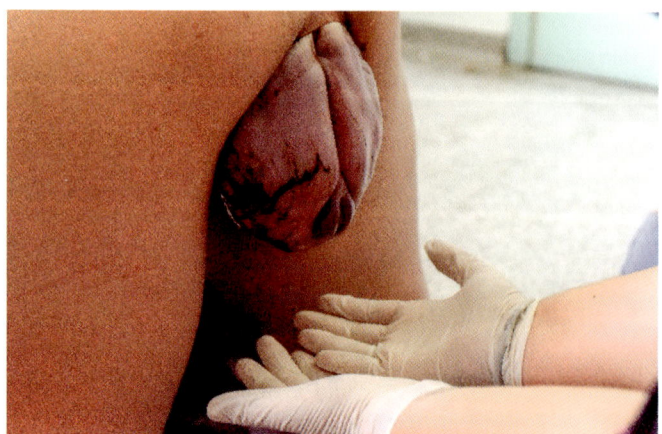
Fabiana Beracochea

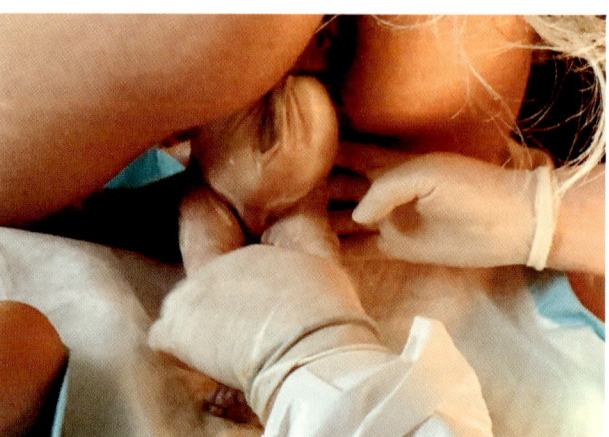
@mamasmidwives

These two pictures above give us a lot of information about what is happening unseen inside the maternal pelvis. As you study this chapter, you'll learn why these two pictures assure us that the arms and shoulders are not trapped.

Another key principle with upright breech birth is that what you see on the outside tells you what's going on in the inside. This is so fascinating! It gets me really excited whenever I teach breech. Why? A breech birth, unlike a cephalic birth, gives you so many external signs and clues of what's going on. You can essentially "read" the baby. The baby tells you what is happening with the next parts that are still hidden from view. You don't really get this with cephalic births, as things are mostly hidden until the very end.

The two photographs below are from different births. Let's talk about what we see and what that means for what is going on inside the mother's pelvis. Take a look first at the one on the left. We see a frank breech baby. The baby is in which position? Sacrum anterior or SA: baby's back (sacrum) facing the mother's front (anterior).

The baby has done its full rotation, which we will discuss later in this less. It has rotated to sacrum anterior and it's coming down. It looks like the legs are out to the back of the knees. So that's what we see on the **outside**.

What does this mean about what's going on in the **inside**? As we'll learn later on in this section, when you see a baby that has rotated to sacrum anterior, this means that the arms or shoulders are not stuck. When you have an arm that is going to cause trouble, it impedes the normal rotation from sacrum transverse to sacrum anterior. If you see the baby rotated to sacrum anterior (facing you if you are behind the mother), that's a sign that everything is normal and that you do not anticipate any problems with the arms.

In these next photos, if you look closely, you can see the tissue of the chest being smooshed together, almost looking like cleavage. We call it "cleavage" or a "chest crease." What does this mean as far as what's going on inside the mother's pelvis? Would you anticipate trouble, or would you anticipate a smooth birth if you saw this?

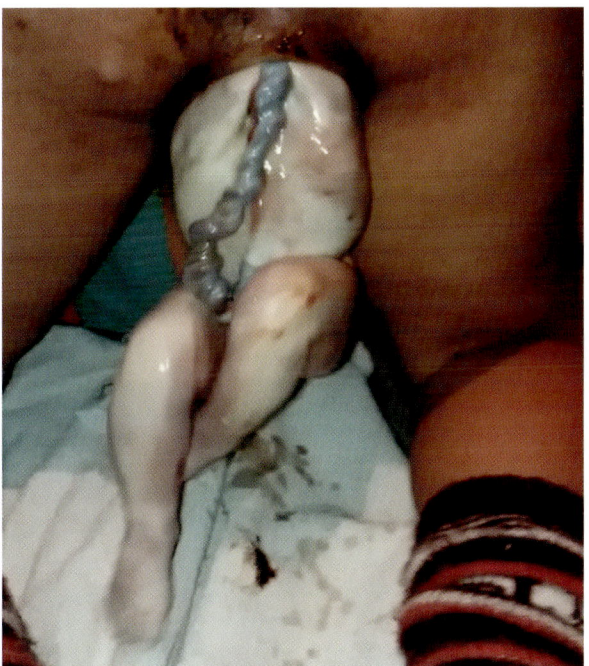
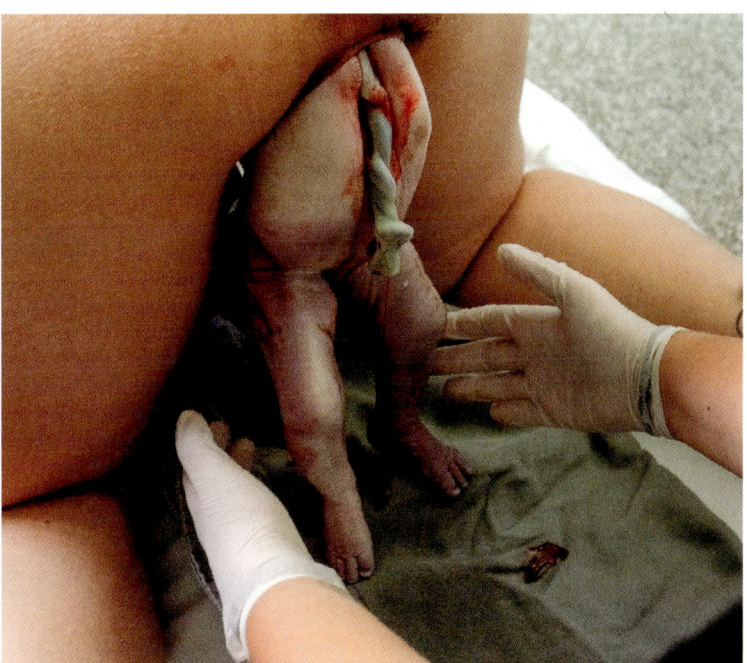

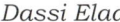
Dassi Elad   *Fabiana Beracochea*

This is a sign that there are **no** problems with the arms, that the arms are not trapped or extended behind the head. Why does the chest crease tell you that?

Think about it in terms of where the baby is: if the arms are folded up near the face, ready to be born rather than being extended behind the head, its forces skin and tissue in the chest to scrunch together, hence creating this chest crease or cleavage that we can see in these photographs. If, however, you have one or two arms that are trapped and extended behind the head, it pulls the tissue of the chest very tight and flat, and there will be no cleavage or chest crease at all. It will be very clear that it's stretched very tightly.

It's amazing that we can know what's happening inside the pelvis based on the clues the babies give us from the outside.

3. Disimpact & rotate

Another key principle is to **disimpact and rotate** when there's a problem. In earlier sayings that some people have been using, especially in the UK, it was "elevate and rotate." It's nice because it rhymes in English. However, we were having issues with trainees hearing the word "elevate" and thinking that meant to lift the baby up (the part of the baby that's outside the mother). That's not at all what we mean!

When we say "disimpact and rotate," what do we mean? You slightly replace the baby back inside the mother and then you rotate the baby off of the obstructed part. Another way of thinking about it could be "replace and rotate," if you like words that sound similar.

Remember, never pull on a breech baby! Instead, disimpact and rotate the baby free of what it's stuck on.

4. Stuck kitchen drawers

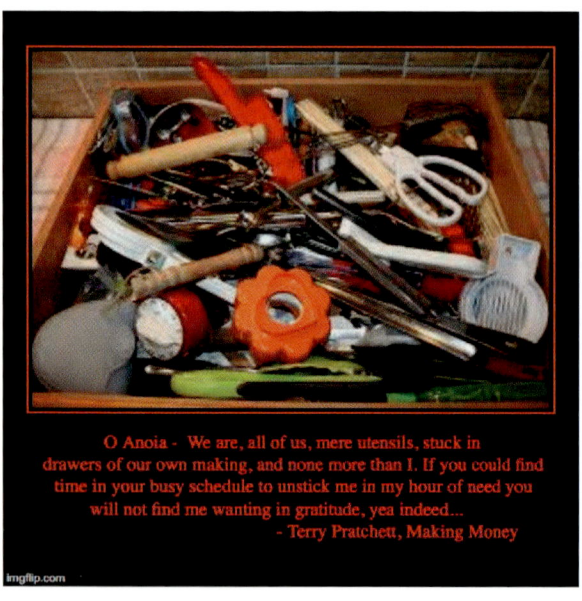

O Anoia - We are, all of us, mere utensils, stuck in drawers of our own making, and none more than I. If you could find time in your busy schedule to unstick me in my hour of need you will not find me wanting in gratitude, yea indeed...
- Terry Pratchett, Making Money

imgflip.com

Mary Cronk was an experienced breech midwife in the UK who died in 2018. She was well known for explaining that a stuck breech baby is like a stuck kitchen drawer. Have you ever had one of those kitchen drawers that's full of utensils, big spoons, and spatulas? Something gets stuck, and you pull it halfway out and it will not move. You clearly can't get it any further out because there's a large object in the way. The way you solve a stuck kitchen drawer is not by pulling harder, but instead by **pushing the drawer back in a little bit**. You put your hand inside and you find the utensil that is holding things up. You wiggle that stuck object out of the way, and then you can pull the drawer out easily.

Obstructed breech birth, in some ways, is a lot like a kitchen drawer. You disimpact and then you rotate. You put the drawer (baby) back inside a little bit, you wiggle the stuck thing free, and then it can come easily.

5. Old dresser drawers

You might also see asymmetry during a vaginal breech birth, due to the baby getting hung up in the pelvis on one side. If you have antique wooden furniture with drawers that open without any complex mechanisms, sometimes pulling on the drawer asymmetrically will get the drawer stuck. It won't move until you put it back in a little bit, wiggle it just right so it's straight, and then it comes out very easily. This often happens with one of the dressers in my own house.

6. Birth stools are useful tools

Andrew Bisits, an obstetrician in Australia, explains how he came to prefer a birth stool over supine positioning (BirthRite video, accessed at www.birthrite.com.au in 2017):

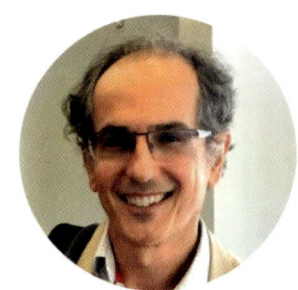

> Initially, I did the breech deliveries in a more traditional sort of lithotomy [on the back] position. And I thought to myself, after all, "This is crazy, you know. There's something that's just not happening right. The position's not helping and I'm not able to help." But then women actually in labor, when they go into the birth stool—and this is when they've changed position a number of times—they say, "Every time I got onto the birth stool, I felt that baby coming down." My own strong impression is that they get up onto the bed, they're fully dilated, and they push and you can't see anything. They get onto the birth stool. Immediately, without any pushing, already you can see the baby coming on to view. And then I suppose the really convincing thing is that I just find on the birth stool the delivery just happens by itself.

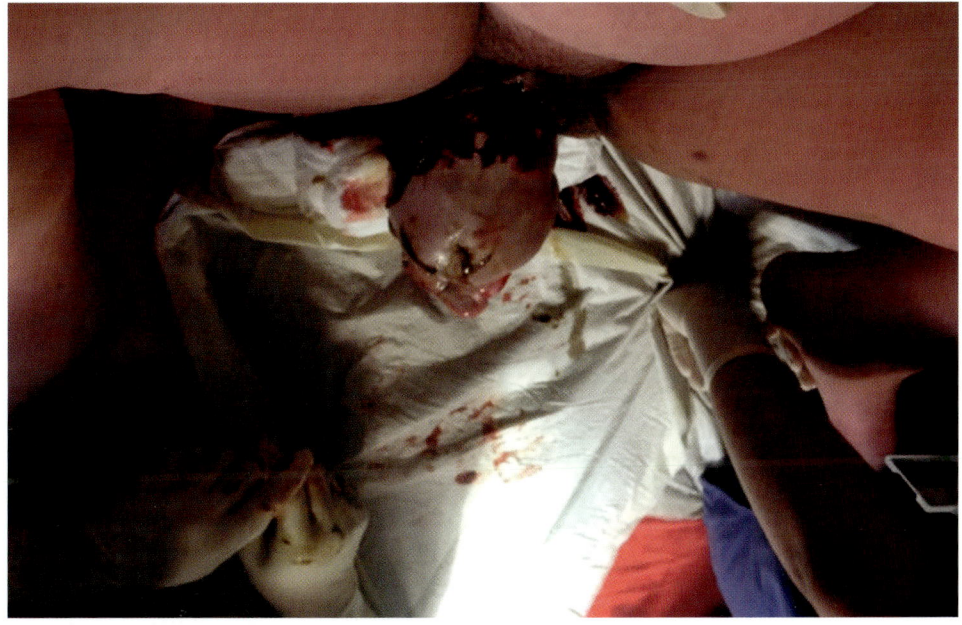

Breech birth on a birth stool

Who "invented" upright breech birth?

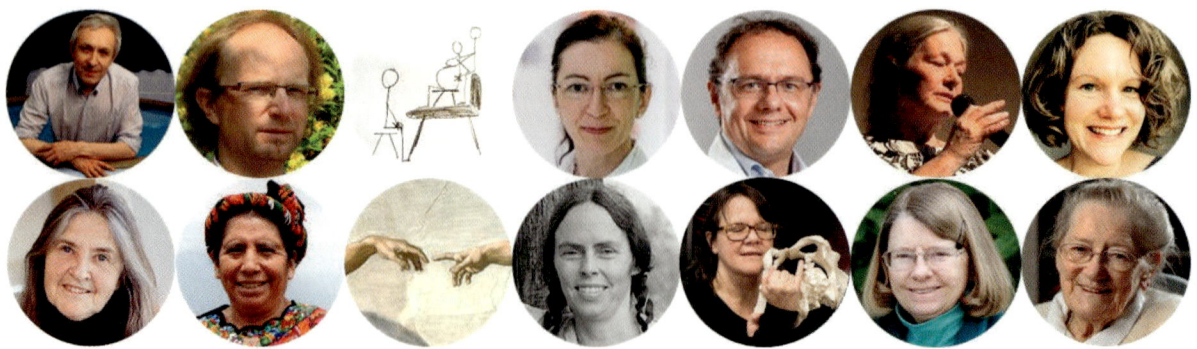

There are people around the world in many different contexts and cultures who have been researching and innovating with upright breech birth. You can see a number of these key actors in the pictures above.

- Michel Odent (France)
- Gerhard Bogner (Austria)
- Burger & Safar (Germany)
- Anke Reitter (Germany)
- Frank Louwen (Germany)
- Jane Evans (UK)
- Shawn Walker (UK)
- Betty-Anne Daviss (Canada), who learned from...
- Guatemalan midwives, who say they learned their techniques from...
- God
- Ina May Gaskin (USA)
- Gail Tully (USA)
- Anne Frye (USA)
- Mary Cronk (UK)

Other names come to mind as well, such as Maggie Banks (NZ) and Gregory White (USA). This is not a comprehensive list, and I apologize if I have left someone out who should have been on it.

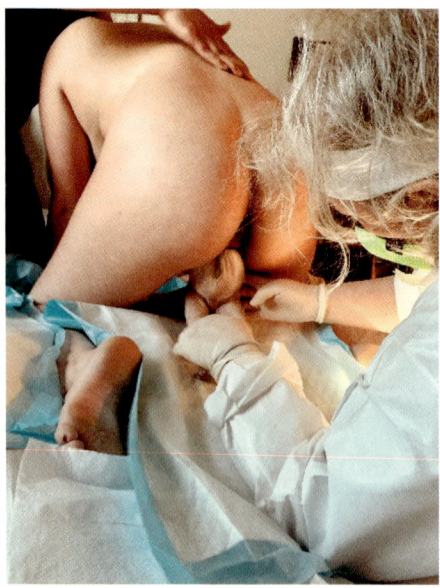
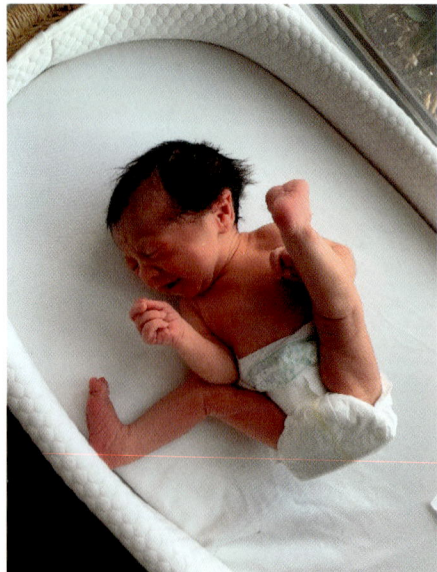
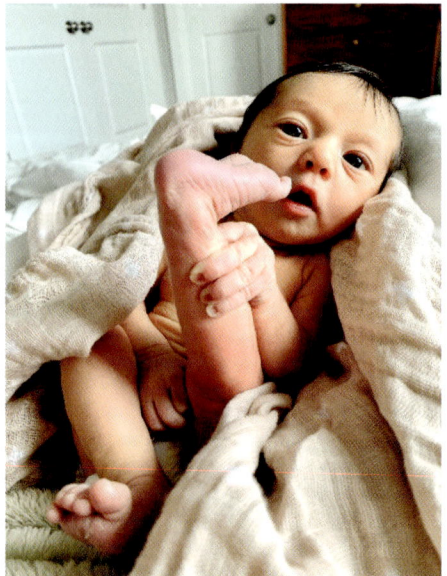

10 mechanisms of upright breech birth

Now we're going to go through the 10 mechanisms of upright breech birth.

1. Buttocks/feet emerge sacrum transverse (ST)

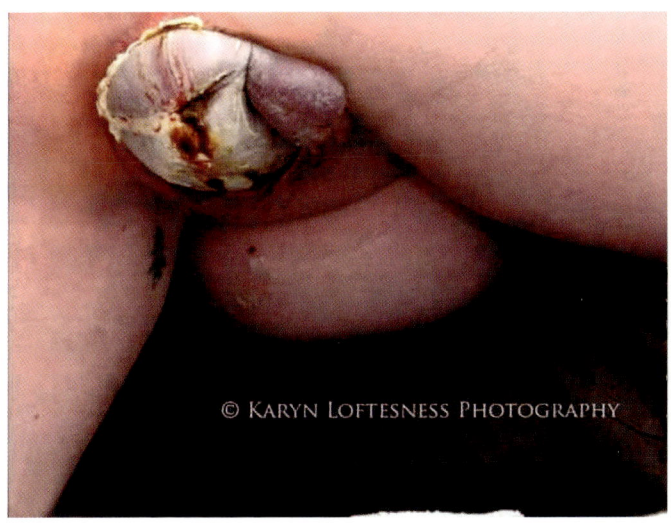 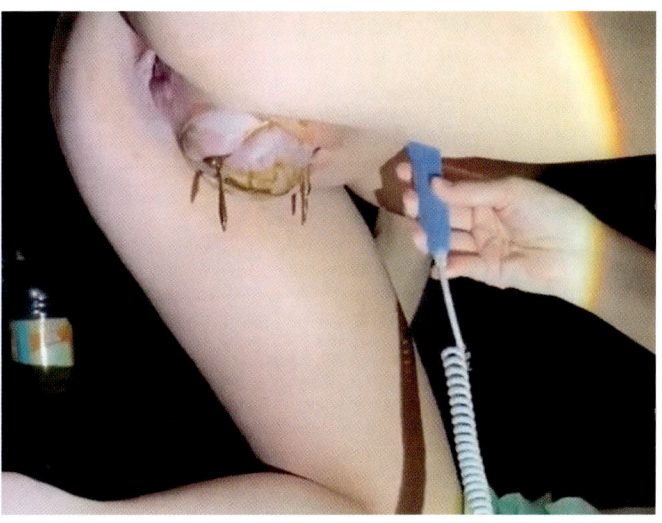

Baby is rumping LST
(baby's back on mother's left side)
Series by Karyn Loftesness Photography

Baby is rumping RST
(baby's back on mother's right side)

The first mechanism of upright breech birth is that when the baby is rumping (which is like crowning, but we call it "rumping" since the rump is coming out), the buttocks or the feet will emerge sacrum transverse. You'll see the baby facing either to one side or the other, and that's totally normal. It would be extremely rare to see a baby rumping fully sacrum anterior.

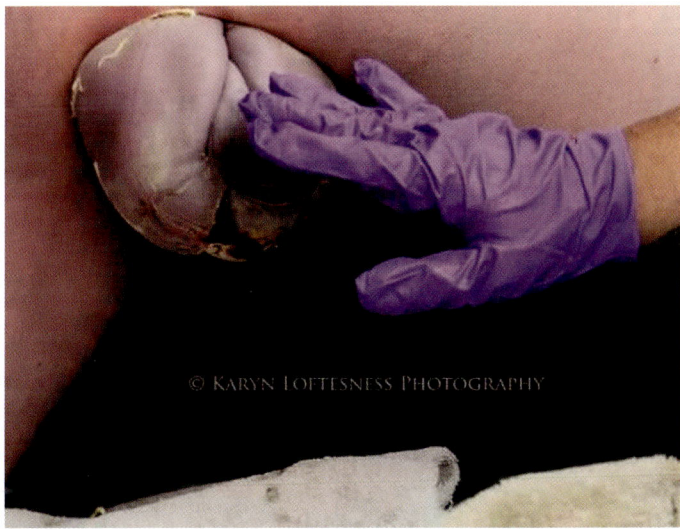 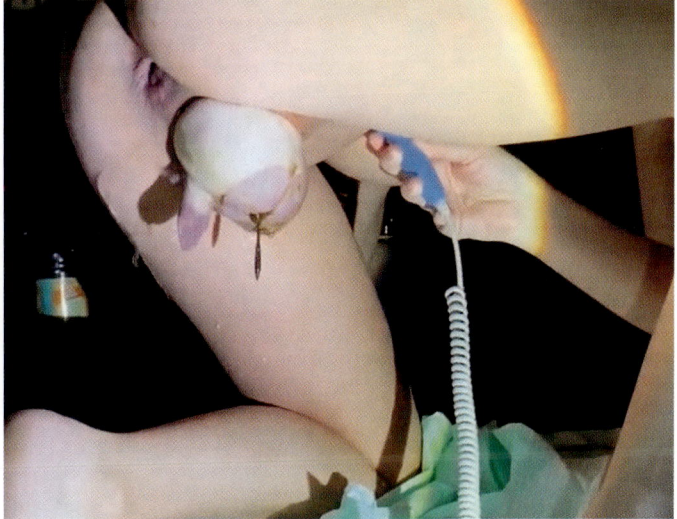

2. Body rotates to sacrum anterior (SA) as trunk is born

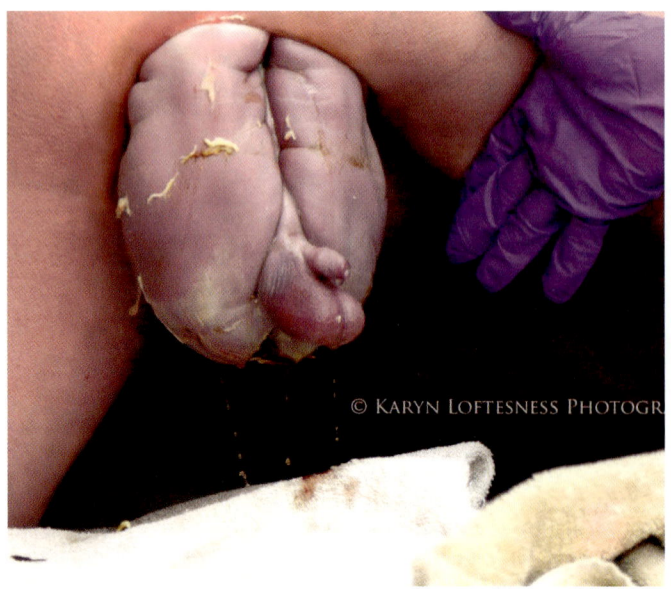
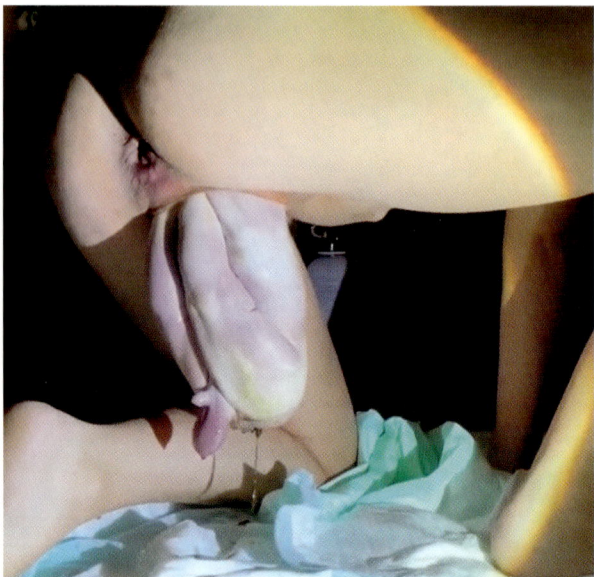

The next step: as the baby comes down and out, the body will rotate to sacrum anterior as the trunk is born. Somewhere between the umbilicus and the nipples, you would expect to see that rotation happen. As you see in the left-hand photo above, the baby has almost finished its rotation, not quite all the way there. And in the right-hand photo, the baby has fully rotated.

(Please note that this is true for frank breeches. However, for complete breeches, they will often only rotate partially to sacrum oblique until the shoulders are out. Dr. Hayes will explain why this happens in one of his lessons.)

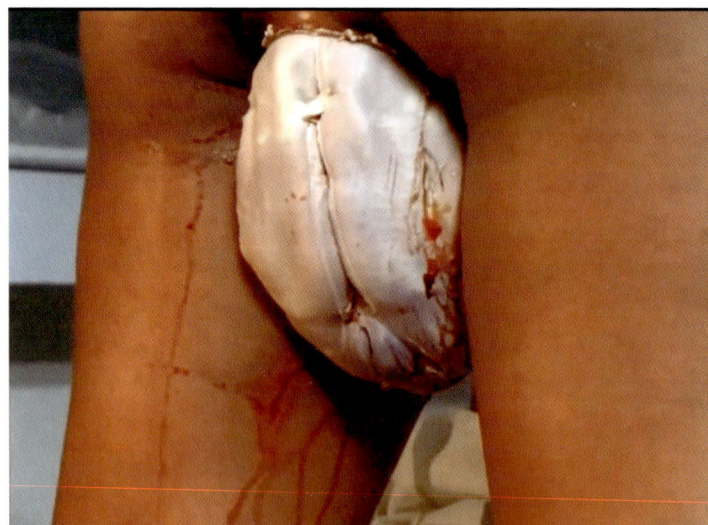
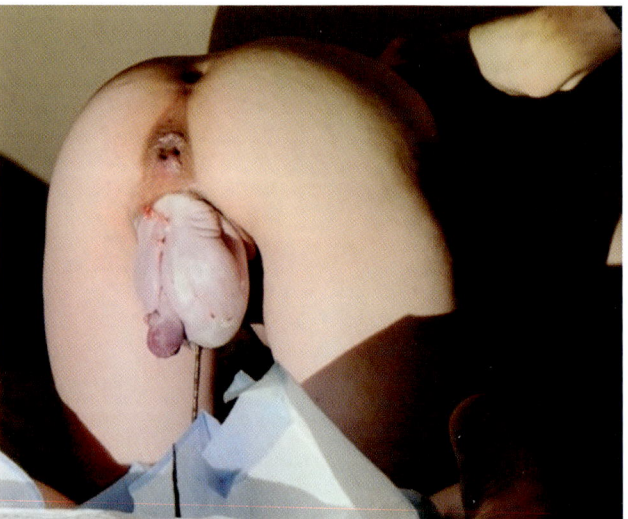

"A Chegada de Thayla"
youtu.be/H4-OwQbZLPw

3. Legs release spontaneously

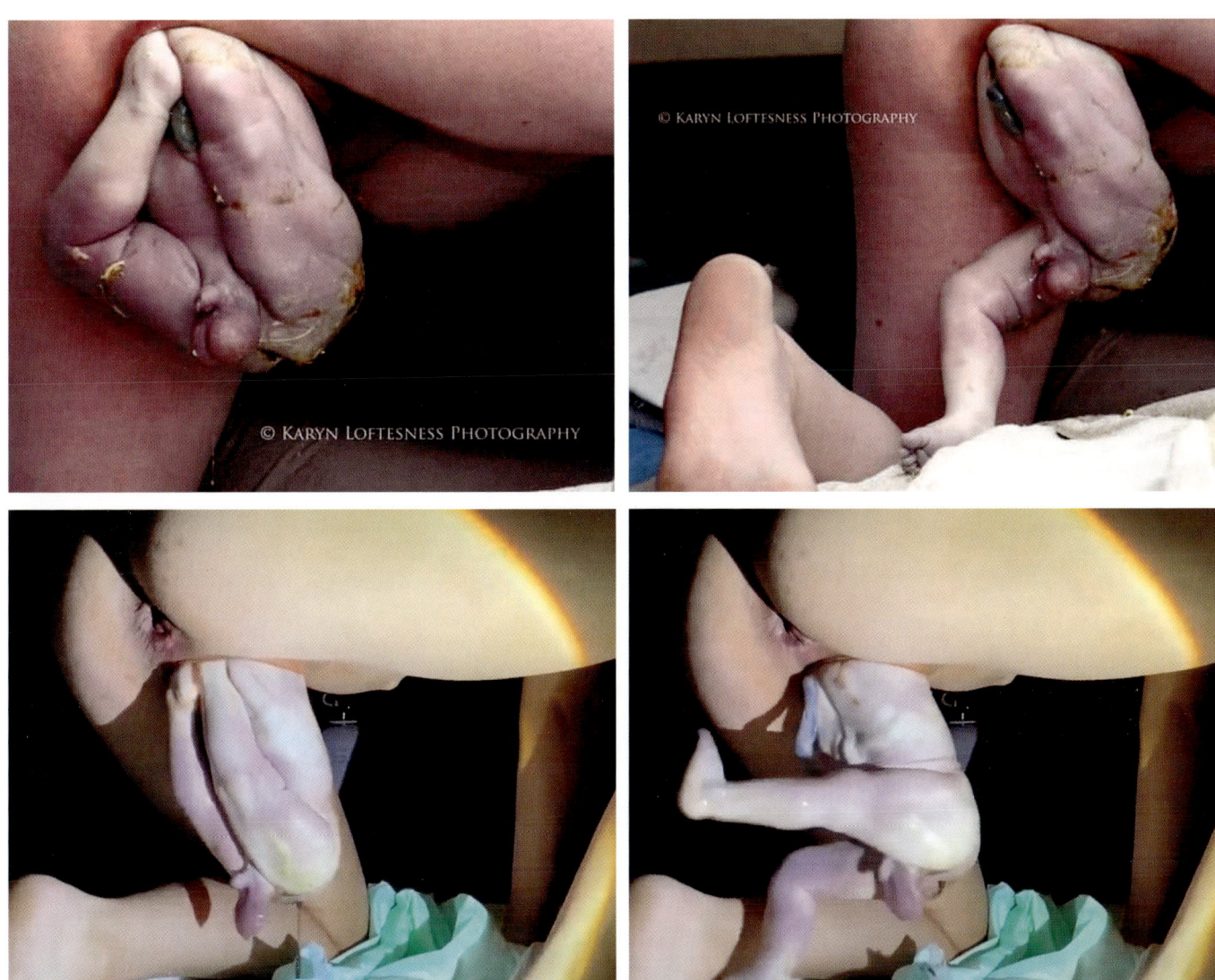

© Karyn Loftesness Photography

© Karyn Loftesness Photography

Play

The next thing you will see in an upright breech birth is the legs will release spontaneously, more or less at the same time, especially if the baby is frank breech. However, this is not necessarily true if the baby is complete or incomplete because the legs might be folded up in non-symmetrical positions. But they will come out on their own. That's the next step in a normal, spontaneous physiological breech birth.

4. "Cleavage" or chest crease = arms are NOT behind head

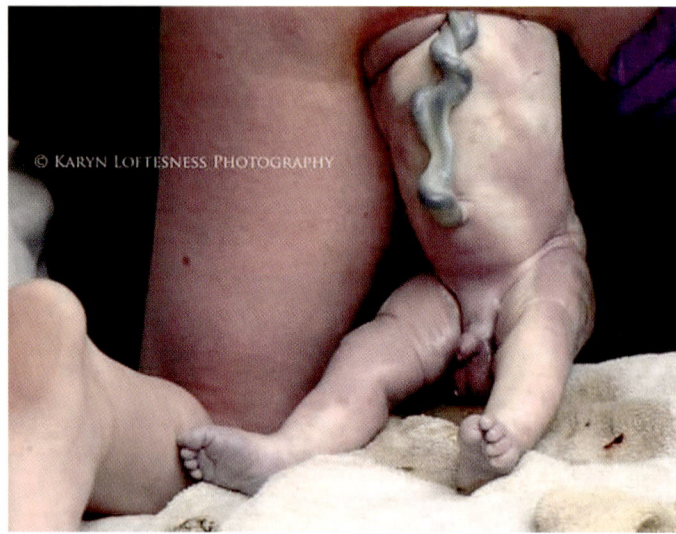 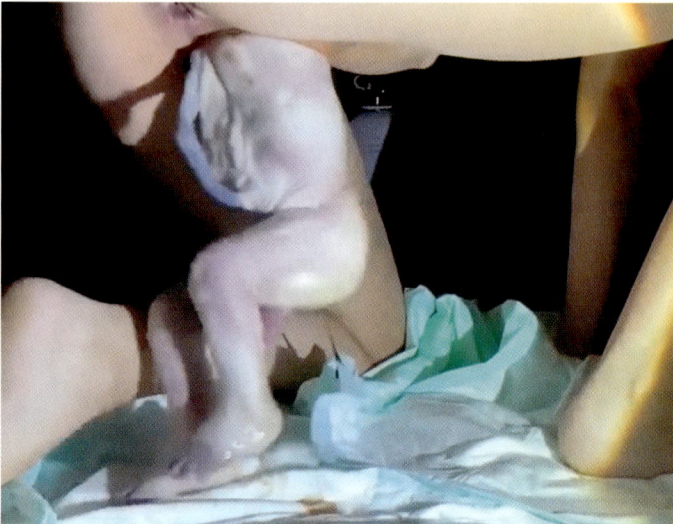

Next, we look for the chest crease or the cleavage, which I mentioned earlier in this section. When you see this nice scrunched-up bunch of tissue on the chest, this means the arms are not extended behind the head. This means you can anticipate a nice, easy release of the arms, likely with the very next contraction.

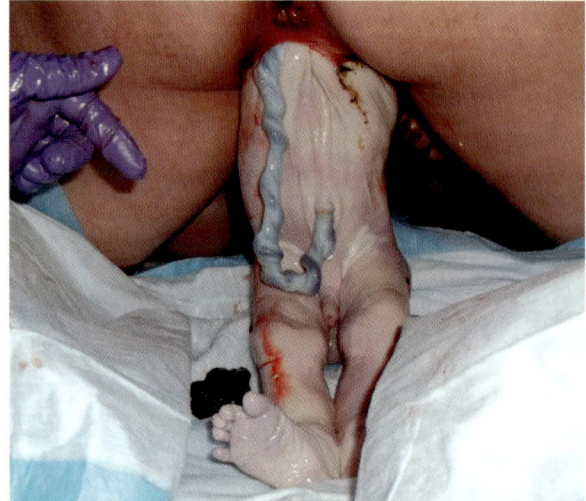 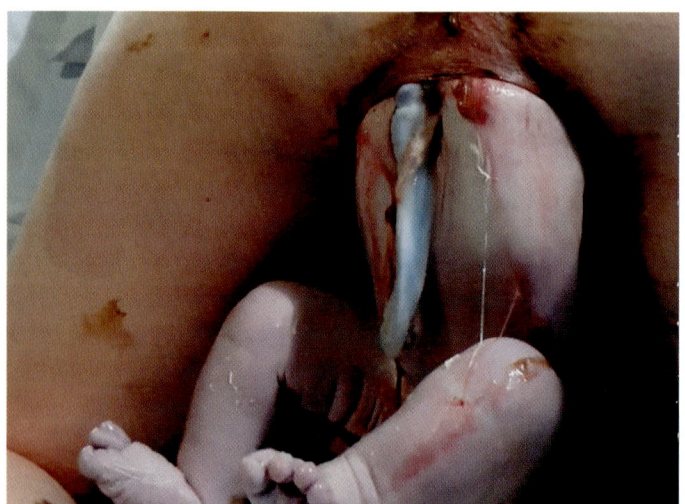

Pamela Qualls

5. Tummy crunches help flex the head

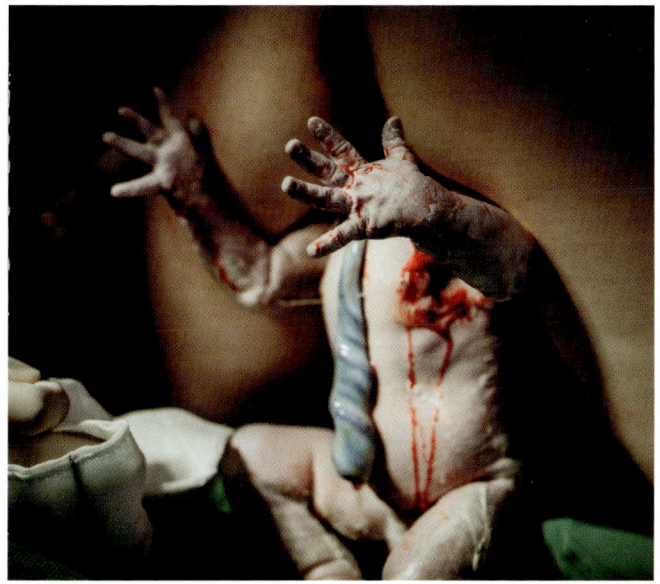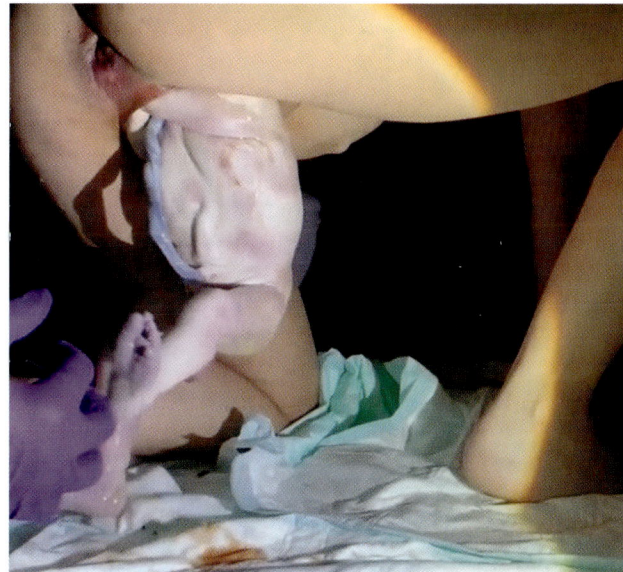

Life & Lens Photography via Facebook

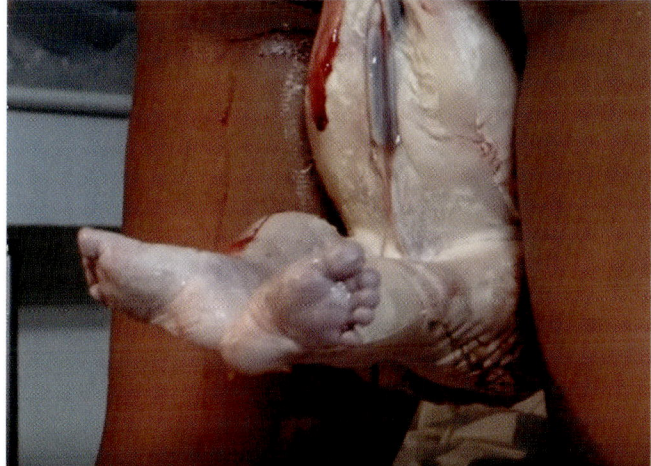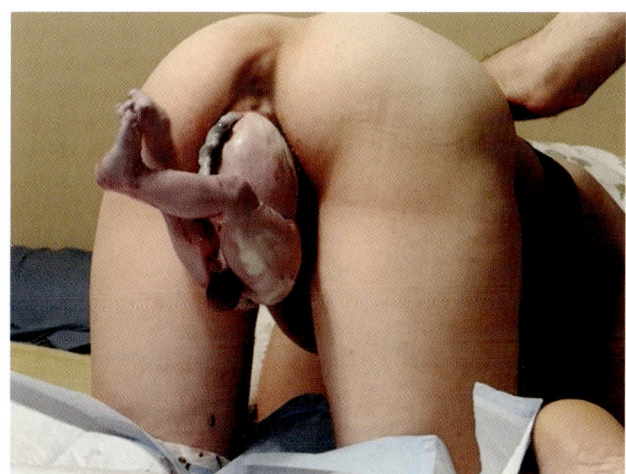

"A Chegada de Thayla"

Next, the baby does tummy crunches, leg lifts, or arm curls once the arms are born. We don't know why the baby does this whole body flexion—probably because it is feeling the effects of gravity for the first time and wants to get back into the fetal position. Unless the baby is compromised, it will usually make these movements after the legs emerge and often again after the arms are out. A baby with poor tone won't be able to do vigorous tummy crunches. That probably explains why a baby with poor tone might take longer to be born, because it cannot assist by pulling its arms down and flexing its head.

Think about this mechanically. When the baby lifts its legs, it contracts the abdominal muscles, curls its spine, and flexes its head downwards towards the chest. Have you ever done sit-ups? Doing so automatically curls your head towards your chest. Having a well-flexed head will then facilitate the birth by presenting the smallest possible diameter in the pelvic outlet.

6. Arms release spontaneously

At this point, the baby has done some nice tummy crunches. The legs are out. The next step is that the arms release spontaneously, more or less one right after the other.

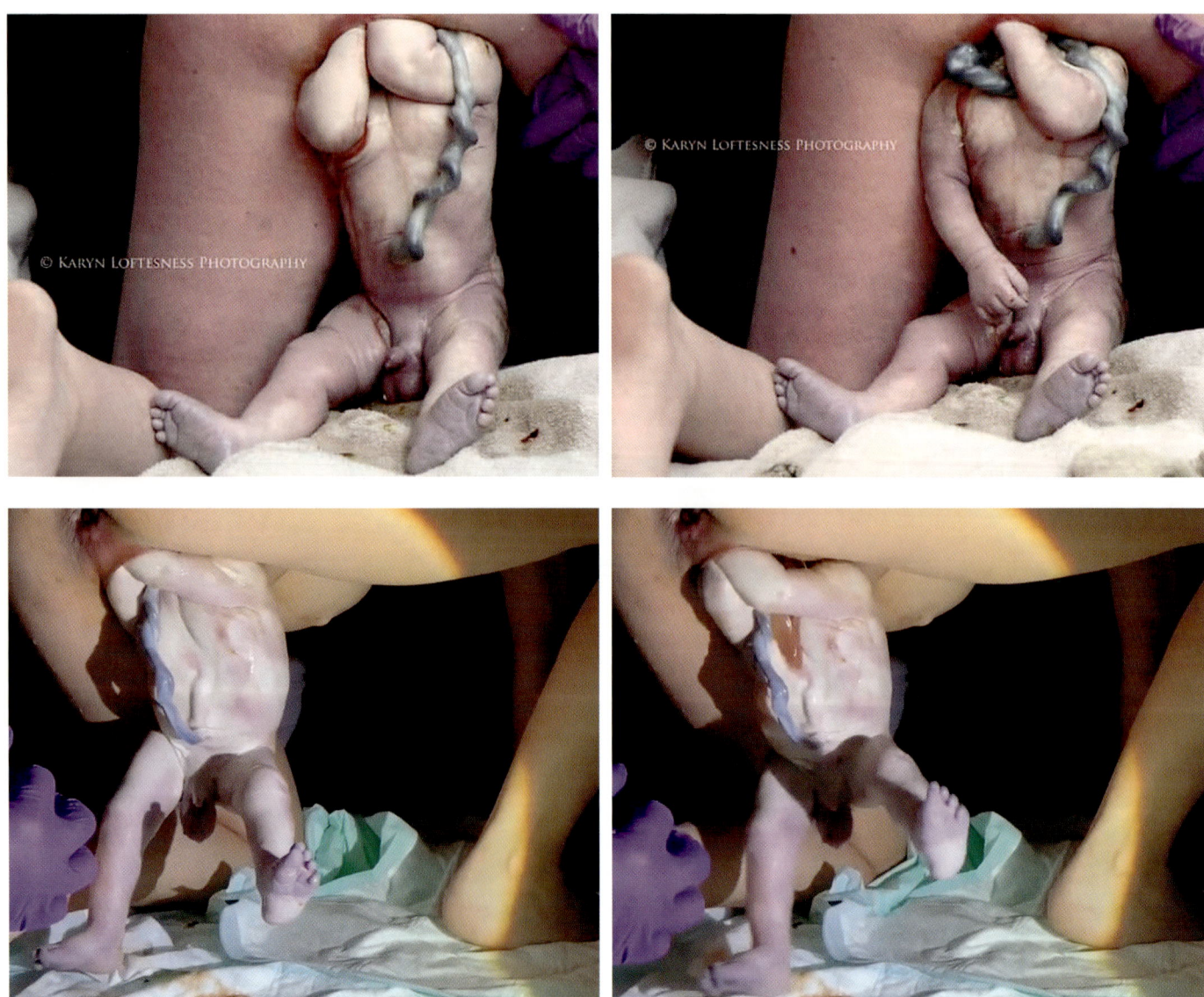

Usually one will roll out, do a little shimmy, and then the other one will roll out right afterwards. It looks something like in these photos above and below. You'll see one shoulder roll and come down, then the other one roll and come down.

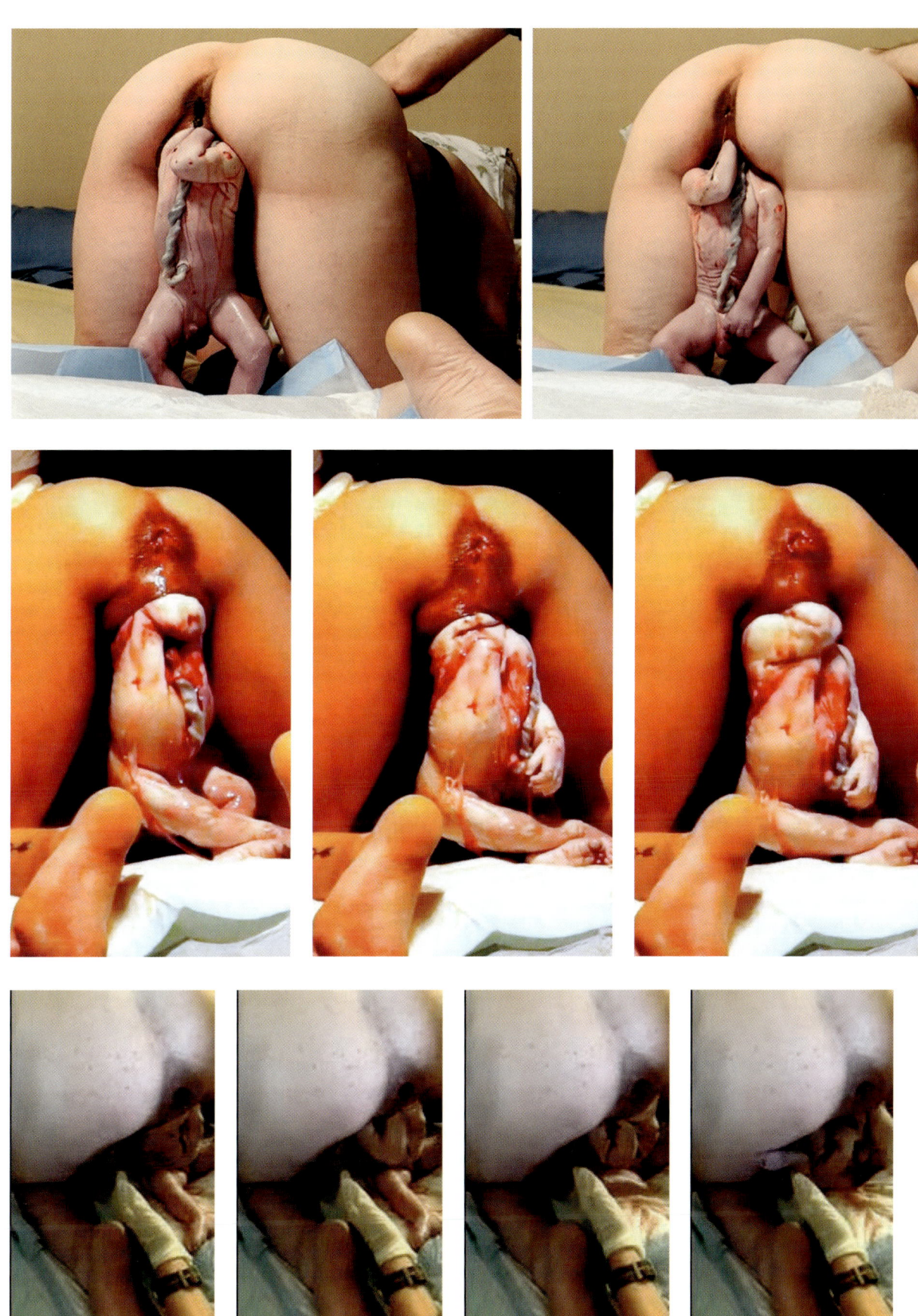

7. Full perineum = head is flexed

Next, take a look at the perineum. You want to see a perineum that looks **full and bulging** rather than **hollow or deflated**. Why? If you have a nicely flexed head, it will bulge the perineum outward because the face is filling up the perineum. In contrast, if you have an extended head, you have a hollow space because the chin has not yet moved down.

Hollow   Full

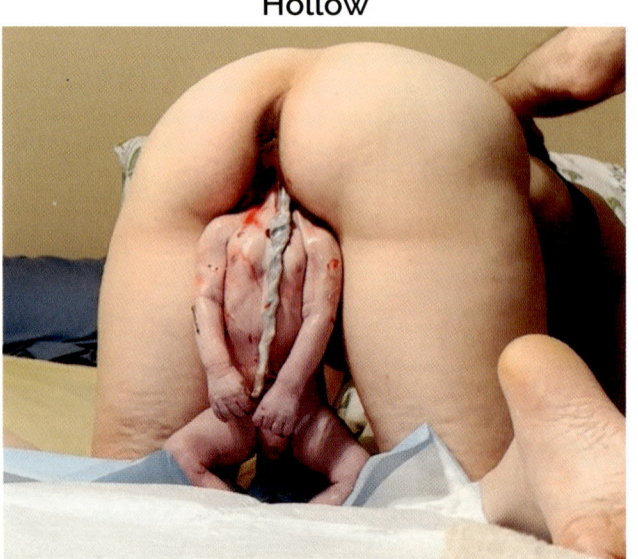 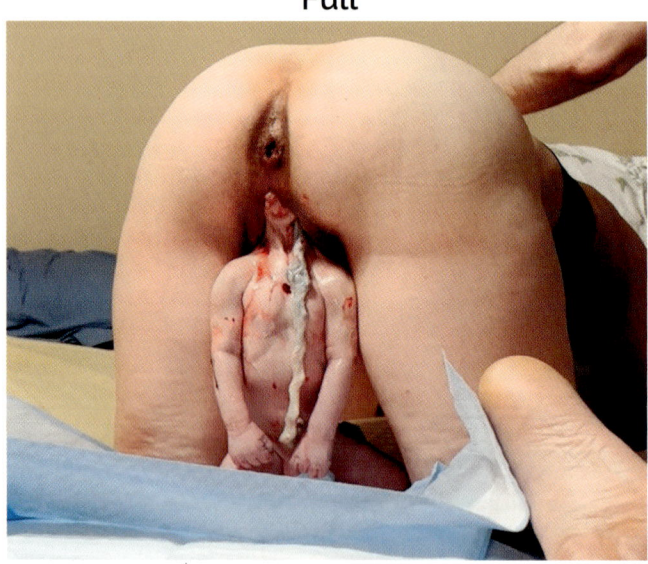

Watch head flexion happen in these images. In the above images, the perineum started looking full once the mother started pushing. A similar thing happened below; immediately after the arms came out, the perineum looked hollow. Fifteen seconds later and with maternal pushing, the baby's head and chin came down. In the 2nd photo on the right, the baby's chin is visible and the nose is poking outwards underneath the perineum, creating a little bulge underneath the rectum. We now have a nice full looking perineum. The head is ready to be born.

Hollow   Full

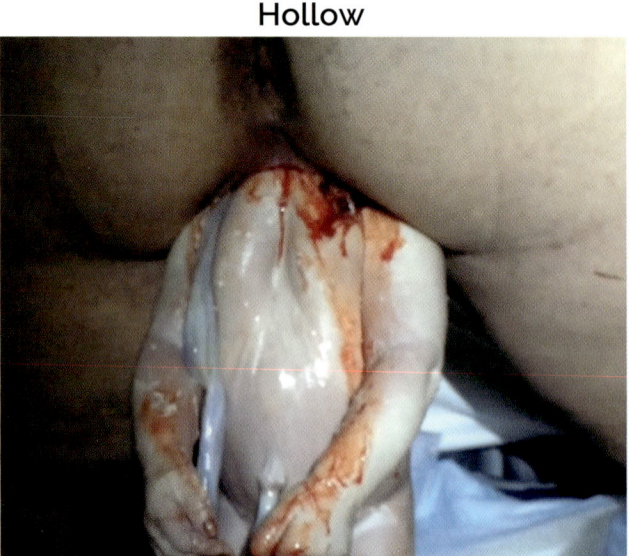 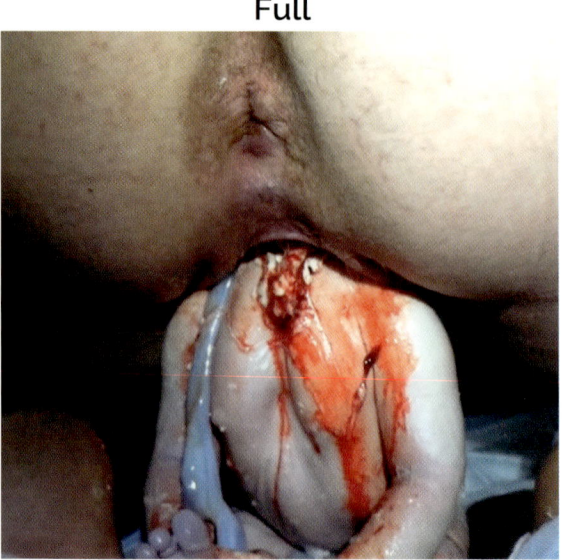

8. Head releases spontaneously

Next, the head releases spontaneously. By time the perineum goes up over the nose, you can expect the rest of the head to fall out. So be prepared to catch once you see the nose!

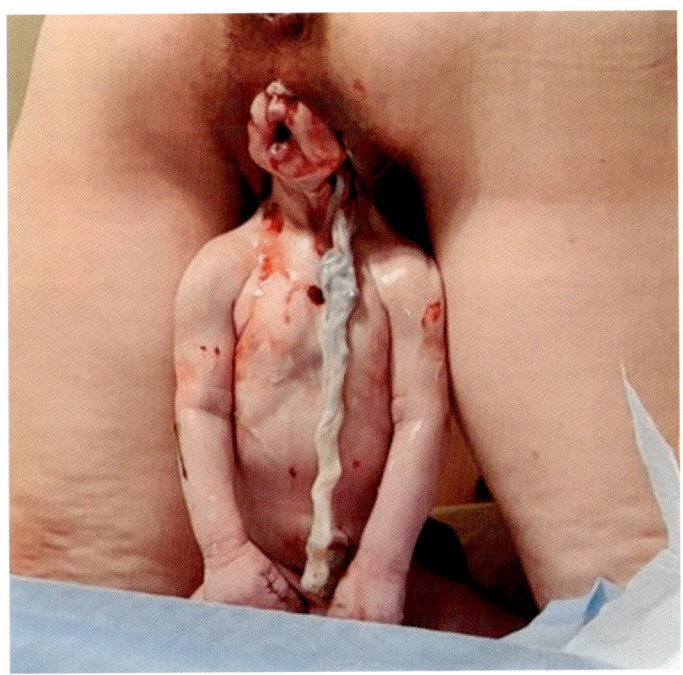 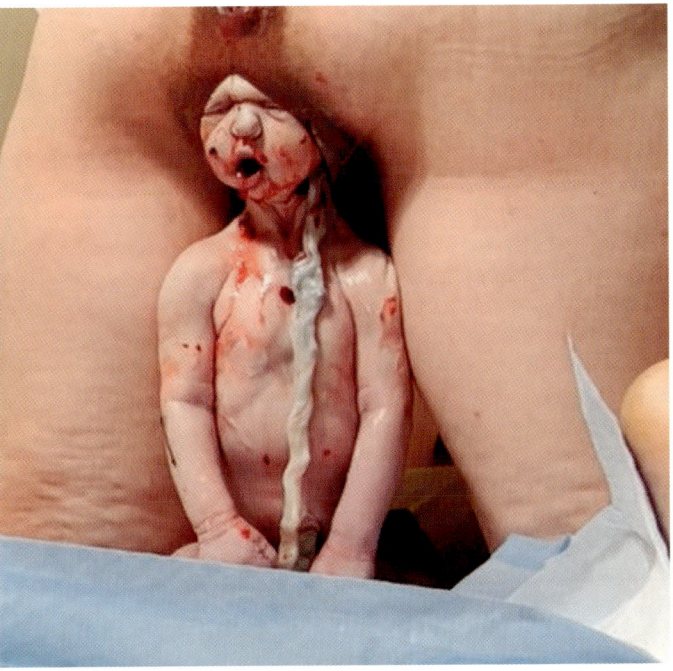

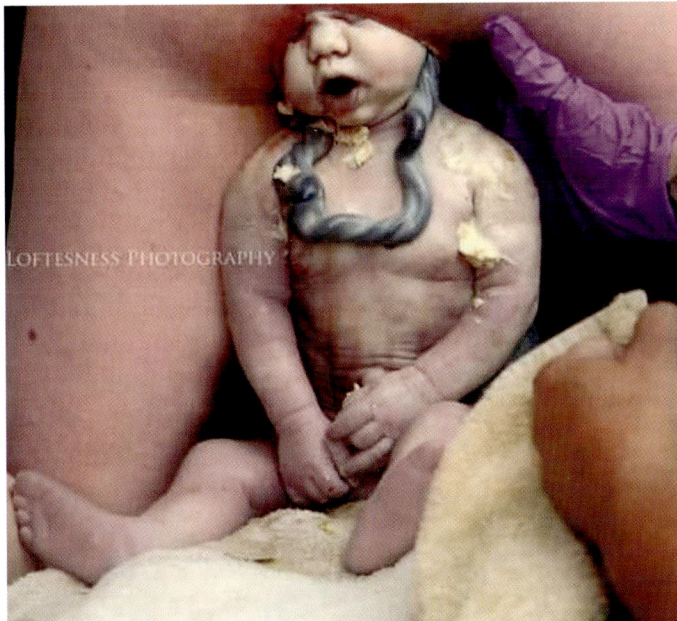 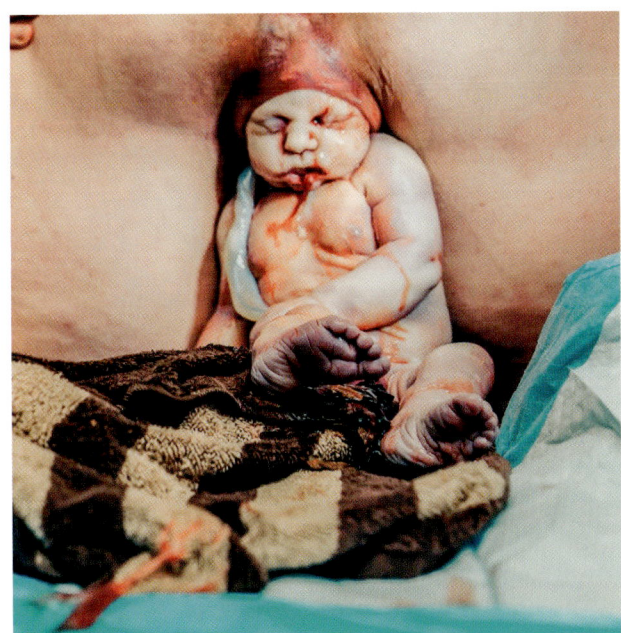

Heather Whitus Photography

But the birth isn't done even though the head is out. What are the last two steps of a normal physiological breech birth?

9. Baby passed to mother

The baby gets passed to the mother. Here's a practical tip. If you're behind the mother and she's on hands & knees or kneeling, you just simply scoot the baby right between the mother's legs. If you go around to either side, the cord is going to get in the way. It sounds obvious, but I've seen some births where the attendant forgets. They start to hand the baby to the mother around one leg or the other. Then the cord gets pulled tight, and they have to go back through her legs.

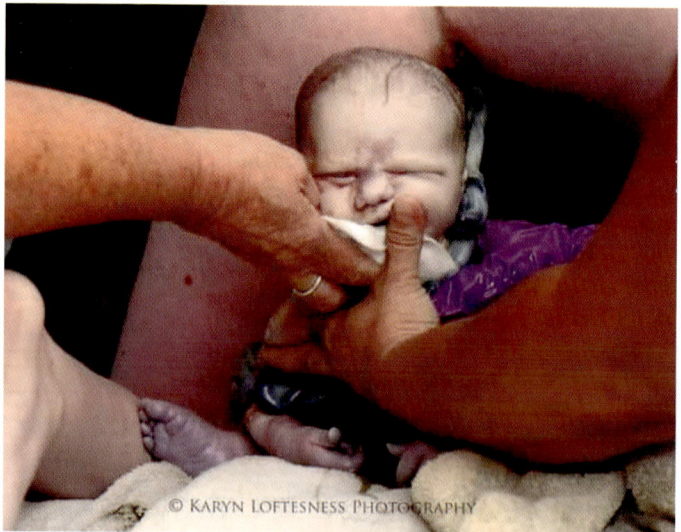
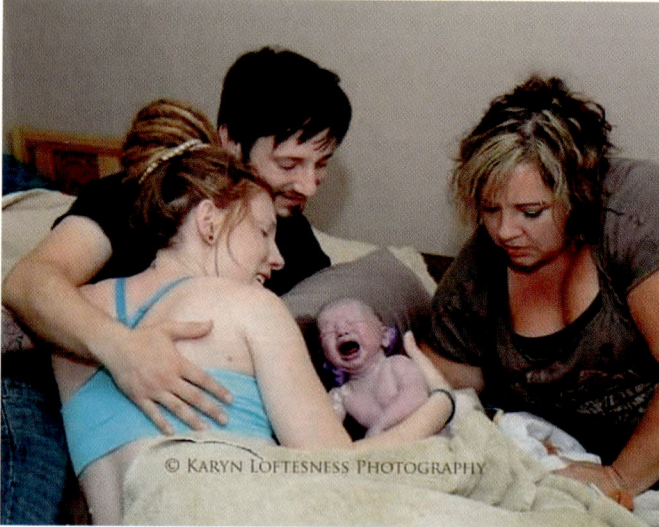
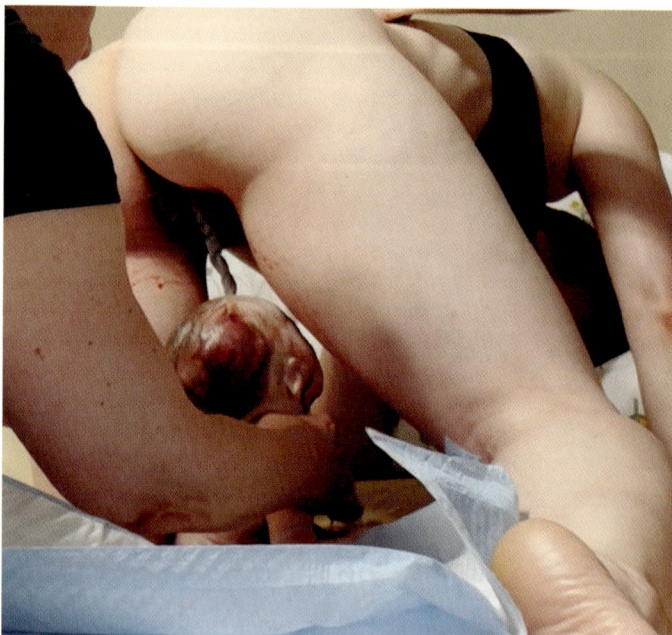
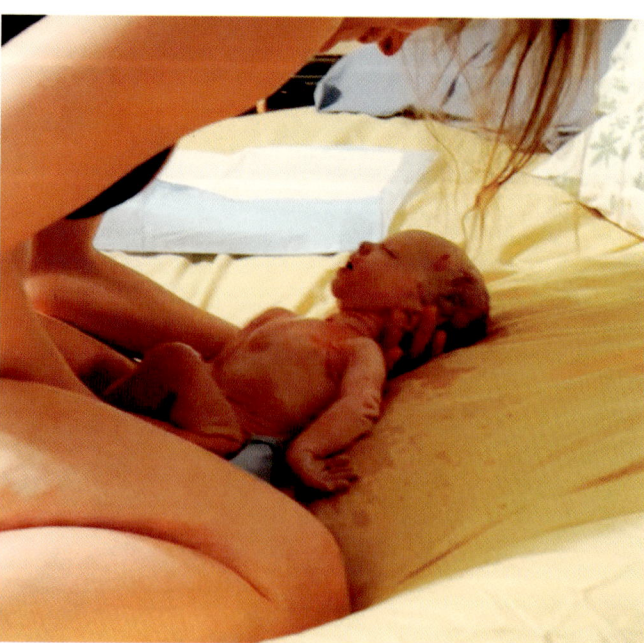

But we're still not done. There's one more step and this one is very important. It's an integral part of the package that we teach when we teach physiological breech birth.

10. Cord intact, even if resuscitating

The last step is leaving the umbilical cord intact (unclamped and uncut) even if you are resuscitating the baby—**especially** if you are resuscitating the baby.

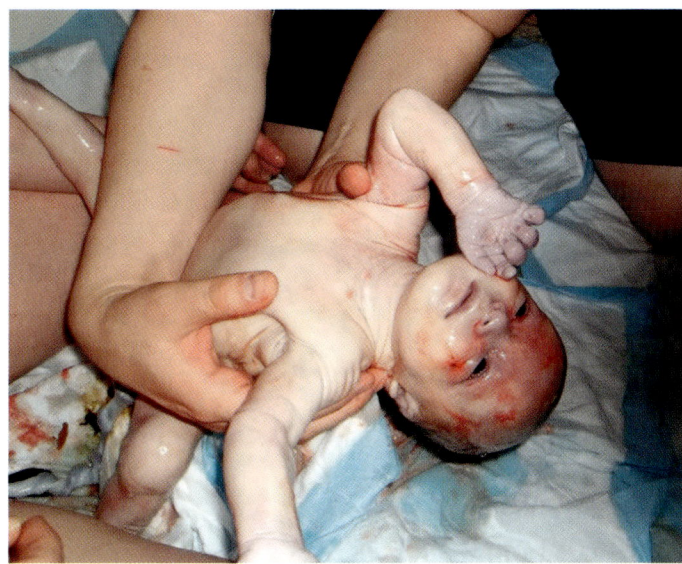

See Ashish et al. Intact cord resuscitation versus early cord clamping in the treatment of depressed newborn infants during the first 10 minutes of birth (Nepcord III)—a randomized clinical trial. *Maternal Health, Neonatology and Perinatology* 5:15 (2019).

Pamela Qualls

There are several high-quality studies on this topic, including a recent randomized controlled trial of resuscitating with or without the cord intact (Ashish et al. 2019). Babies do worse if you cut the cord when you're resuscitating versus if you leave the cord intact.

We ought to be actively working on reorganizing our birth practices and, if need be, reworking our birth spaces so that we can resuscitate with the cord intact. In order to facilitate this, providers will need to learn how to resuscitate with the cord intact. They will need mobile equipment that can be brought right to the bed or birth pool. It may require conversations with the pediatric team if you are not the one doing the resuscitation. But it's imperative that you keep the baby's lifeline and oxygen supply intact while you are resuscitating.

This concludes the lesson on physiological breech birth. We have learned the ten normal mechanisms, which tell us what we should be seeing when everything is normal. Next is a lesson about maneuvers for breech birth with a focus on upright breech maneuvers. How do we help babies when they get themselves stuck?

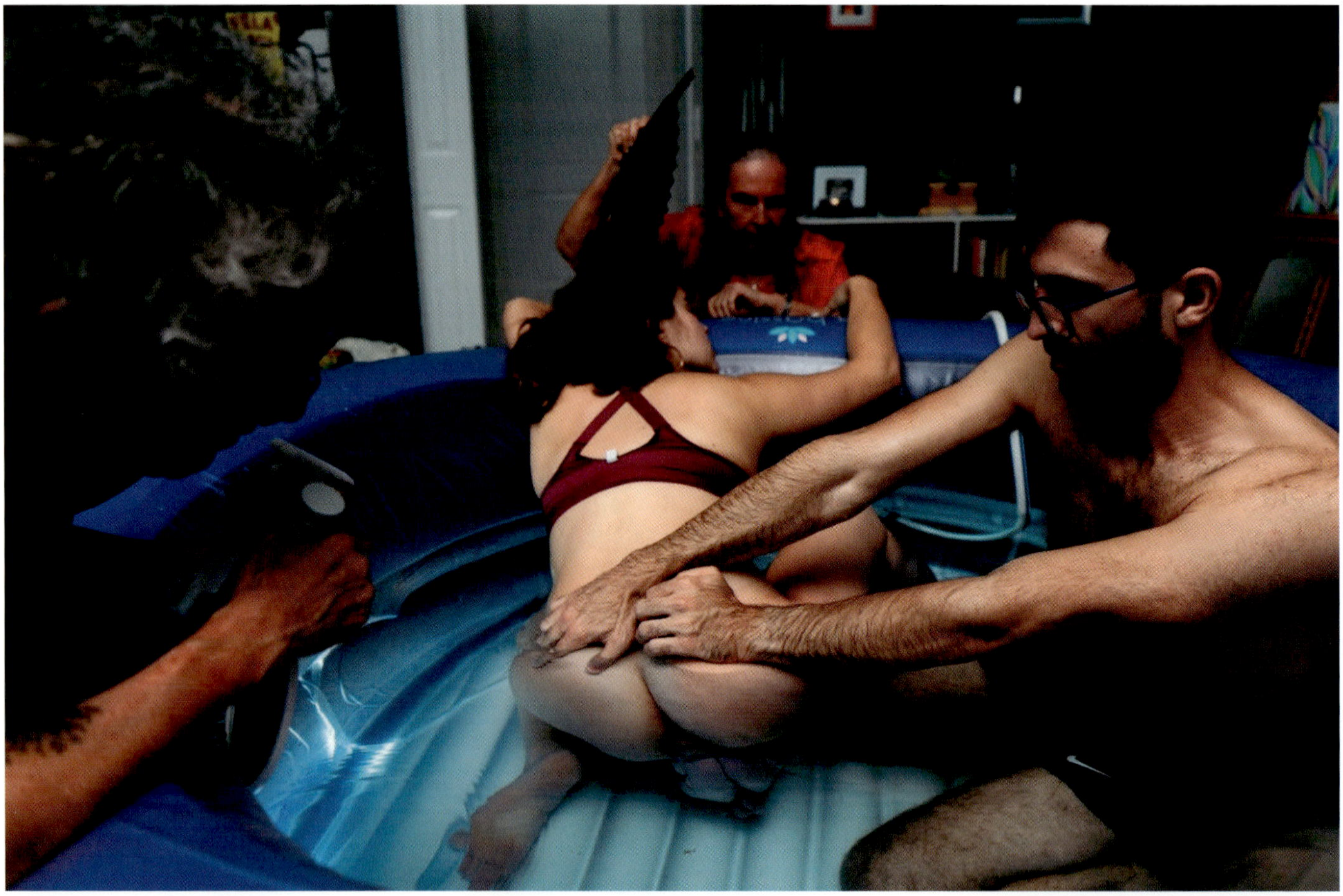

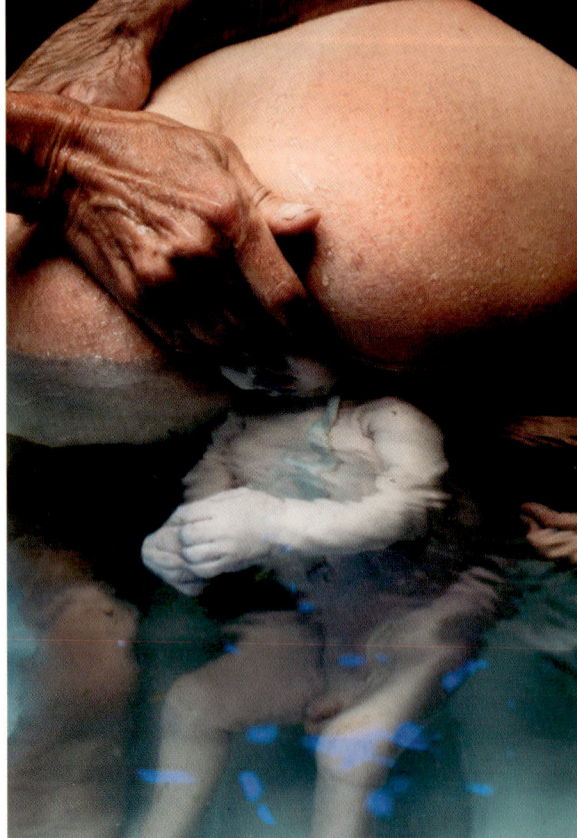

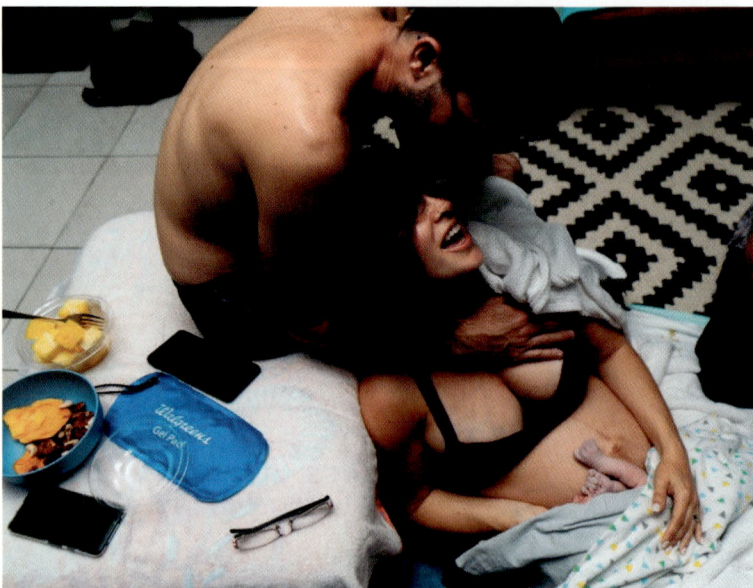

Mary Beliz, birth photographer: marybelizphotos.com
Fadwah Halaby, midwife: midwife360.com
Barbara Harper, water birth educator: waterbirth.org

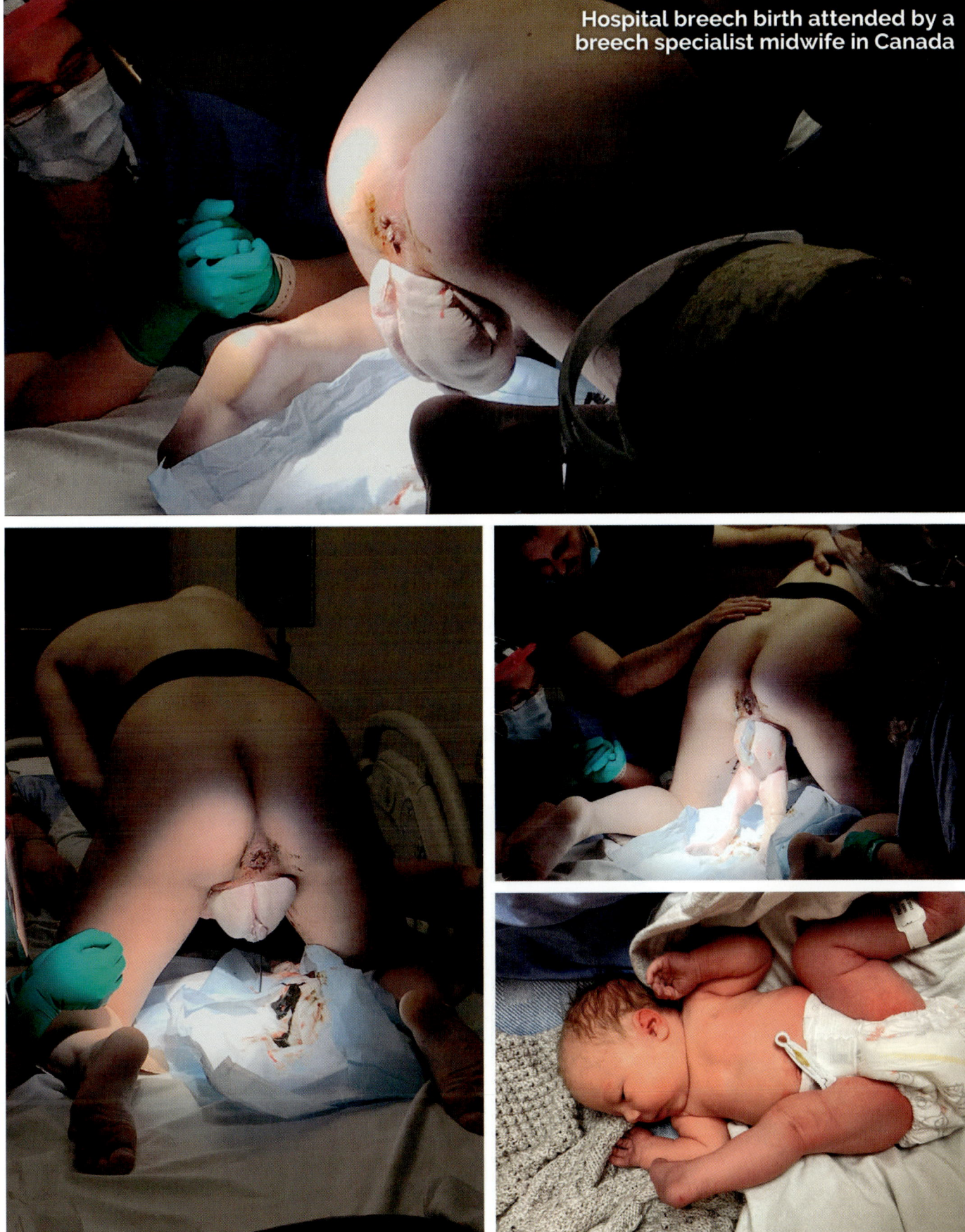

Hospital breech birth attended by a breech specialist midwife in Canada

Cassidy Piney

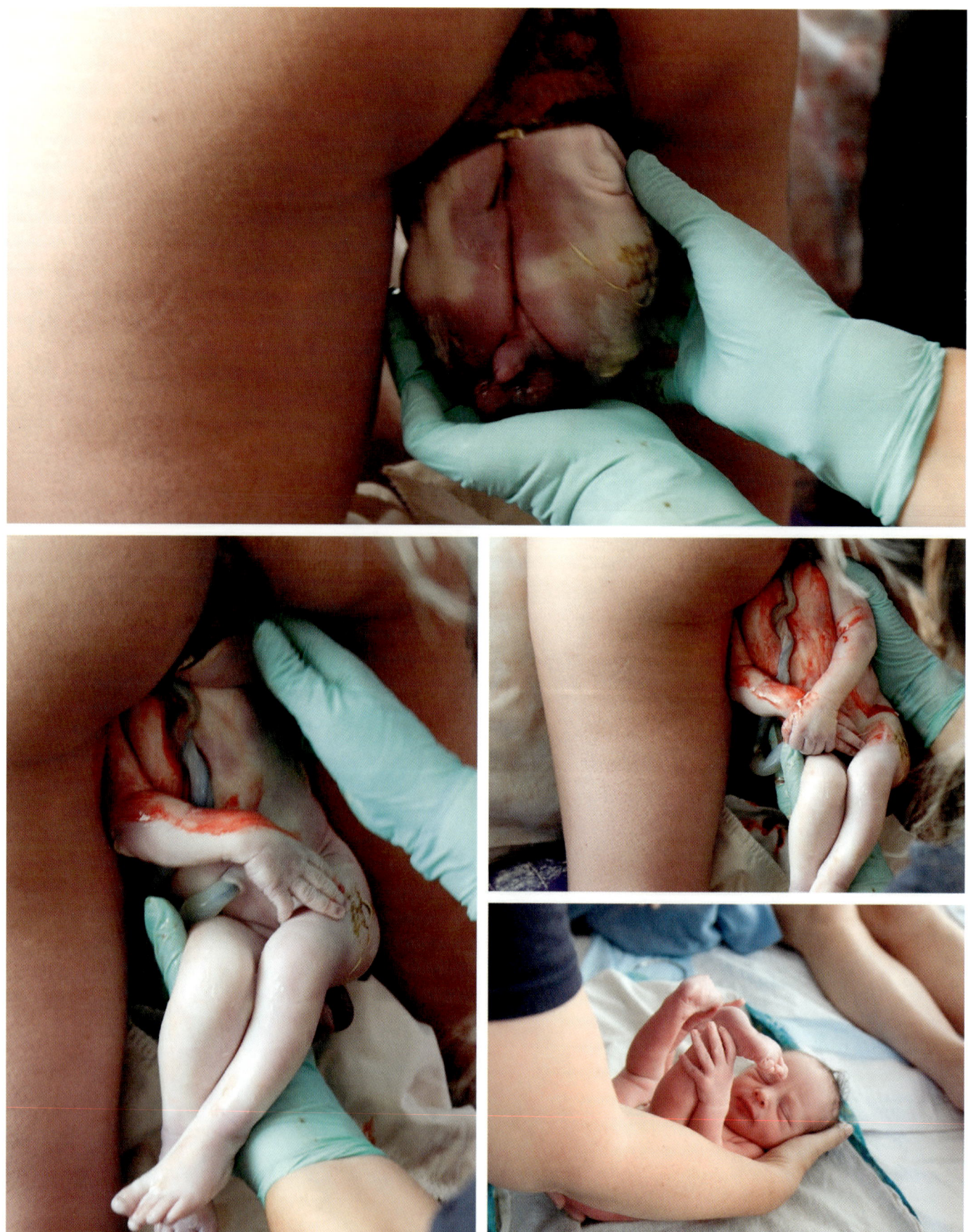

Undiagnosed frank breech. Jamilah Pemberton. Midwife: Sunshine Tomlin, Photographer: Jesse Malley

Lesson 6: Maneuvers for Breech Birth

By Rixa Freeze, PhD

In the last lesson you learned about the normal physiology of vaginal breech birth. In this lesson, you will learn about the maneuvers specific to upright physiological breech birth. In addition, we'll review a few of the older maneuvers that we still use today when women are in supine (on the back) positions. Think of this lesson as an encyclopedia. It's good to be familiar with them all, but for your own clinical practice, we recommend mastering a smaller subset of maneuvers first (see Lesson 10).

Each maneuver is listed in order of the body part it is helping to free. Please consult your handouts as you are studying this lesson. These can be found at the beginning of this guide.

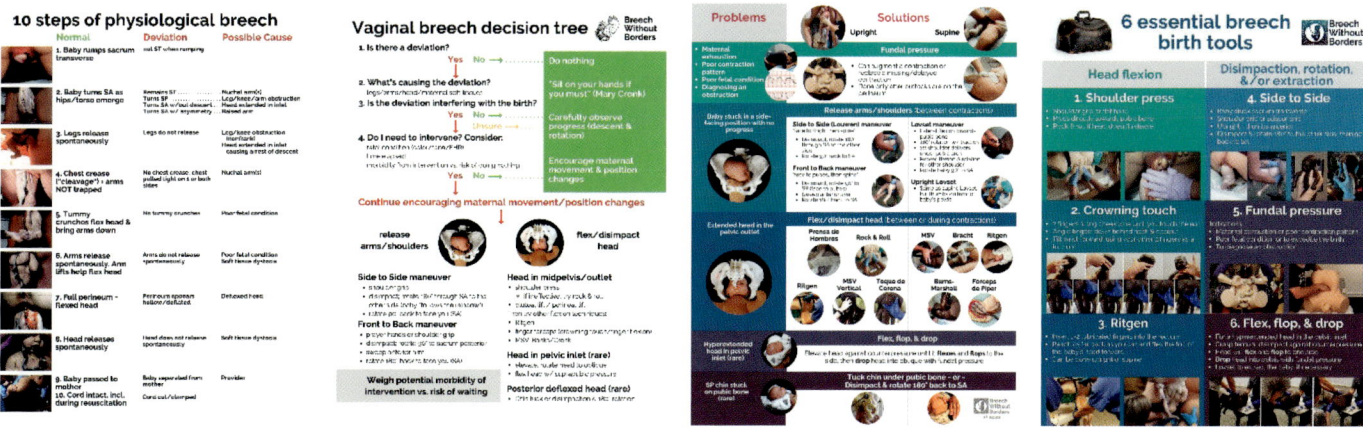

First, we will discuss **maternal movement and positioning**. This is an important and valuable tool, because the people you care for should be free to move about as they please. We presume that encouraging maternal movement and positioning are part of your practice.

Next, we'll learn about maneuvers used to free **arms and shoulders**: nuchal arms, arms up behind the head, etc. Then we'll learn maneuvers used to free the **head**, which may be deflexed or hyperextended, usually in the pelvic outlet and on rare occasions hyperextended in the pelvic inlet or a cervical head entrapment. We'll talk about strategies for correcting a **sacrum posterior rotation**.

And finally, we'll talk about some **soft tissue maneuvers**. These are less about maneuvering the baby and more about maneuvering the maternal soft tissues to help the baby come out. This is something you do at the very end when the baby is held in by skin and muscle.

6a: Maternal movement and positioning

When the mother is upright, mobile, and free to move, she herself can do many things to facilitate the baby being born. Maternal movement and positioning should be your first line of intervention if something seems awry. Carefully assess the situation: Does the baby need more room in the pelvic inlet or in the outlet? Does it seem like something is stuck on one side? Would an asymmetrical lunge of some sort be useful? Do you want to try Walcher's, which opens the inlet? Do you want to try squatting, which opens the outlet? Do you want to try standing, to see if the baby could benefit from more gravity?

Helping free a baby's arm by changing positions

The photos below come from a midwife-attended hospital birth in New Zealand. The mother was a family doctor (GP) having her 2nd baby. Notice the baby hanging asymmetrically with its right arm extended. The midwife suggested a shift to a squatting position, which allowed the baby to rotate slightly oblique, making more space for the baby's arm to descend. Then the midwife suggested standing up, which brought significant descent with the assistance of gravity acting on the baby. The baby's raised arm was born alongside the head.

Hands & knees	Squatting	Standing
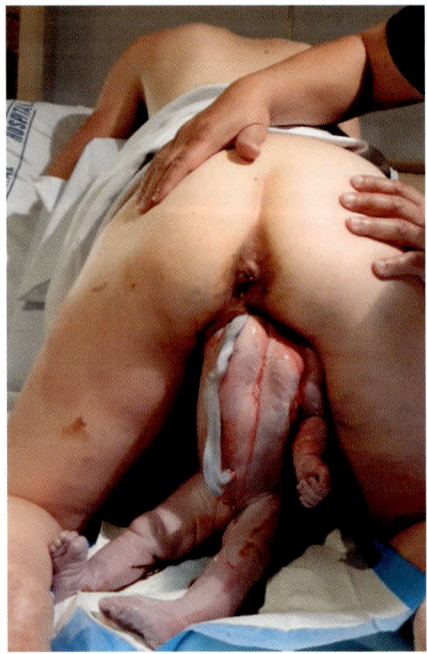	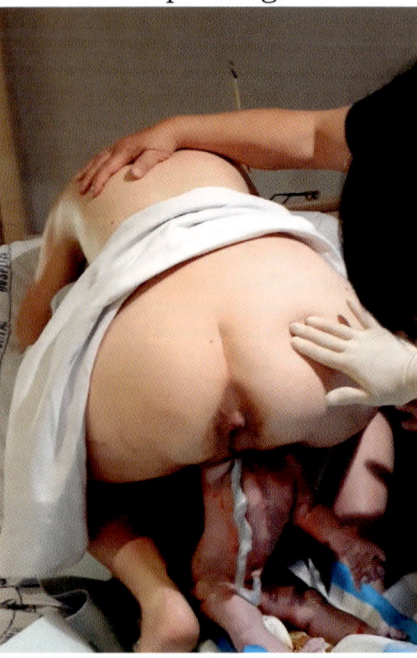	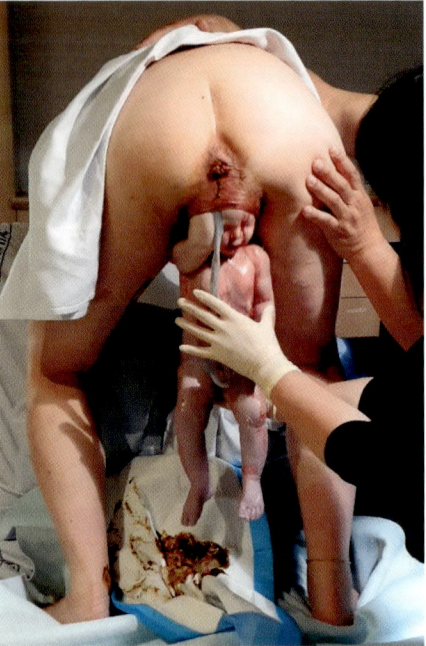

Positions to open the inlet

Walcher's

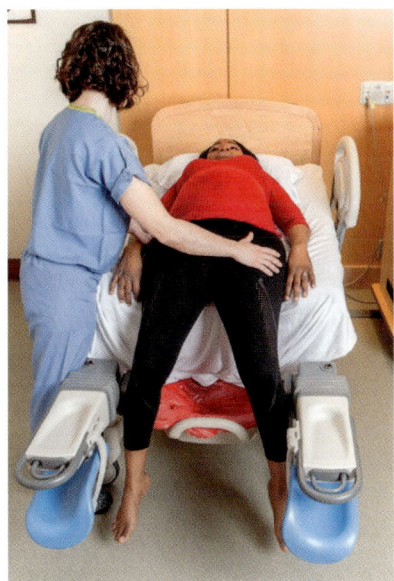

*From Spinning Babies®
Photo by Megan Crown, Property of
Maternity House Publishing, Inc.*

Modified Walcher's (in a birth pool)

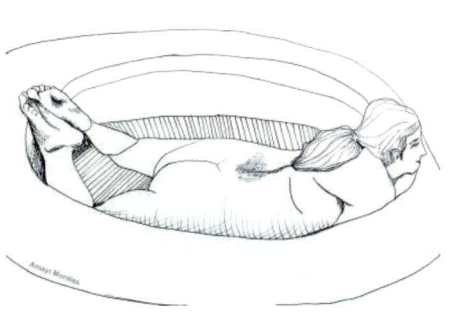

from artofopening.com

Abdominal lift & tuck

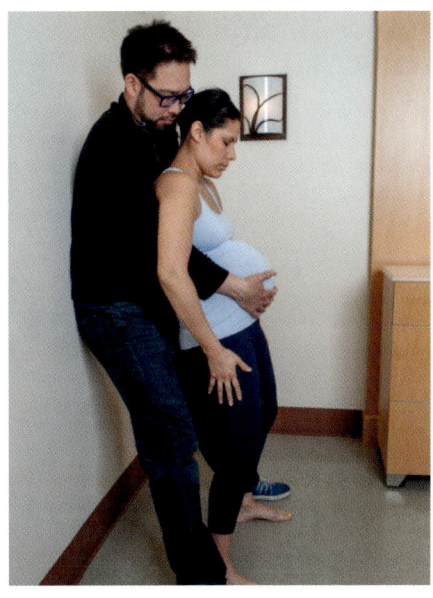

*From Spinning Babies®
Photo by Megan Crown, Property of
Maternity House Publishing, Inc.*

Positions to shift the pelvis or open the outlet

Asymmetrical lunge

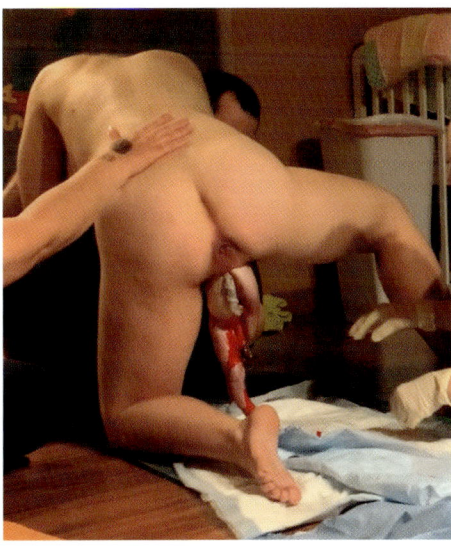

Standing squat

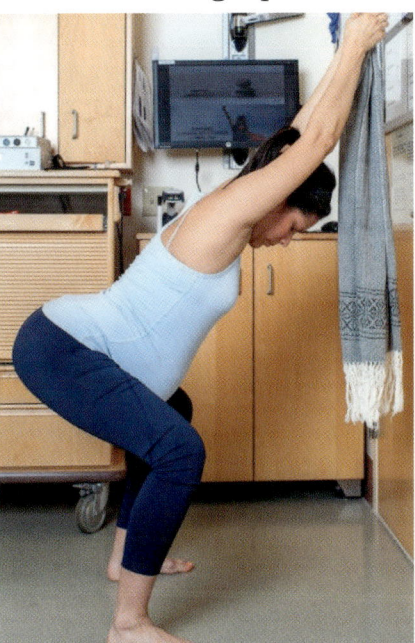

*From Spinning Babies®
Photo by Megan Crown, Property of
Maternity House Publishing, Inc.*

Deep crouch

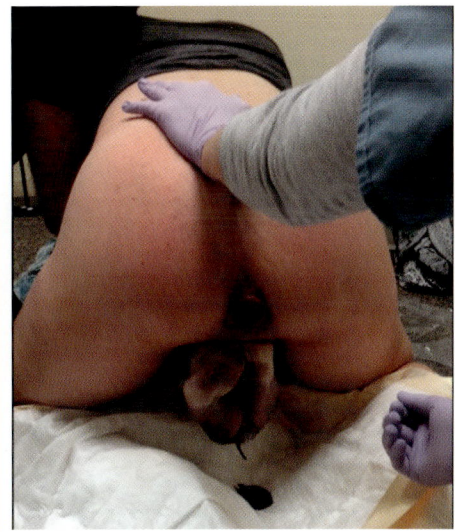

Knees together vs. knees apart

If you want to open the pelvic **inlet**, have the mother put her knees apart with her feet together. (You may note that is a common supine birth position in hospital beds—and it is often counterproductive because it closes the pelvic outlet!) If you want to open the pelvic **outlet**, put the knees together and the feet apart. This opens the outlet due to internal rotation of the femurs.

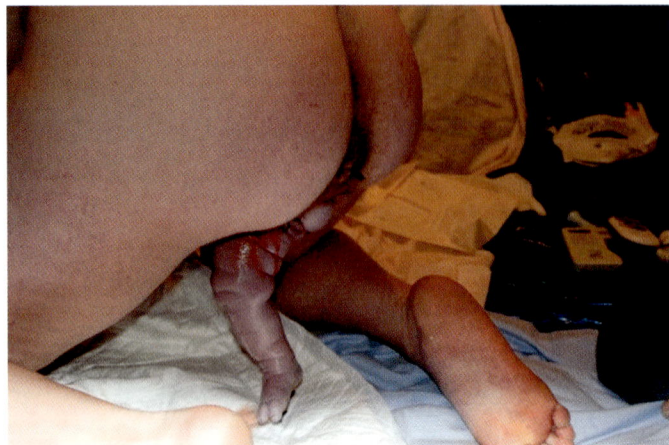
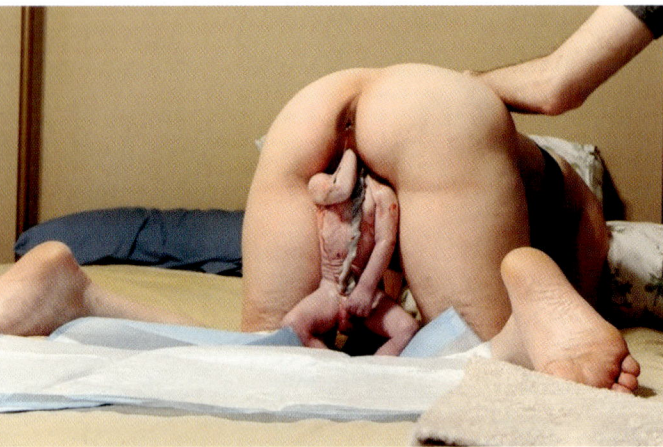

Knees apart, feet together
Joy Horner

Knees together, feet apart

There are many other maternal positions besides the ones shown above. Sometimes just *changing* positions is more important than which position the mother chooses. Encourage the mom to try different things, such as squatting, wriggling her bottom, circling her hips, or bending forward and backward.

Baby on a bike?

I learned something very interesting from Sister Morningstar, a Cherokee midwife. She learned this from traditional Mexican midwives. They would say, "When you have a breech baby, the baby comes out riding a bike, looking for the floor." She explained it to me: when the baby comes out, it is kicking its legs, almost looking like it is riding a bike.

Remember when we talked about the baby doing tummy crunches? The Mexican midwives were describing these kinds of movements: flexing and lifting and kicking the legs. The Mexican midwives would say, "The baby rides a bike looking for the floor." The women were usually in a deep squat, so the baby was very close to the floor.

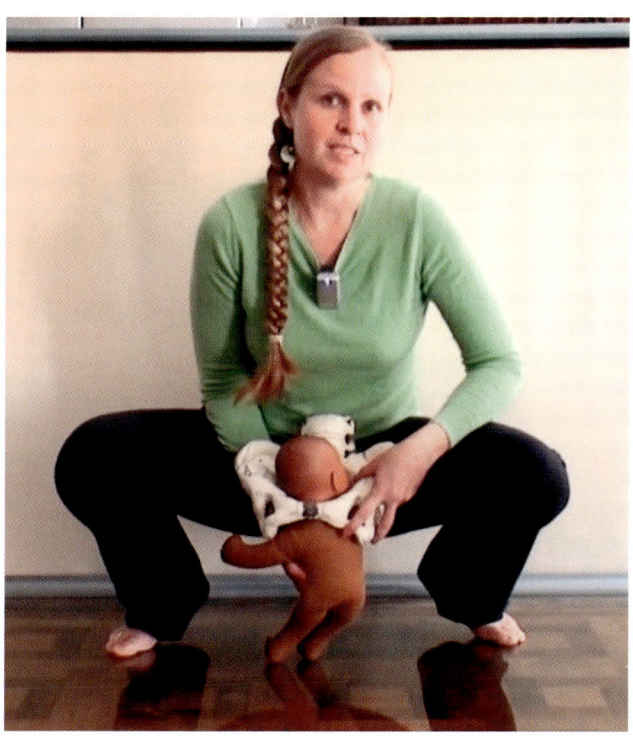

Imagine me being in a deep squat. After the baby's legs come out, it kicks its legs and the legs hit the floor. Babies have something called a standing reflex: when their feet hit a surface, they instinctually push against it and straighten their legs.

If the baby is low enough to the floor that it can actually push against the floor, and the baby is still inside the mother like this, it essentially can disimpact itself. This would help the baby to help free itself from any obstructions.

I love learning things like this because it makes me realize how these processes are so deeply rooted in anatomy and physiology. Our cultures can define how we act in labor and maybe even the positions we assume, if we've been taught to do certain things or not. But when it comes down to the physiology of breech birth, there is something very universal about it.

Squat

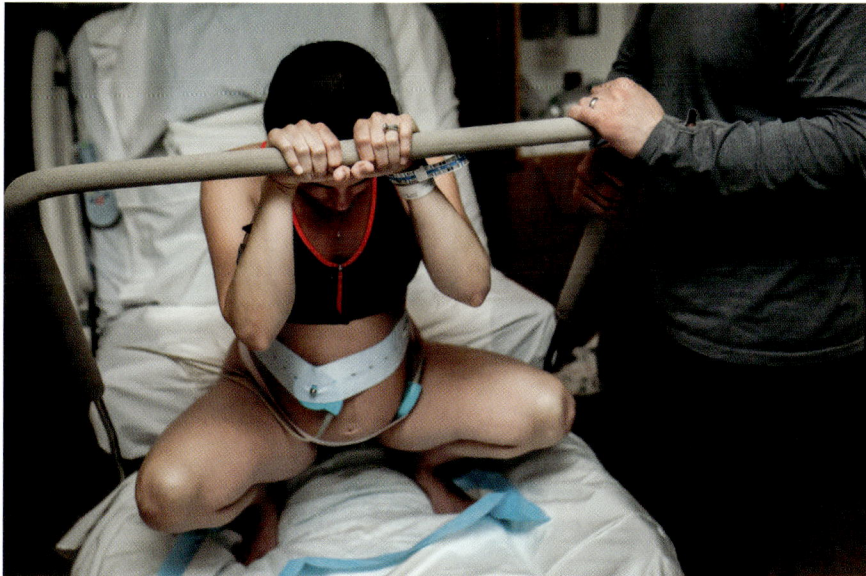

Hospital VBB
Denver Birth Photography
monetnicole.com/stories/vaginal-breech-birth-baby-jack

Supported squat

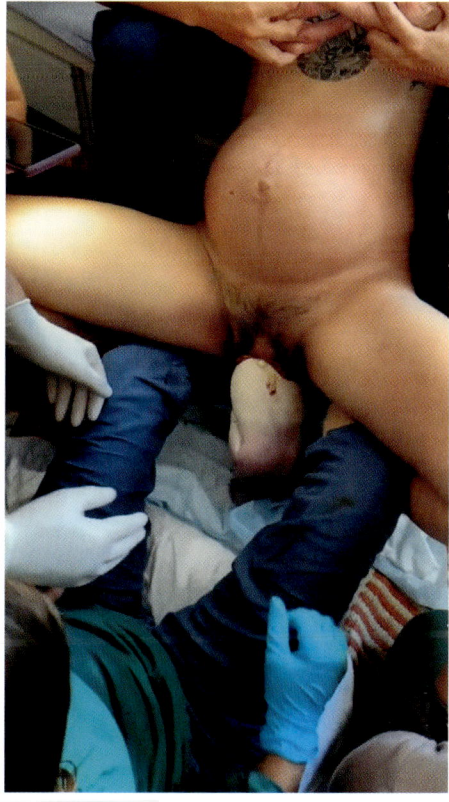

6b: Stuck arms and shoulders

As we talked about earlier, in a physiological breech birth, you should not pull on the baby. Pulling is the opposite of what we want to do. (Pulling should not be part of your obstetrical vocabulary at all, unless you're doing one very specific maneuver—Løvset.) However, with everything else in physiological breech birth, the approach should be to **disimpact and rotate**. You slightly replace the baby back inside the mother to disimpact what is stuck and then rotate it off the impaction.

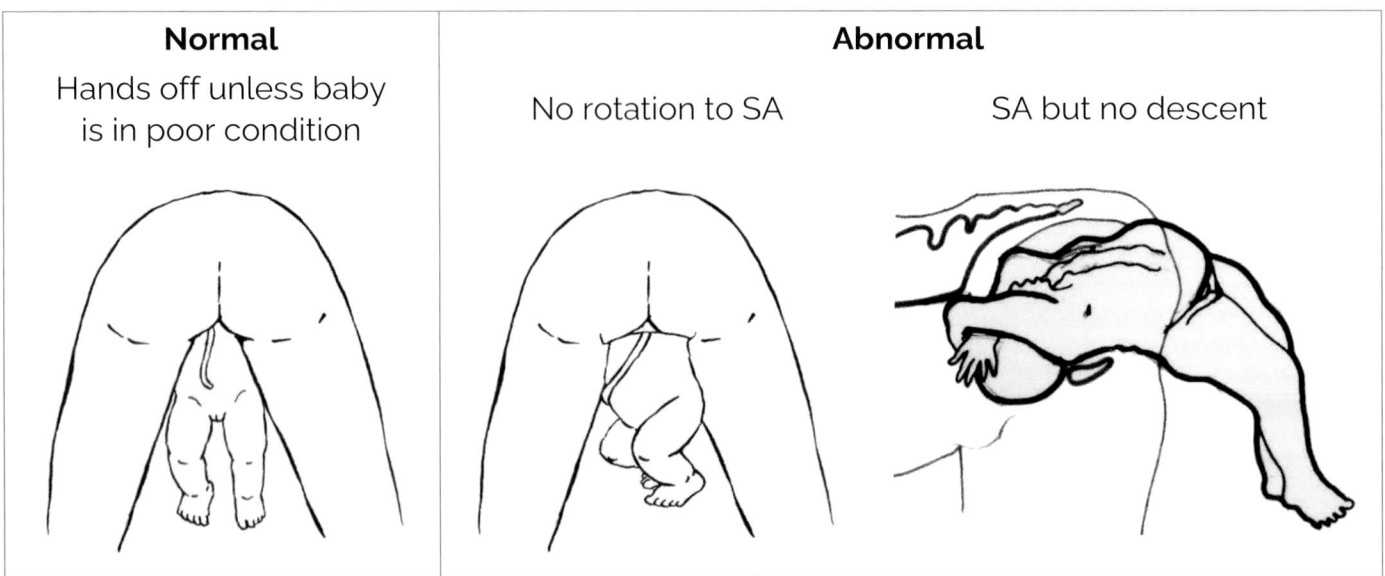

Normal	Abnormal	
Hands off unless baby is in poor condition	No rotation to SA	SA but no descent

The table above shows normal versus abnormal in a physiological breech birth. The two illustrations on the left are from Dr. Frank Louwen's study of upright breech birth in Frankfurt, Germany (2017). On the far left, the illustration shows a baby that has rotated normally to sacrum anterior (facing straight towards you, if you are behind the mother). This indicates that the baby's arms or shoulders are not stuck in the pelvis and is a sign that everything is normal. You don't need to do anything at this point, assuming that the baby's color, tone, and heart rate are reassuring.

What are signs of abnormal? The illustration in the middle shows a baby stuck in a side-facing (sacrum transverse) position. This is a classic sign that the baby's arms or shoulders are stuck somewhere. You will see no further movement from this position, despite strong contractions and obvious efforts on the mom's and the baby's part to move.

The illustration on the far right shows an uncommon situation that is also abnormal. Thie illustration comes from Gail Tully, a midwife in Minnesota, USA, who encountered this situation in her practice. The baby's arms may be crossed above the head, impeding further descent. Or the head may be hyperextended and trapped in the pelvic inlet. The baby will rotate to sacrum anterior but will remain quite high and will not descend any further.

1. Side to Side maneuver

The first main rotational maneuver for freeing trapped arms in an upright breech birth is the Side to Side maneuver, also known as the Louwen maneuver. This was developed by Dr. Frank Louwen and Dr. Anke Reitter of Frankfurt, Germany. This is an adaptation of the Løvset maneuver, which you will see in old obstetric textbooks. Dr. Louwen was familiar with Løvset, but then he started doing breech births in an upright position. He used some of the ideas from Løvset, but with a different application and different set of techniques.

Indications for a rotational maneuver: the baby is stuck in a side-facing position (sacrum transverse). If the baby does not descend any further, despite a strong contraction, this means that one or both arms are stuck. It is now time to intervene.

These photos below show a baby stuck in a side-facing RST position. They were taken 1 minute apart. Descent was arrested at the position of the second photo.

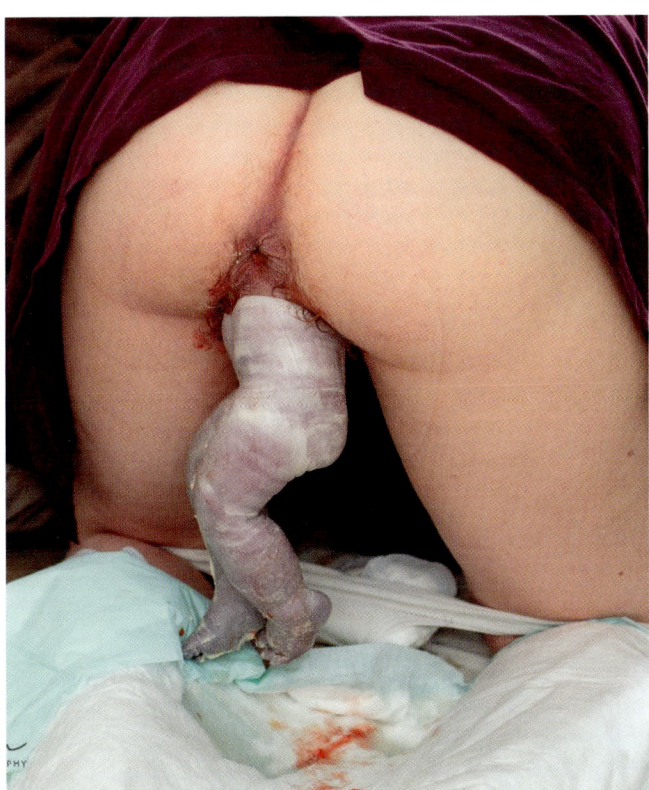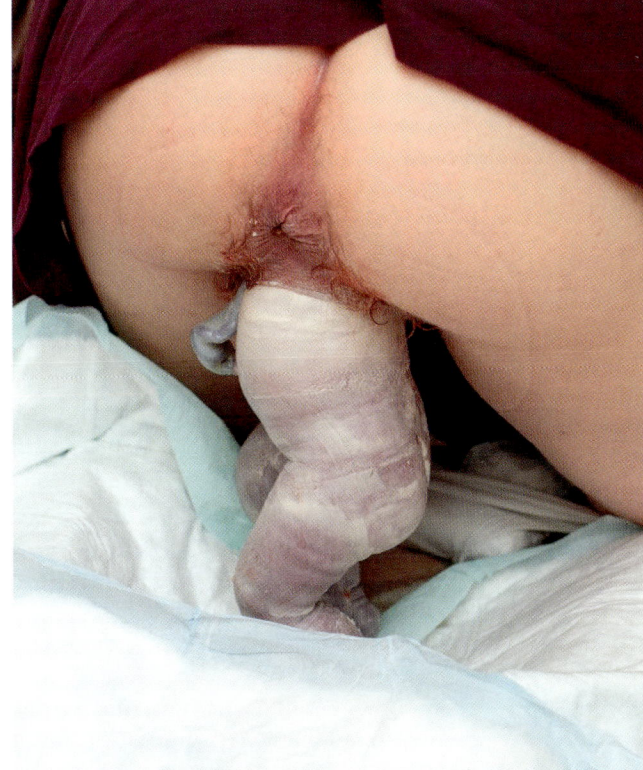

Melanie Ellison Photography

To do the Side to Side maneuver, you can do a shoulder grip or a scissor grip.

Shoulder grip:

You reach in and grab the baby via the shoulders, one hand on each shoulder, going up under the armpits. Your thumbs will be on the front of the shoulder and your other fingers on the back of the shoulder.

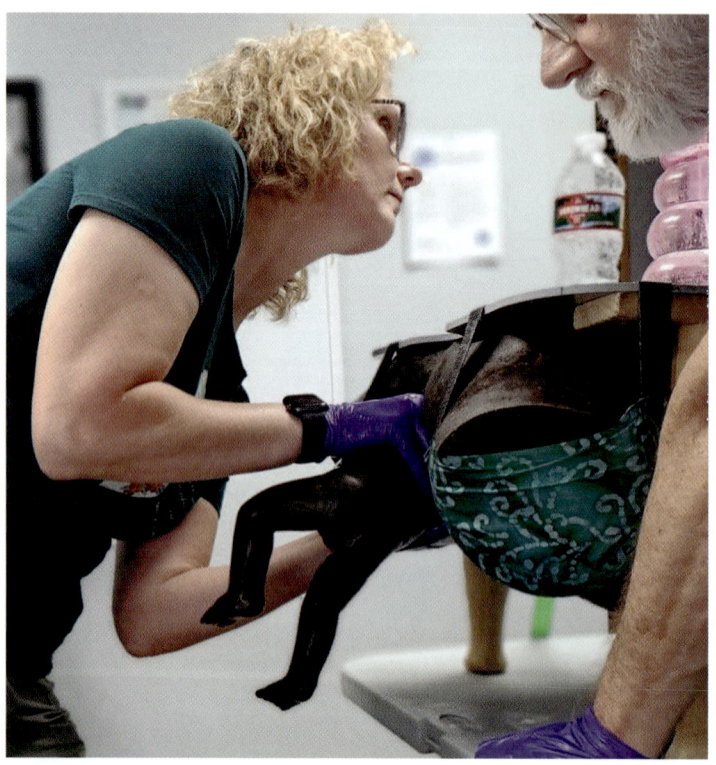
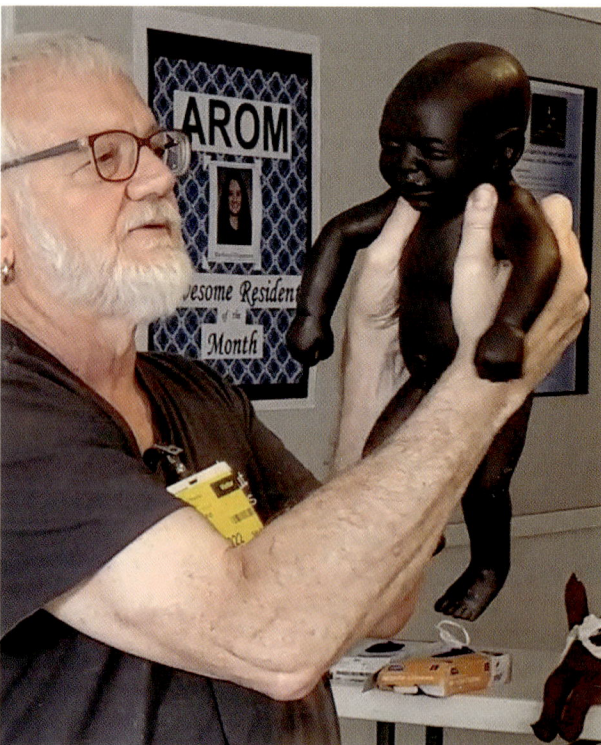
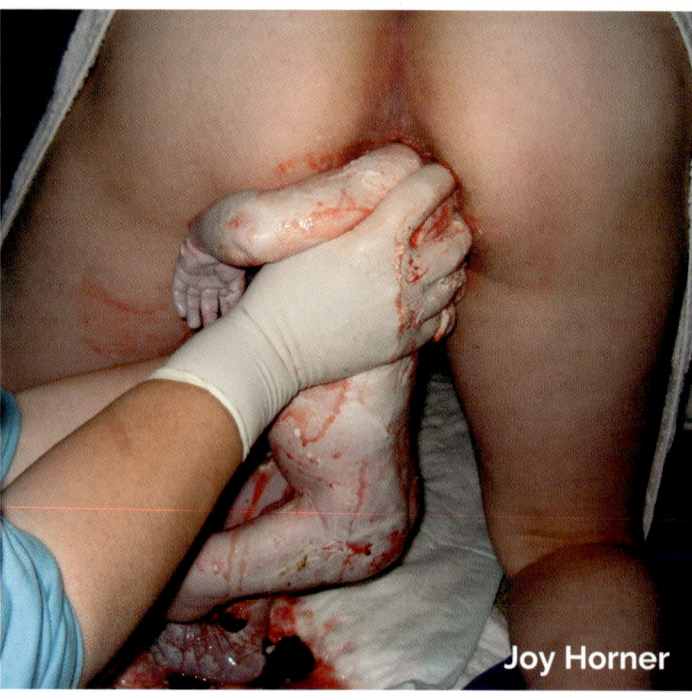
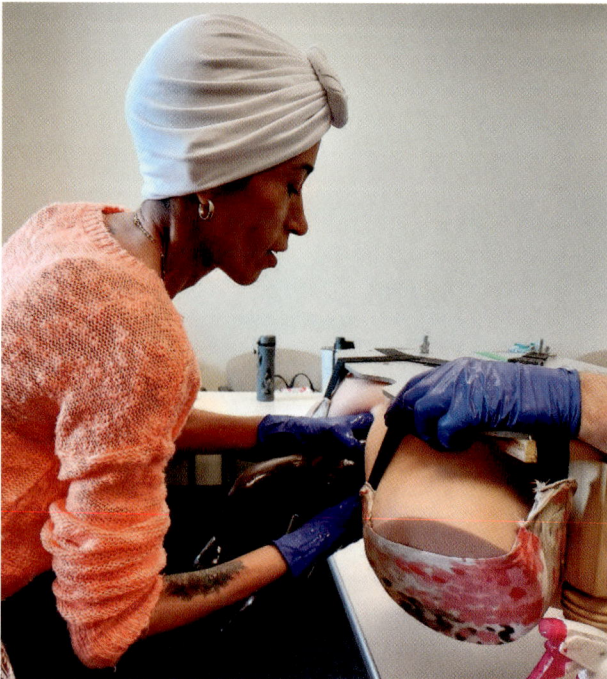

Joy Horner

Scissor grip:

As another option, you can reach in with your first and second fingers making a "V" that goes underneath each armpit. The scissor grip takes up less room laterally inside the mother.

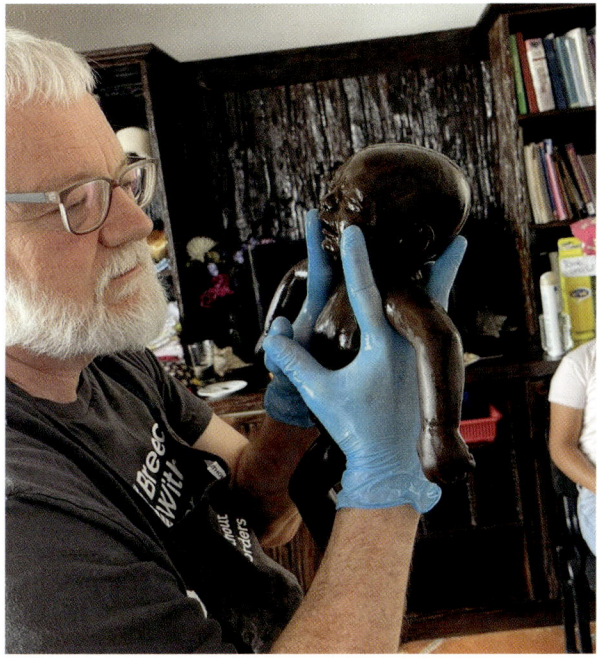 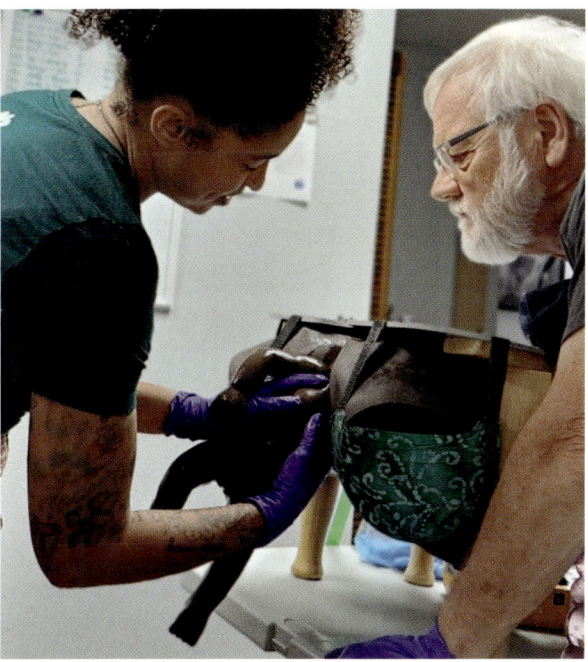

How does this maneuver work? You disimpact the baby, and then you rotate the baby approximately 180° so the baby faces the mother's other thigh. Next you rotate the baby 90° back so the baby faces the mother's spine (sacrum anterior). This will free the stuck arms and bring them near the face.

When you do the rotations, the baby should always be facing towards the mother's back half, never towards the mother's front half. Think of your baby as following a rainbow from one side to the other, and then back to the middle.

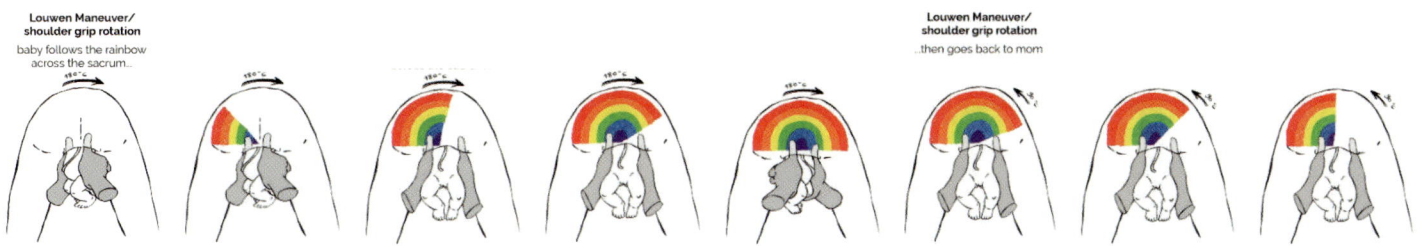

On the next page you will see the steps of the Side to Side Maneuver.

To review, you turn the baby to the mother's other side, and then you turn back so the baby faces the mother's spine. One of our midwife students likes to describe it as "**Face to thigh, then spine**."

Steps of the Side to Side maneuver

View from mother's front		View from mother's back
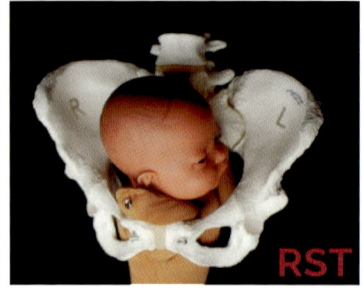	Baby is stuck in a side-facing position.	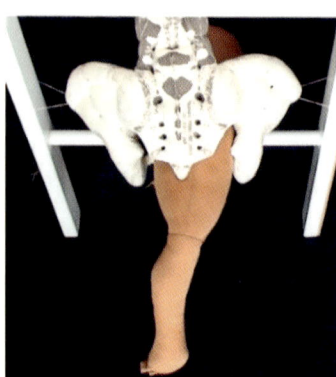
	1. Grab the baby with either the shoulder grip or the V grip. Disimpact the baby. In this picture, the baby is facing RST (the baby's spine towards the mother's right thigh).	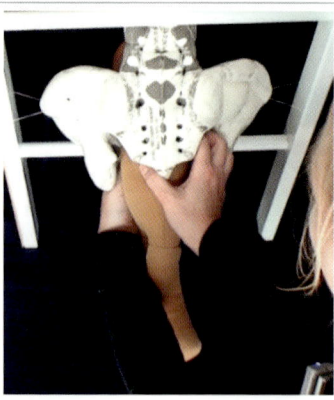
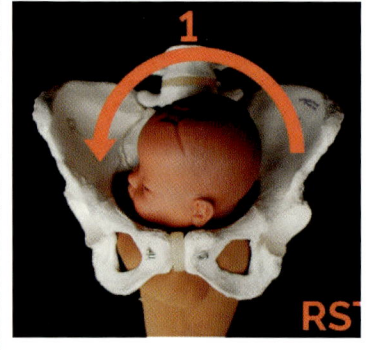	2. Rotate the baby ~ 180° to face the other side. Always rotate the baby's face past the spine—never past the pubic bone! We have now rotated the baby to LST (the baby's spine facing the mother's left thigh).	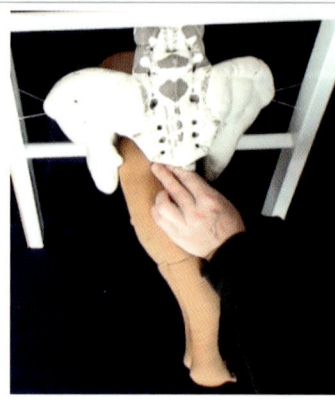
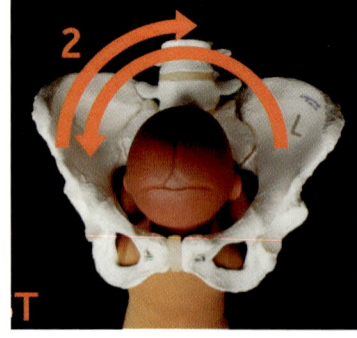	3. Next, rotate 90° back so the baby faces the mother's spine. Normally this will bring both arms in front of the baby's face. You can ask the mother to push, or you can gently sweep each arm out, supporting the baby's bottom with your other hand to avoid pulling down on the baby.	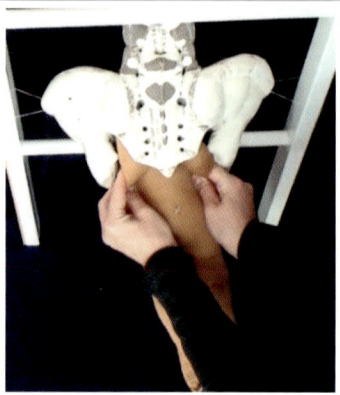

2. Front to Back maneuver

The other main rotational maneuver in upright breech birth is called the Front to Back maneuver. It also helps free stuck arms. Here is what a stuck anterior arm can look like:

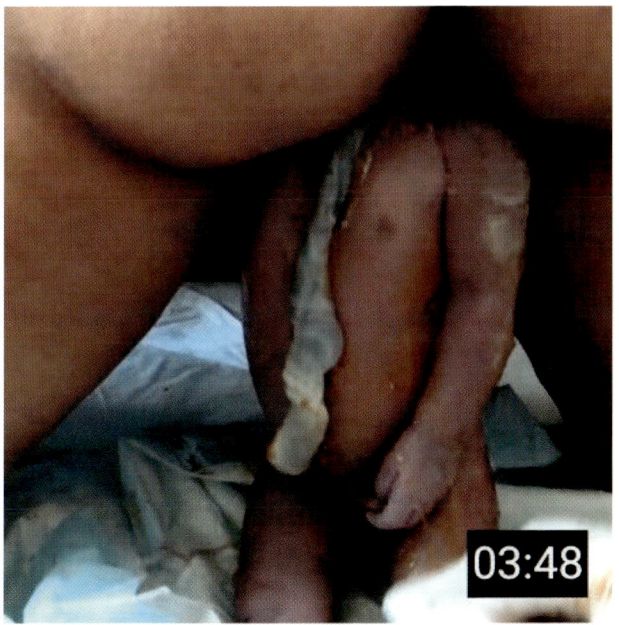

This picture comes from a midwife before she attended our workshop. The baby came down and descended pretty well, still facing sacrum transverse (towards the mother's left thigh). The posterior arm was born, but the anterior arm (in other words, the arm facing the mother's pubic bone) was clearly stuck. If you look closely, you can see the baby's underarm showing. It's clear that this baby is stuck and that the arm is pulled tight behind the head. You also see absolutely no cleavage on that one side where the arm is stuck. It's flat, and you can almost see the shoulder blade sticking out behind the baby.

This baby did come out shortly afterwards. The midwife was able to sweep down the anterior arm, rotate the baby to SA, and free the head with a shoulder press (which we will teach later in this lesson). The baby did need some resuscitation, but otherwise did fine and recovered right away.

Here is another picture of a trapped anterior arm with the posterior arm out.

To resolve this specific situation, you can use the Front to Back Maneuver. In this maneuver, you grip the baby either with a **shoulder grip** (which we explained in the section above) or with a **flat hands grip**.

Melanie Ellison Photography

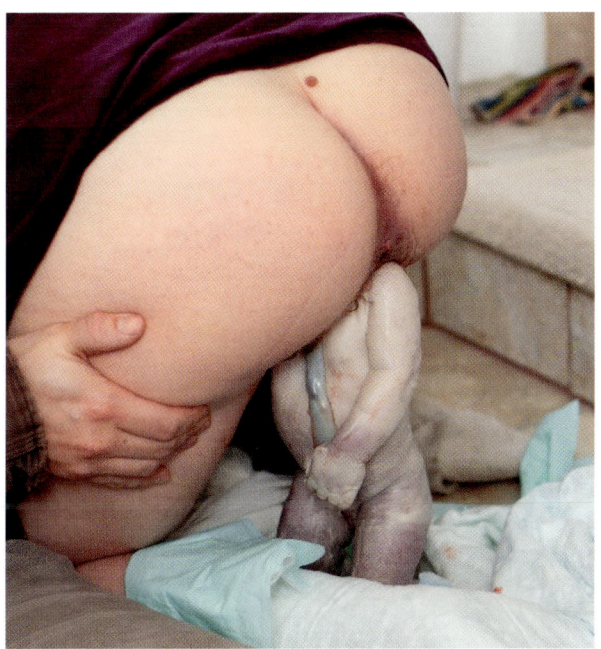

Flat hands grip:

These pictures below show the **flat hands grip** (sometimes referred to as *prayer hands* or *namaste hands*). Place the flat of each hand on the baby's back: one hand on the baby's chest and the other on the baby's back. Keep the thumbs straight, flat, and parallel to your fingers. Do not poke the baby's abdomen with your fingers or thumbs! Your hands will go surprisingly far inside the mother. You may even be able to feel the baby's chin and/or the back of its head.

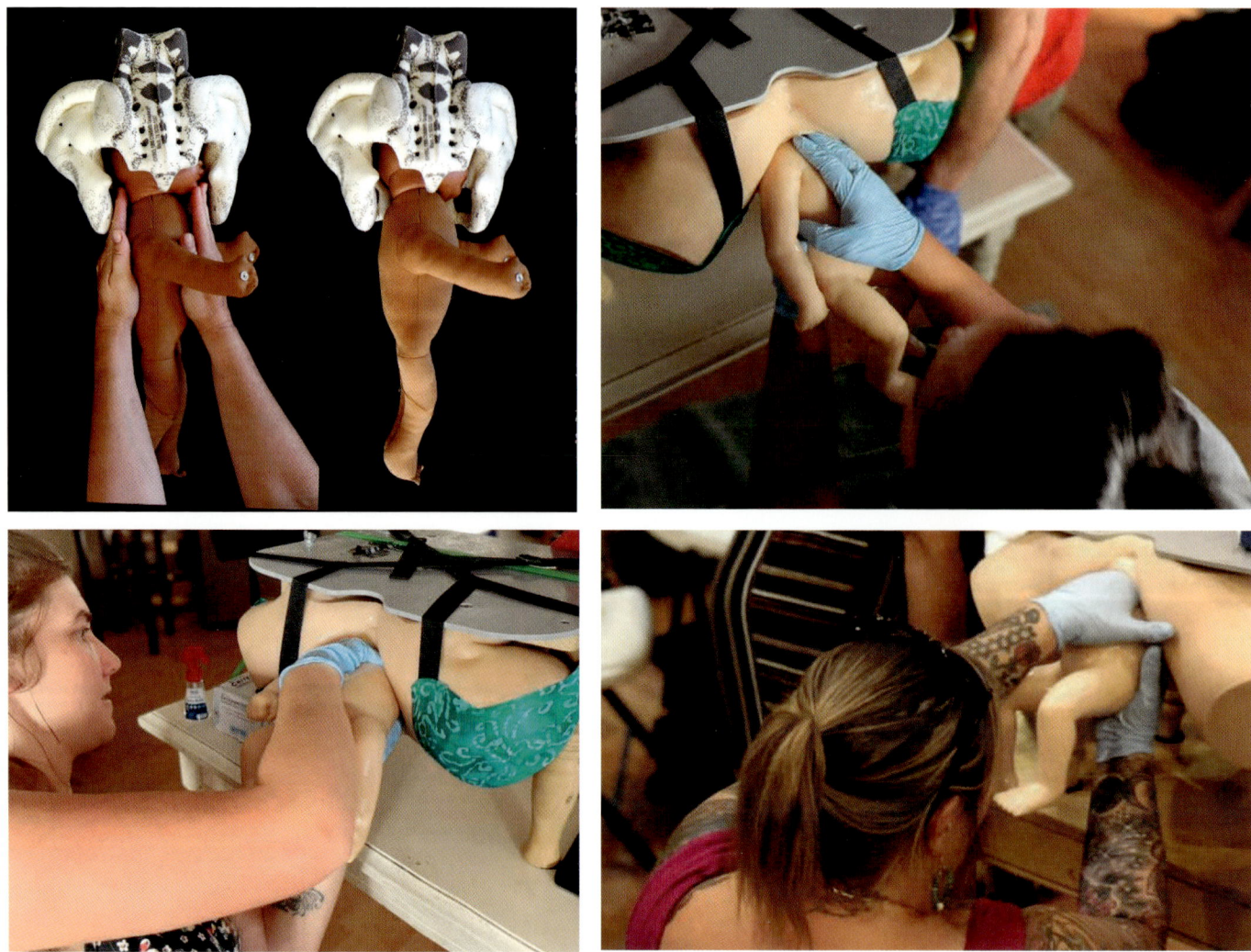

You can also grip the baby's shoulders. This works especially well if the posterior arm is already born since 1 of the 2 shoulders is already out. This is called a **shoulder grip**, which we discussed earlier in the Side to Side maneuver section.

Steps of the Front to Back maneuver:

View from mother's front   **View from mother's back**

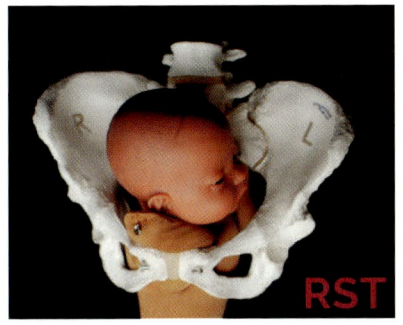

Before the maneuver begins, the baby is stuck in side-facing position due to a trapped anterior arm (the arm that faces the pubic bone).
In this example, the baby is RST (baby's back is facing the mother's right).

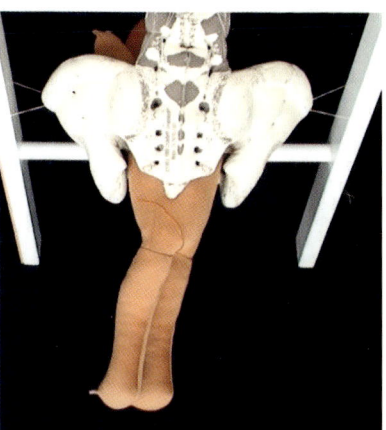

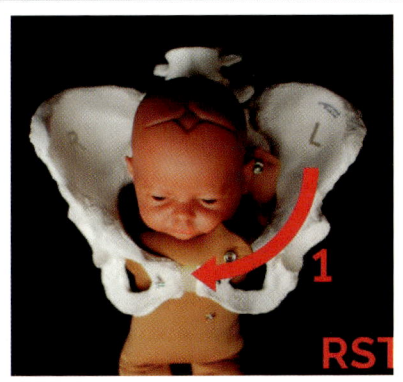

1) First, you disimpact and then turn the baby 90° to face the mother's pubic bone (SP or sacrum posterior). (This is arrow #1.)

See how this helps bring that arm in front of the face?

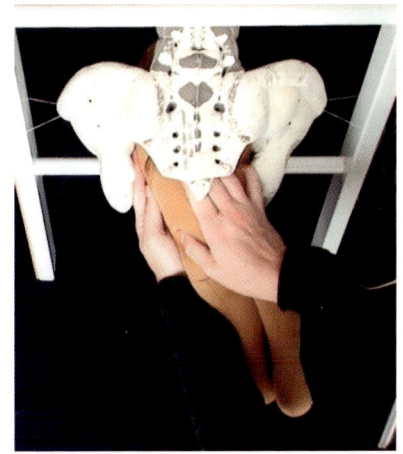

2) Next, if possible, gently sweep down the anterior arm from underneath the pubic bone and across the baby's face. This is usually done with your bottom hand.

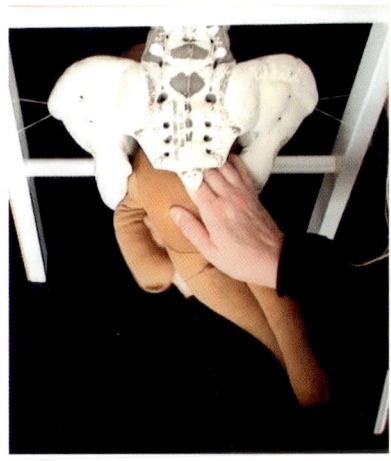

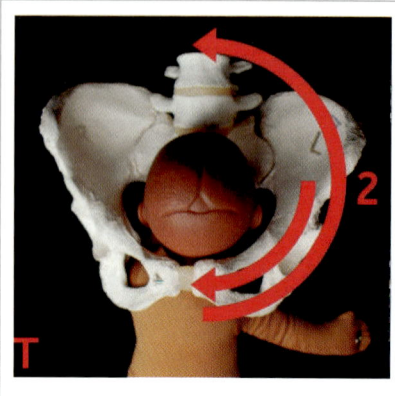

3) Finally, you turn the baby 180° back to face the mother's spine (back the way you came from). In other words, turn the baby back to face you (assuming you are behind the mother).
This rotation is arrow #2.

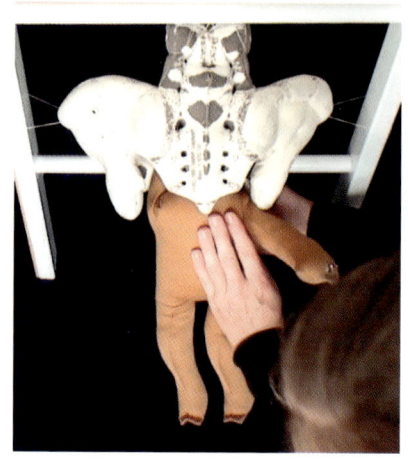

4) The baby's other arm (the one that was originally facing the mother's spine) will either birth on its own, or you can gently sweep it down. Support the baby's bottom with your other hand to avoid pulling down on the baby.

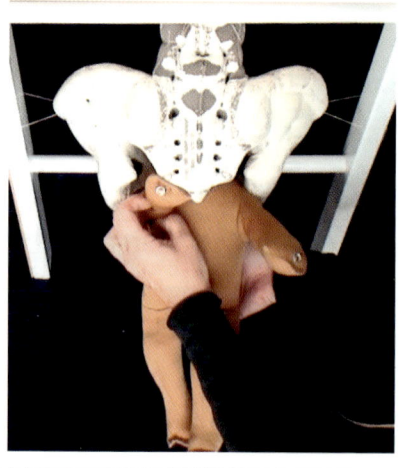

To review, you turn the baby to the mother's front, bring down the anterior arm, and then turn the baby to face the mother's back, hence the "Front to Back" maneuver. One of our midwife students likes to describe it as **"Face to pubes, then spine."**

If the posterior arm is already born, then I would suggest using the shoulder grip rather than the prayer hands grip. Why? You have a much better grip when you can grab the shoulders.

3. How to sweep down arms

You may need to sweep down arms, whether independently or as part of a maneuver. If you do this improperly, you risk breaking the arm. Reach up and around the back of the shoulder, then follow the arm down to the elbow. Bring the elbow towards the midline of the baby and then down. This will sweep the arm across the baby's face and then down. This illustration shows a supine arm sweep, but the principle is the same with upright births (medicalguidelines.msf.org). To avoid pulling the baby's body down, put gentle counterpressure on the baby's bottom (under the buttocks or between the legs) with your free hand while sweeping the arm with your other hand.

4. Løvset maneuver

So far, we've talked about two main maneuvers for an upright breech birth if one or both arms are stuck: the Side to Side and the Front to Back maneuvers.

However, it's also important to understand the Løvset maneuver. It's still in common use today in most places that do breech birth on the back. This maneuver is very different than the two upright physiological maneuvers. Remember how we say, "Never pull on the baby—no traction"? You have to ignore that when you're learning Løvset! This is a maneuver that is *meant* to be done with traction (pulling). It's a corkscrew maneuver where you simultaneously pull on the baby while you're turning and corkscrewing the baby out.

Steps of the Løvset maneuver

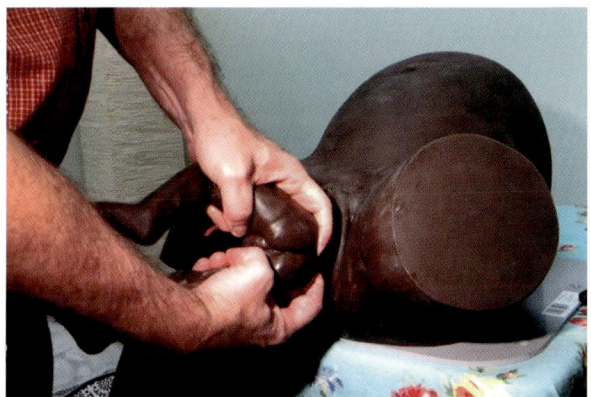

The first step in Løvset is to grab the baby's pelvis. If the mother is lying on her back, your thumbs and/or forefingers will go on the back of the baby's pelvis. This ensures that you rotate in the correct direction.

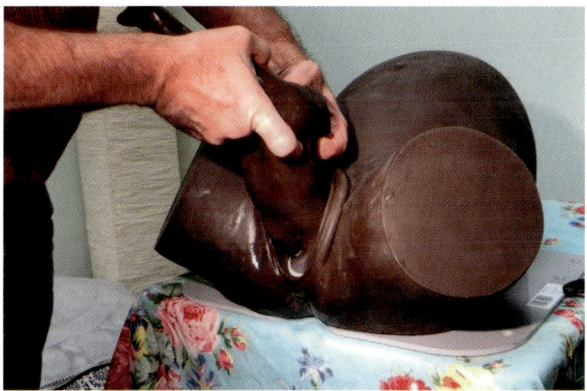

Next, flex the baby sideways (laterally) towards the mother's pubic bone. Remember how the sacrum curves? This curve points the way that you should flex the baby.

This flexion pulls the posterior arm and shoulder very low into the sacrum.

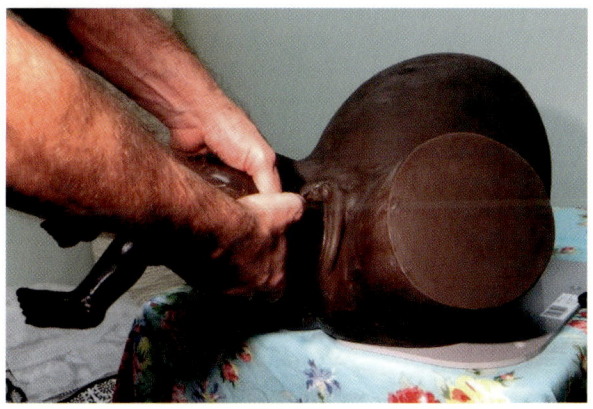

With thumbs on the back of the baby's pelvis, rotate the baby 180°. Pull straight back towards your own torso as you rotate.

This rotation will take the shoulder (which is now low in the sacrum) and corkscrew it down and out underneath the pubic arch.

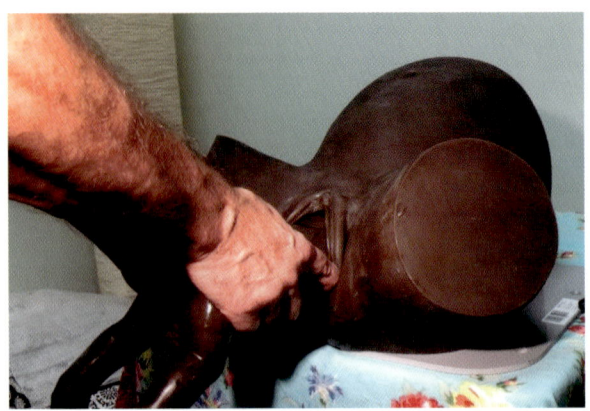

Midway through the first 180° rotation

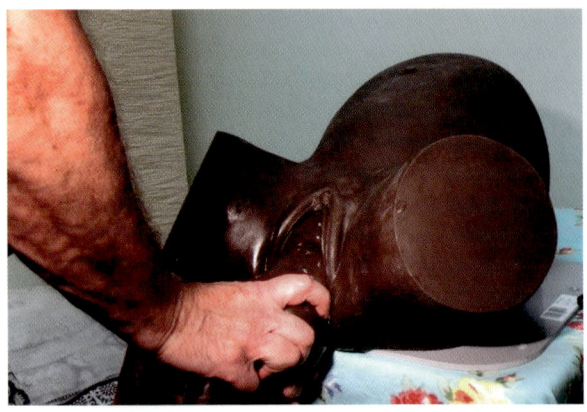

The first 180° rotation is complete; notice the shoulder appearing under the pubic arch.

Remember, the mother's pubic arch is higher than the sacrum. When the first shoulder is flexed low into the sacrum and then rotated 180°, it will deliver under the pubic arch.

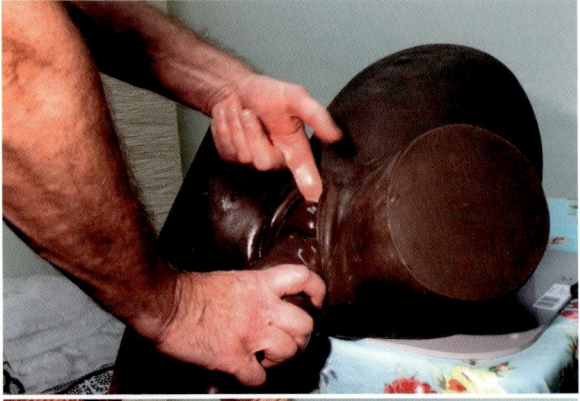

You can release the first arm/shoulder at this point.

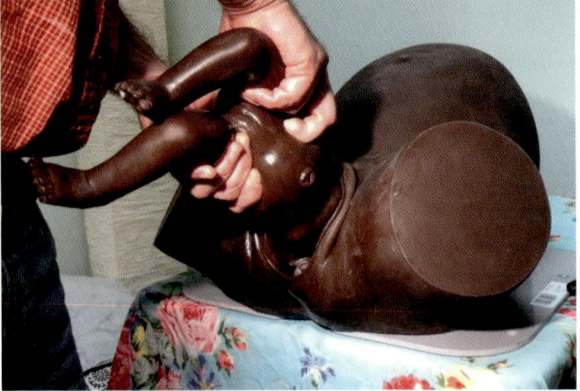

Next, flex the baby towards the mother's pubic bone. Follow the direction of the sacral curve.

This brings the 2nd shoulder low into the sacrum.

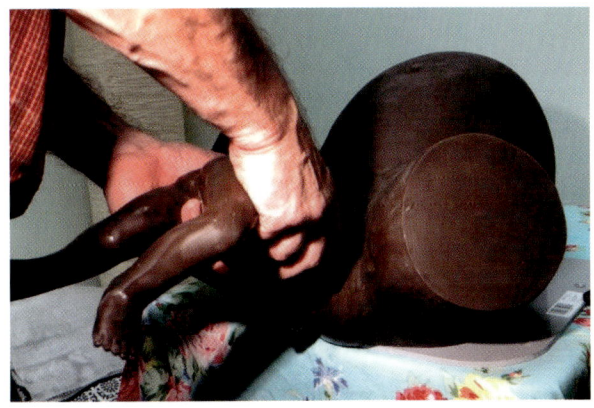

Do a 2nd 180° rotation back the way you came from. Pull straight back towards your own torso as you rotate.

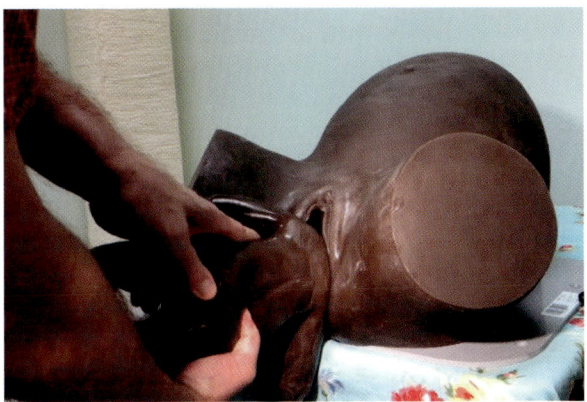

The baby is now fully rotated 180° back to where it started from. Both shoulders should have delivered.

You may need to help deliver the 2nd shoulder/arm under the pubic arch.

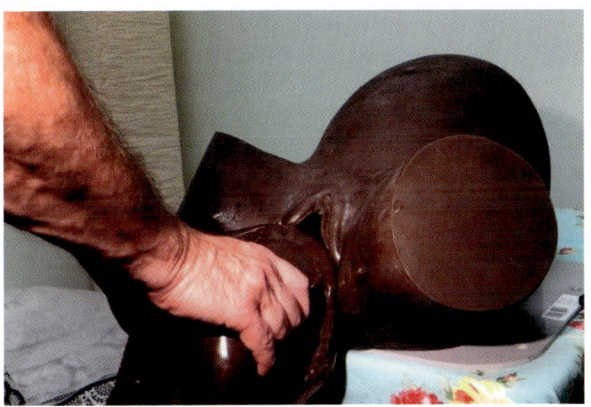

Rotate the baby's body 90° back to sacrum anterior (baby facing the mother's spine).

You have completed the Løvset maneuver.

The Løvset maneuver assumes an impaction of the anterior shoulder behind the symphysis pubis. It is an extraction maneuver and is designed to remove the baby.

Now you have both shoulders out. The baby's head typically will be somewhat deflexed because you have been putting traction on it. At this point, the classic follow-up to the Løvset maneuver is to do the Mauriceau-Smellie-Veit (MSV) maneuver (illustrated below), which we will discuss in the section about freeing trapped heads.

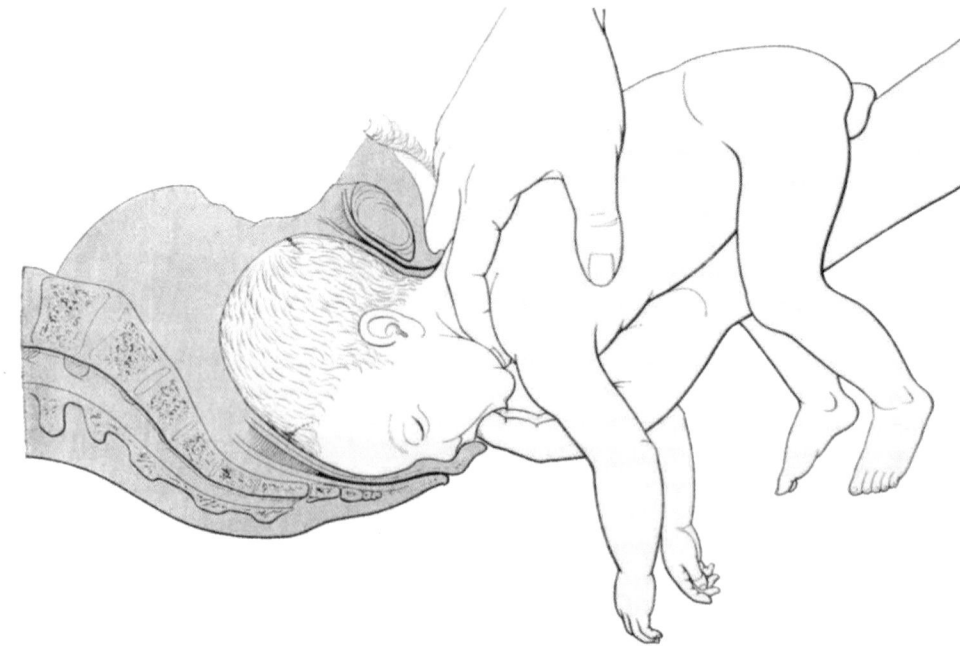

Now I'm going to show you the Løvset maneuver turned 180° around, with the mother upright. It's very unlikely that you would need to do the Løvset when a woman is upright, because we have two other very effective maneuvers (Side to Side and Front to Back). However, it's good to learn upright Løvset just in case.

Steps of the upright Løvset maneuver

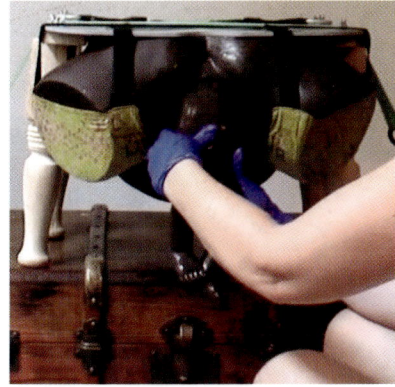
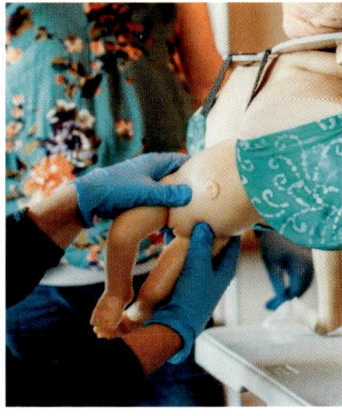

Grab the front of the baby's pelvis with your thumbs. Keep your hands on the pelvis and legs only—never on the soft parts of the abdomen!

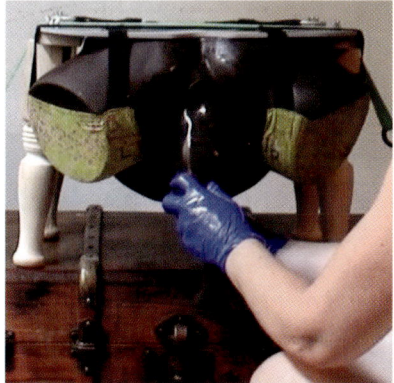

Flex the baby towards the mother's pubic bone (following the direction of the sacral curve).

This flexion pulls the posterior arm and shoulder very low into the sacrum.

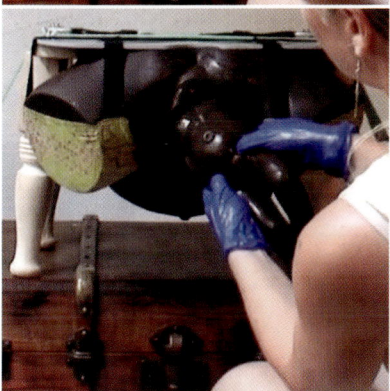

With thumbs on the front of the baby's pelvis, rotate the baby 180°. Pull straight back towards your own torso as you rotate.

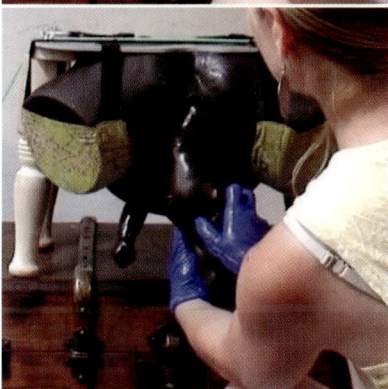

Next, flex the baby a second time towards the mother's pubic bone. Follow the direction of the sacral curve.

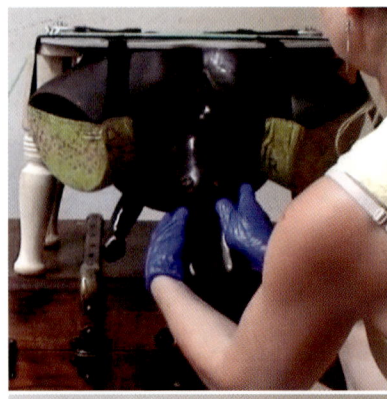

Do a 2nd 180° rotation back the way you came from. Pull straight back towards your own torso as you rotate.

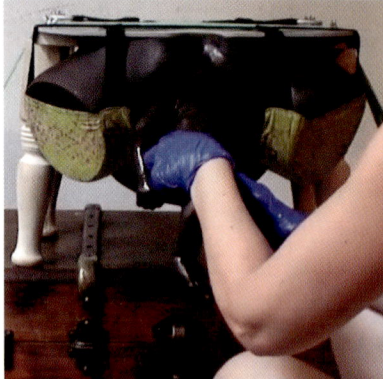

Midway through the 2ⁿᵈ 180° rotation.

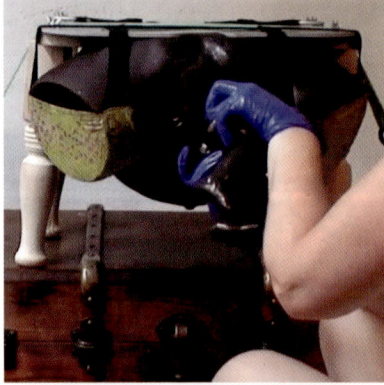

The baby is now fully rotated 180° back to where it started from.

The 2ⁿᵈ arm/shoulder should deliver under the pubic arch. You can help release it if necessary.

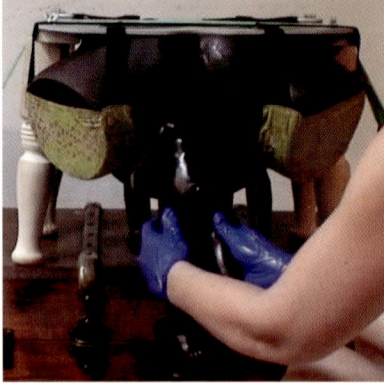

Rotate the baby's body 90° back to sacrum anterior (baby facing the mother's spine).

You have completed the upright Løvset maneuver.

You now know three main strategies for freeing tapped arms: Side to Side, Front to Back, and Løvset, plus arm sweeps when indicated.

6c: Freeing a trapped head

Now the baby is out except for the head. What if you have a head that is stuck? Normally it will be stuck because it's deflexed enough to keep the diameter of the head from coming through the maternal pelvis. This is where we have some very effective tools, especially if you're doing upright physiological breech birth.

How can you tell if the head is deflexed?

The perineum will look **hollow and deflated, rather than full and bulging**. Here is an illustration of what it looks like inside the pelvis. You will feel a "bird's beak" on exam. When you do an exam, you feel a sharp, pointy thing under the perineum, if you can feel it at all. That's because you're feeling the baby's chin pointing upward.

Deflexed head: Upright   Deflexed head: Supine

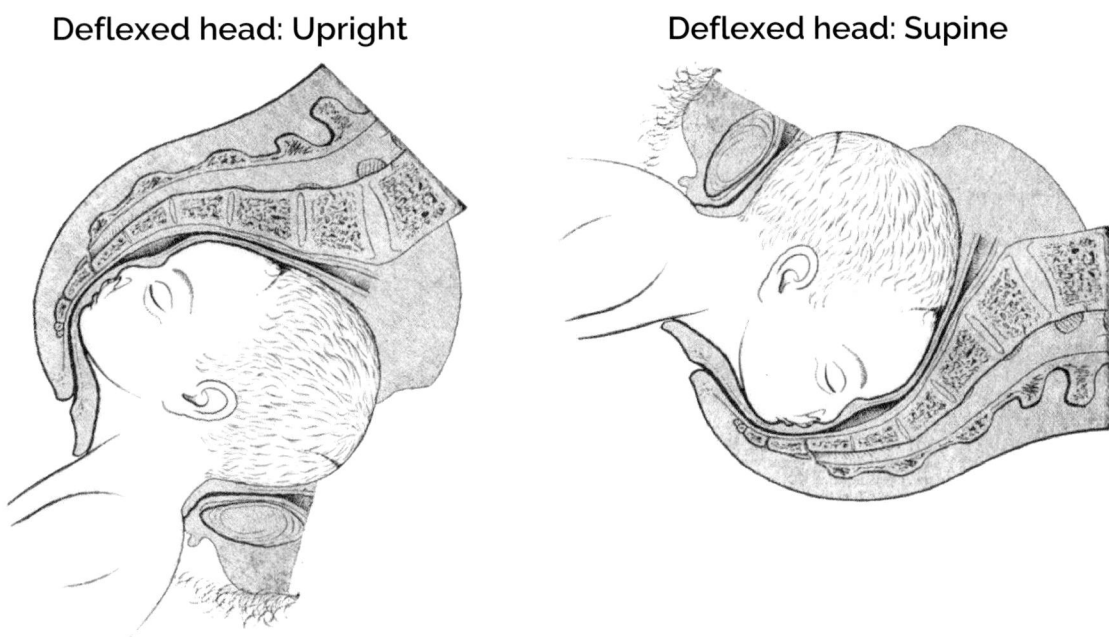

1. Shoulder press

The most important technique for freeing a head during an upright beech birth is the shoulder press. The shoulder press is beautifully elegant because it helps the head flex without the need for an invasive maneuver like the MSV (Mauriceau-Smellie-Veit), which was shown earlier.

Let me explain the mechanics behind the shoulder press. You have a baby that is out except for the head. The head is not adequately flexed to fit through the pelvic outlet. You want the head to flex because a flexed head presents a smaller diameter through the pelvic outlet.

The mother's pubic bone is right behind the occiput (the back of the baby's head). The shoulder press simply pushes the baby straight back towards the mother's pubic bone. This pushes the occiput against the pubic bone and flexes the head. It's very simple and very elegant.

Note that the direction of the force should be pressing the occiput directly towards the pubic bone. Be sure not to pull down on the shoulders; that will extend the head and make your situation worse.

These three photos below show a shoulder press on a baby that had been losing tone. In the first picture, the chin has just cleared the perineum. In the second picture, the nose has emerged. The midwife continued the shoulder press until the head was born.

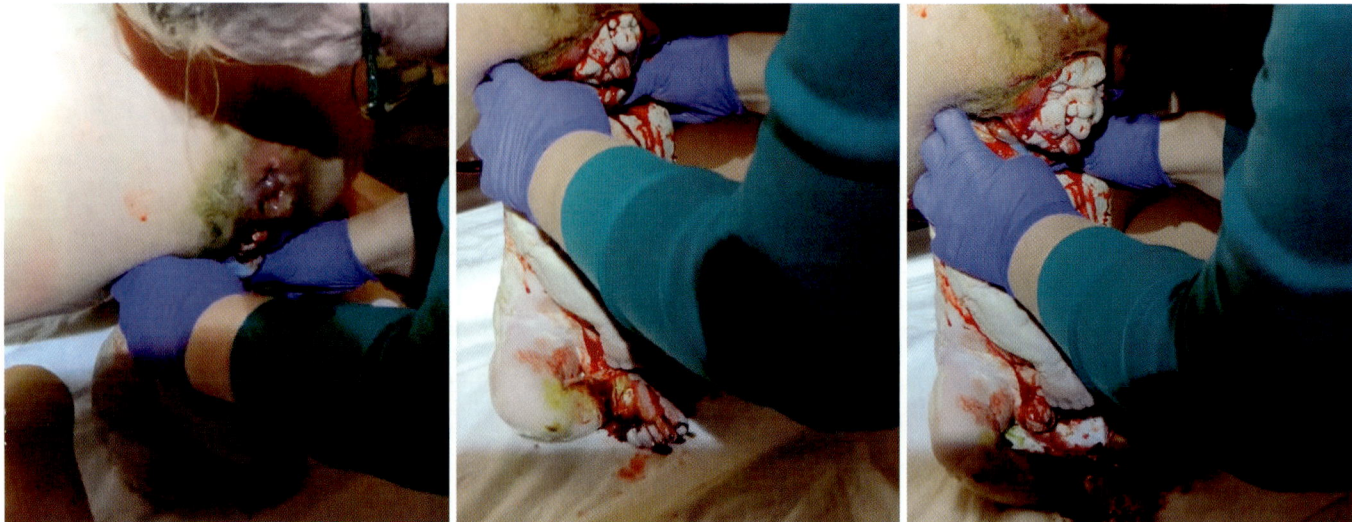

To do a shoulder press, there are two main techniques, both of which are effective.

Technique #1: Grab both shoulders

One way is to grab both shoulders with your thumbs in the front and your fingers on the back of the shoulder blades. **Do not press on the clavicles or push your thumbs into the sternum**; instead, grab the entire shoulder girdle: thumbs on the front of the shoulders, fingers on the back. Press the baby straight back towards the mother's pubic bone.

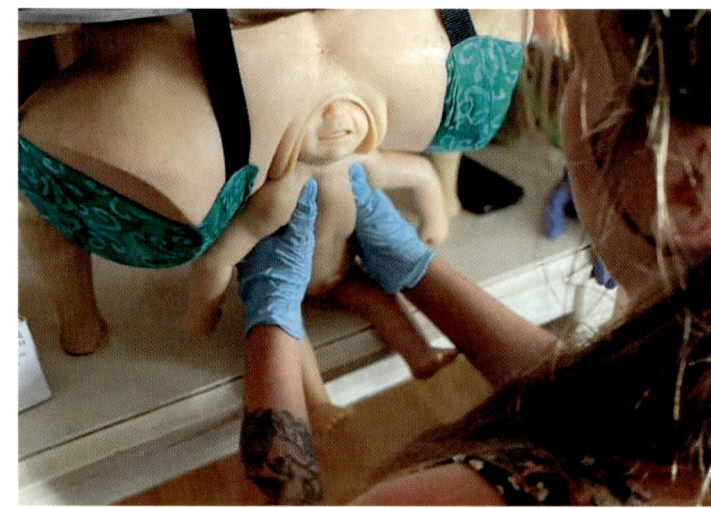

You can grab by going underneath the armpits, as we see in this picture with our simulator, or you can grab the shoulders from above, as the midwife did in the pictures above.

Technique #2: Flat hand press

A second technique (the one we prefer) is to put the flat of your entire hand against the baby's chest. Press firmly backward towards the mother's pubic bone. You can see how the baby's neck would fall right into the crook between my finger and my thumb. See the pictures below for proper hand placement. A one-handed shoulder press is useful because it frees the other hand for another maneuver, if necessary.

Flat hand press: Note how the baby's chin descends as the head flexes

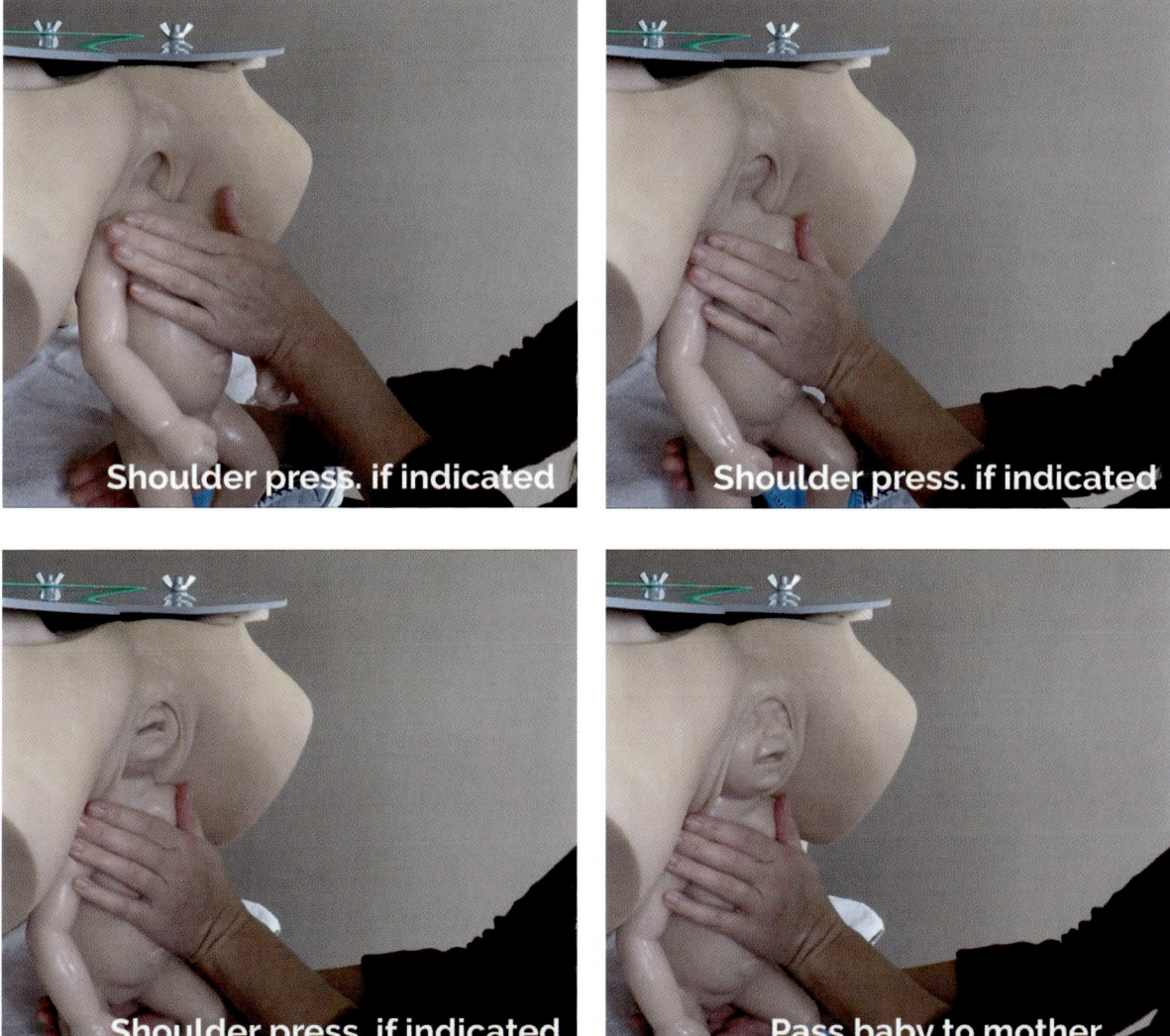

Whichever way you do the shoulder press, you will need to press very firmly. It may surprise you how much force you need to help the head to flex.

Is the head straight?

What to do if the shoulder press doesn't bring the baby out? First, check to be sure the head is aligned straight towards the mother's spine. If the head is turned to one side or the other, it will be hard to flex. You can gently turn the head back into the proper position with a finger on the side of the chin or cheek.

Dorsal lithotomy variant of the shoulder press (Burns-Marshall)

It is theoretically possible to adapt the Burns-Marshall maneuver to add an upside-down shoulder press at the end (or add a Ritgen, which we will learn later in this lesson). The Burns-Marshall maneuver is where you let the baby hang until the nape of the neck is visible, then you grab the baby by the feet and gently pull the baby up in the curve of the sacrum. That extends the baby's neck, and the baby in turn responds by trying to flex its head. Once the baby is in position D, you could add the shoulder press if the head does not release on its own.

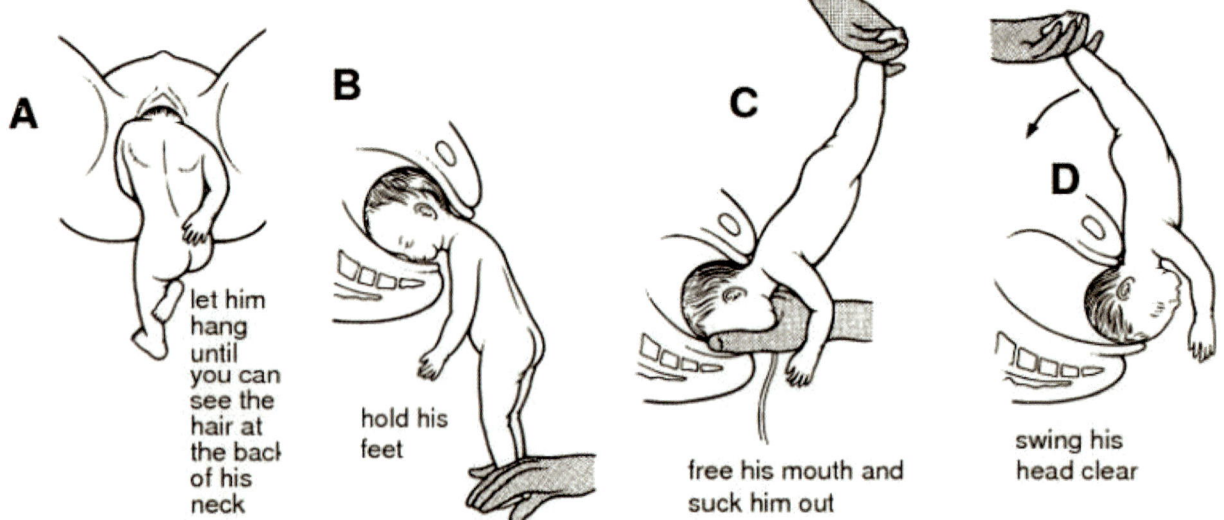

Image found online; original source not available

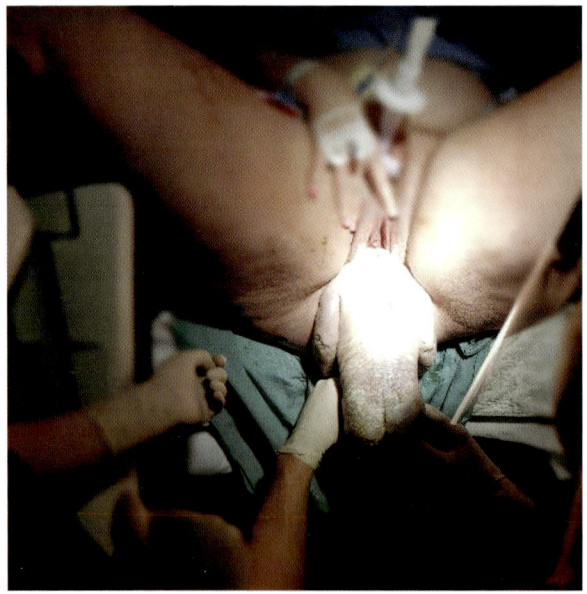

Left: Letting the baby hang until the nape of the neck is visible (step A of the Burns-Marshall maneuver)

Abby

Burns-Marshall with shoulder press

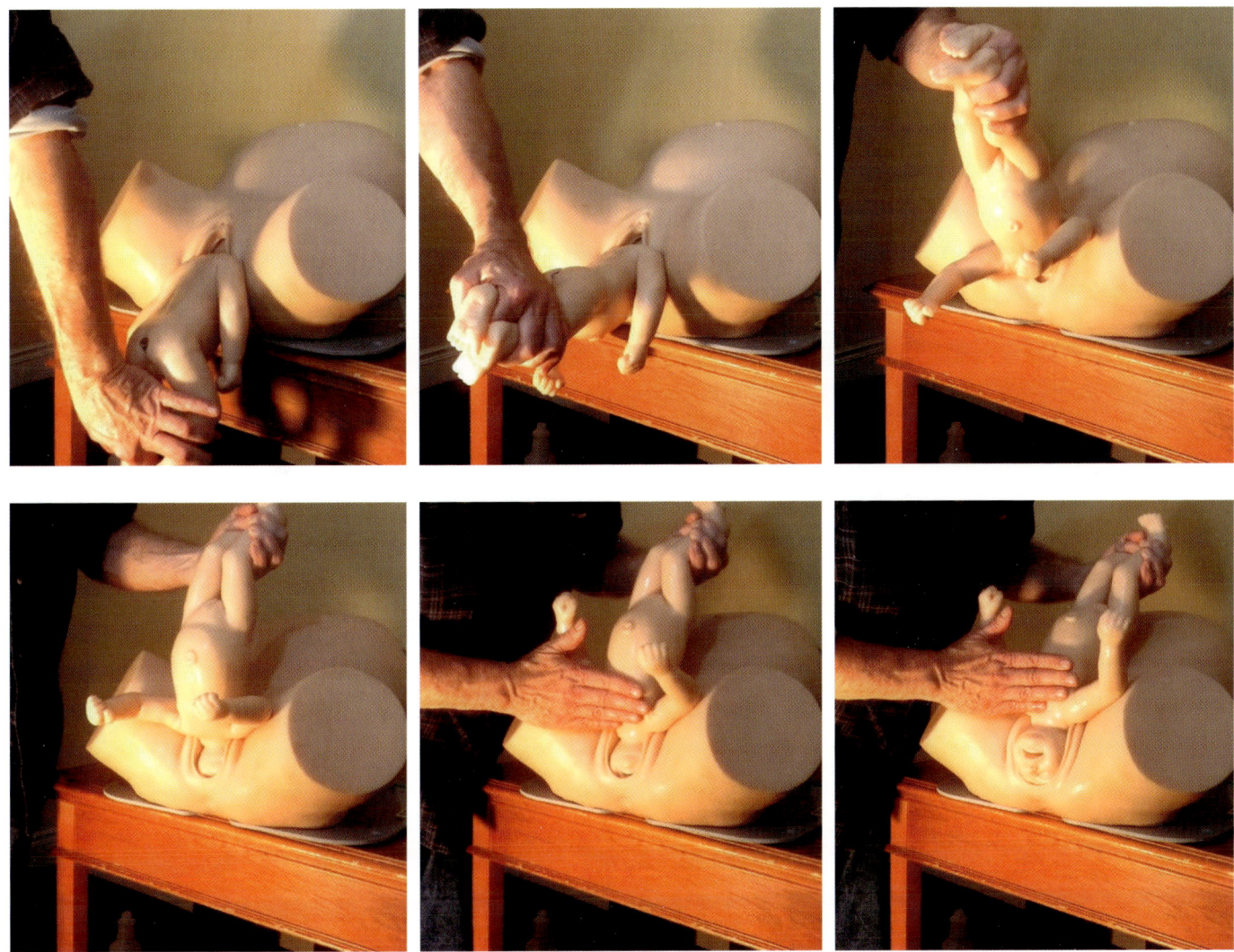

2. Rock & Roll

If you have a particularly tight perineum, a particularly stuck or extended head, and you're putting a significant amount of pressure on the baby's chest and not getting as much flexion as you want, you can significantly improve the effectiveness of the maneuver by pressing, releasing, pressing, releasing. This is called the Rock & Roll.

You have to find the right amount of force and rhythm. If it's too fast or too slow, if it's too gentle or way too hard, it won't work. But there is a sweet spot where it's just fast enough and just enough force that doing these short bursts of shoulder press will bring that baby out. Give it a try for 5-10 seconds after the shoulder press. If it doesn't work, move on to another flexion maneuver.

3. Ritgen

Let's say the Rock & Roll doesn't work. What could you do next?

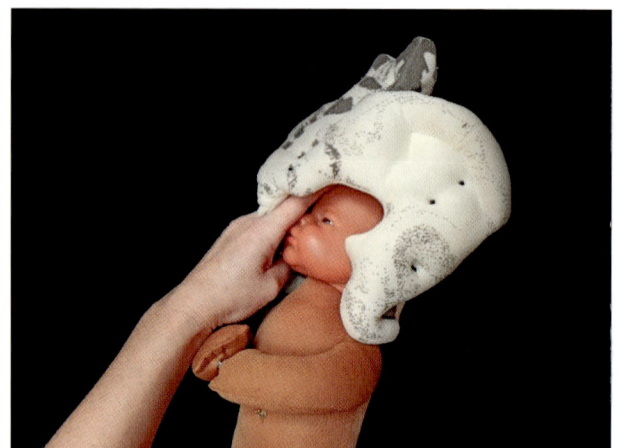

The Ritgen maneuver involves placing two fingers into the mother's rectum. This allows you to reach to the top of the baby's head and flex it forward. Obviously, it's probably not going to be the most comfortable thing for the mother. However, at that point, nothing is going to be comfortable. Explain to the mother what you need to do. We recommend trying the Ritgen maneuver before doing something much more invasive, such as the MSV (Mauriceau-Smellie-Veit).

Be sure your hands are gloved and your fingers are well-lubricated. Gently insert 1-2 fingers into the rectum as far back as you can. This will allow you to reach far back on the top of the baby's head and bring it forward.

The photo on the left shows Dr. Hayes doing a Ritgen maneuver to release the head. The woman is sitting semi-reclined on her partner's legs. This was preceded by a Bracht maneuver due to poor fetal tone. The photos on the right show an upright Ritgen on our simulator.

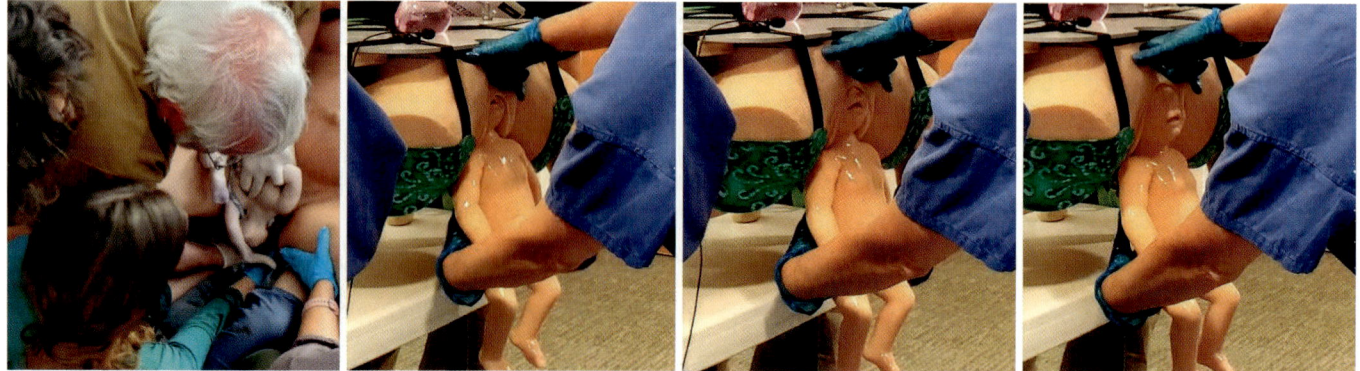

4. The Crowning Touch

Betty-Anne Daviss has developed a technique called "the Crowning Touch." Insert two fingers along the cheekbone to the ear, then angle your fingers downward and continue to the back of the baby's head. Your ring and pinkie fingers will remain on the outside. Next, tilt your wrist forward, using your last two fingers as a fulcrum. This will flex the baby's head forward while simultaneously pushing the baby's chest towards the pubic bone. The Crowning Touch seems to have eliminated the need for forceps. In a series of 1,026 upright breech births, 4% used the Crowning Touch and none required forceps (Daviss et al. 2021).

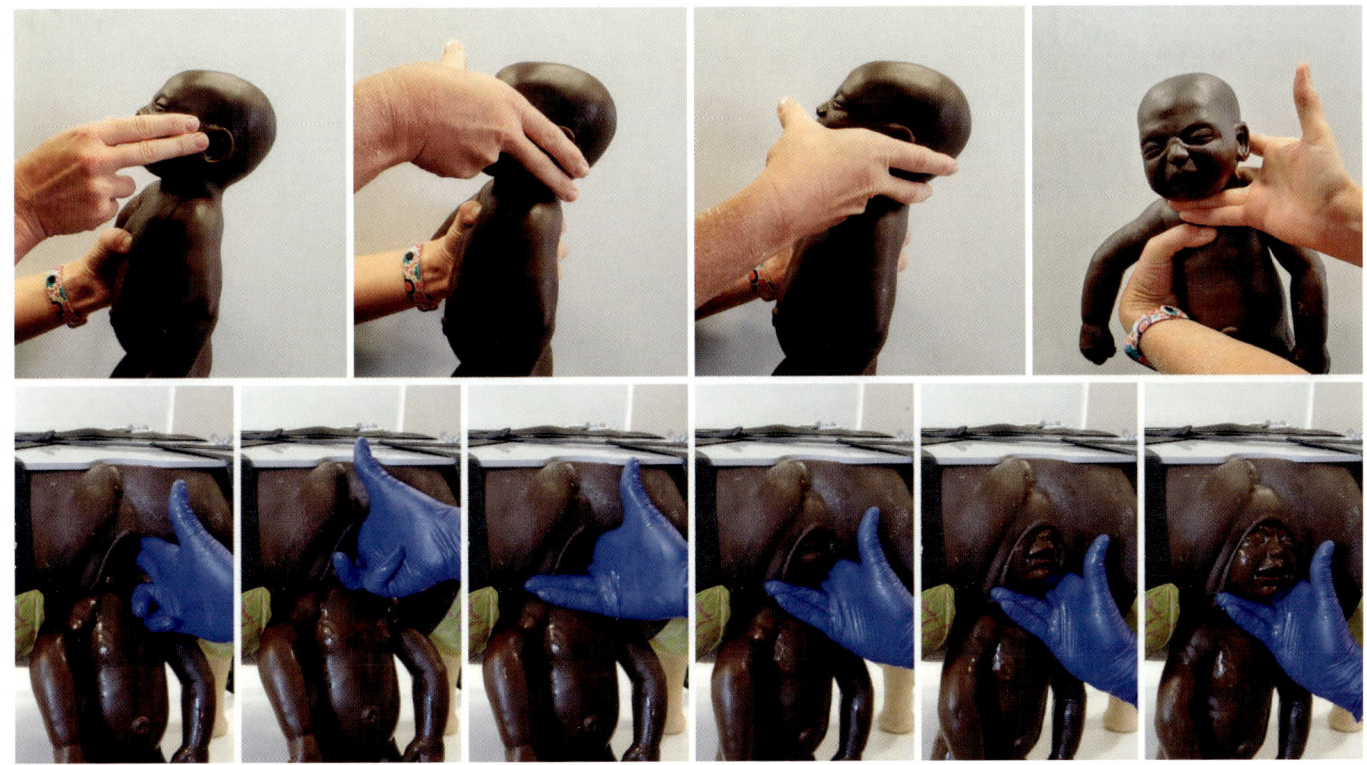

5. Finger flexion

Gail Tully, a midwife in Minnesota, has used a two-handed flexion technique along the temporal bones, which she calls "finger flexion." In her words: "The baby's head is released by placing your fingers on the temporal bones, then gently flexing the head. For stargazer babies: Reach up to the chin, slightly turn the baby's head to the oblique to bring the head down, then turn the baby's head back to the AP diameter." (2016 Amsterdam Breech Conference, breechwithoutborders.org/amsterdam5)

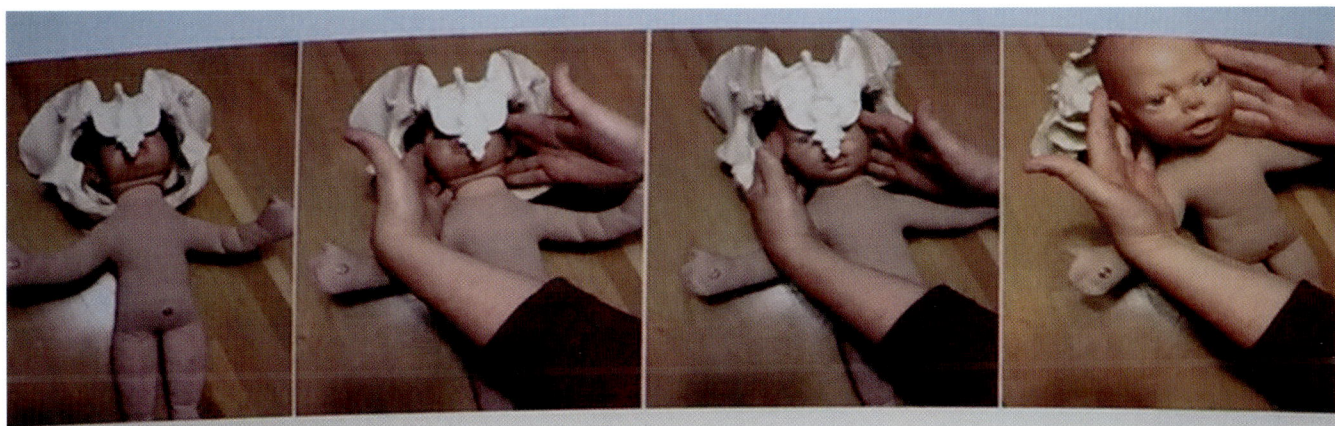

6. MSV (Mauriceau-Smellie-Veit) maneuver

This is a very common maneuver used in supine breech births since the early 1600s. It uses two hands to help flex the baby's head. One hand goes behind the baby's occiput and pushes upwards. The other hand goes on the baby's face (mouth and/or cheekbones) and pulls downwards. Usually, an assistant does suprapubic pressure during the maneuver; maternal pushing will also assist your efforts.

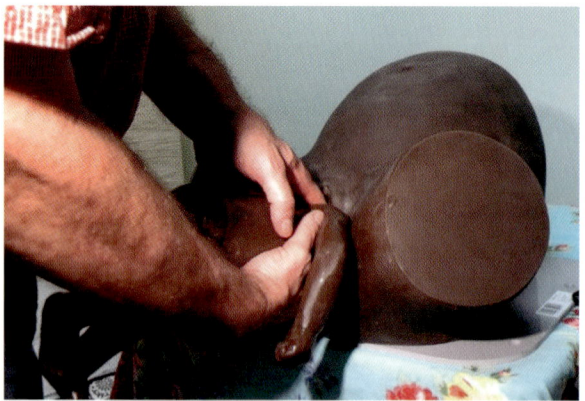

With one hand, put two fingers on the back of the baby's occiput. With your other hand, put two fingers on the baby's malar eminences (cheekbones) and/or one finger in the mouth and flex the baby's head so its chin tucks into its chest. Some people put a finger in the baby's mouth instead of on the cheekbones; others do both the mouth and the cheekbones together. Be careful not to poke the baby's eyes!

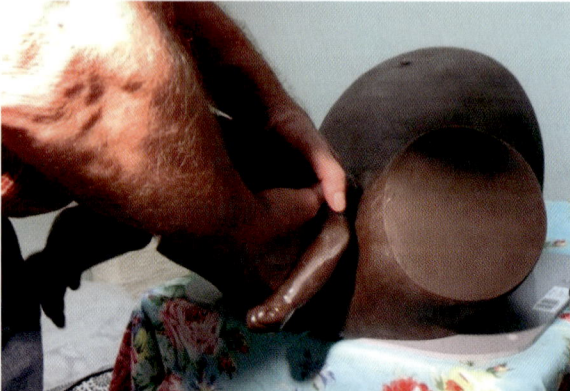

As you are flexing the head, guide the baby to follow the sacral curve.

In a supine birth, this means lifting the baby upward towards the mother's belly.

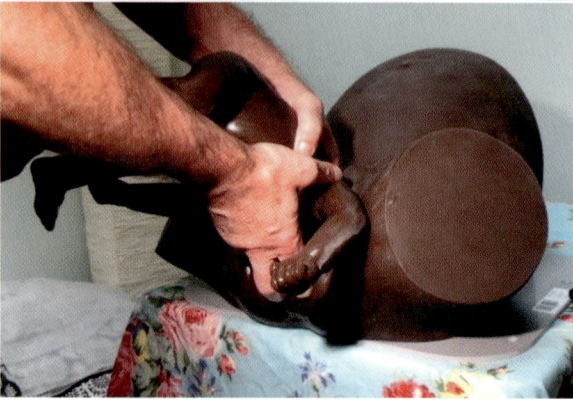

Gently maintain that position as you continue flexing the head and pivoting the baby around the mother's pubic bone.

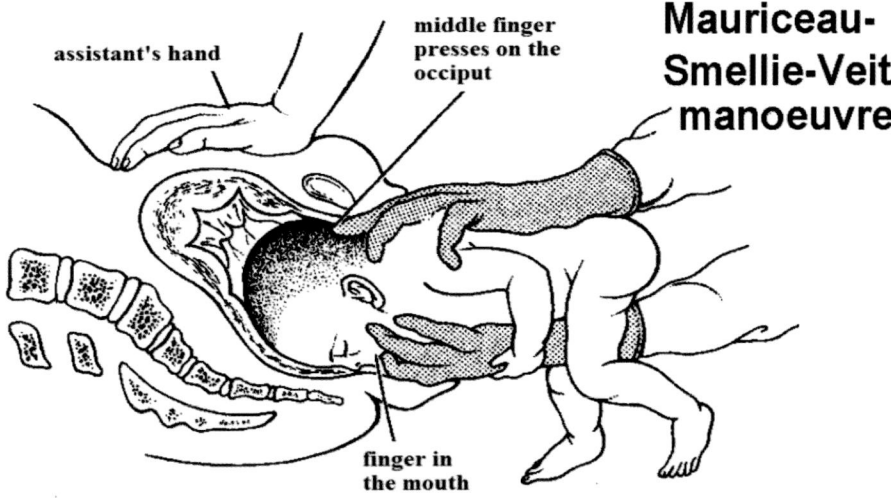

Image source unknown

7. Gentle upright MSV technique

We have already shown you how to do the MSV when the woman is on her back. It's also possible to do this maneuver when the woman is upright. Some people call it the MSV-Cronk or MSV-Banks, named after the midwives who wrote about it.

Kristine Lauria, a midwife who worked in Amish communities for many years before serving overseas with Médecins Sans Frontières, has developed a very gentle way to do MSV with the mother upright.

She places her **middle finger on the back of the baby's head** (occiput). With her other hand, she places her **first finger inside the baby's mouth**. The palm of her hand is against the baby's chest, which allows her to feel the baby's heartbeat as she is doing the maneuver. In this picture, we are discussing this technique while she was halfway around the world working in a refugee camp.

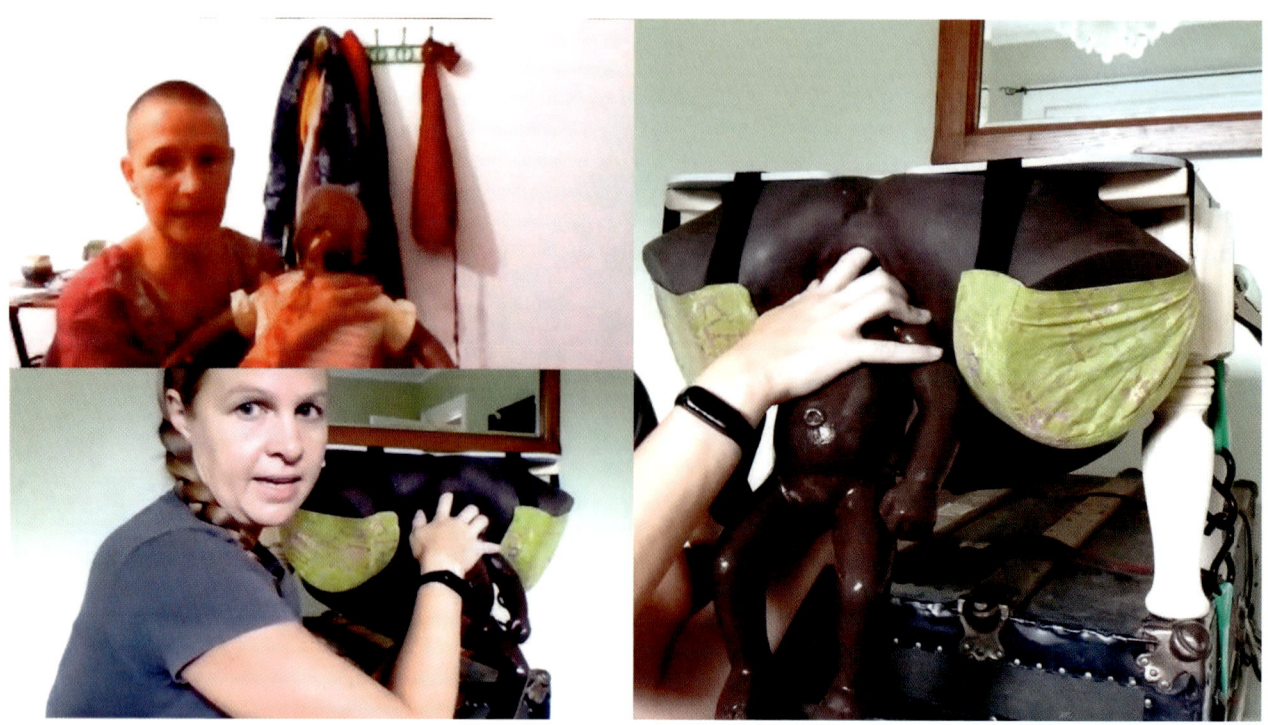

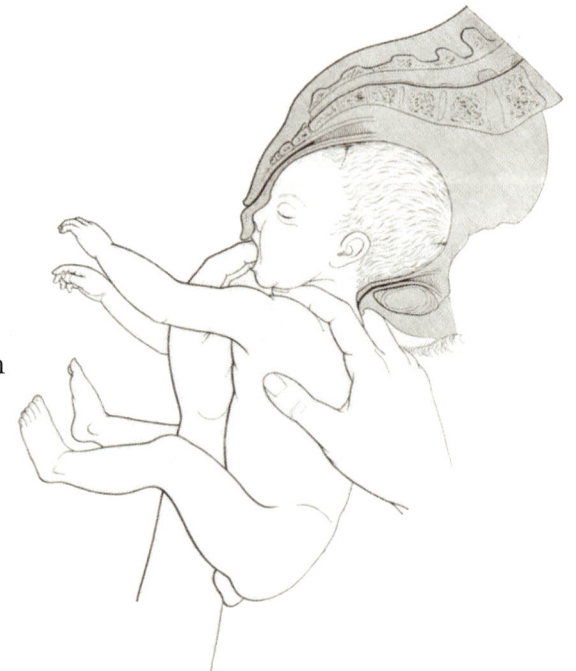

She gently pushes upward on the back of the baby's head while pulling downward on the mouth. Watch as the baby's head flexes and descends.

Note how much easier it is to do the MSV when the mother is upright rather than on her back. The baby naturally follows the curve of the sacrum and dangles while you do the maneuver. You can also see very well what is happening. But when the mother is on your back, you have to lift the baby's body up and around while you are doing the maneuver. Another good reason to encourage women to stay upright!

Steps of the gentle upright MSV maneuver

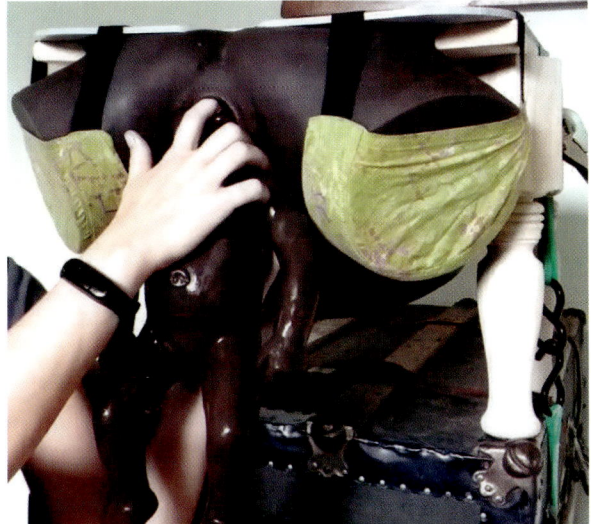

I am starting to flex the head with both hands.

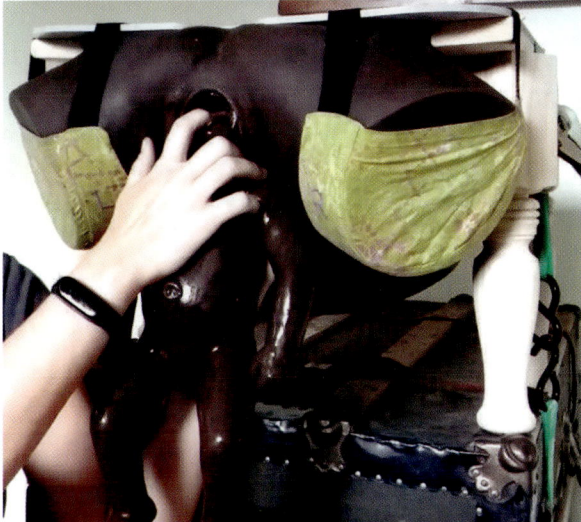

I am gently pushing upward on the back of the head while pulling downward on the baby's mouth.

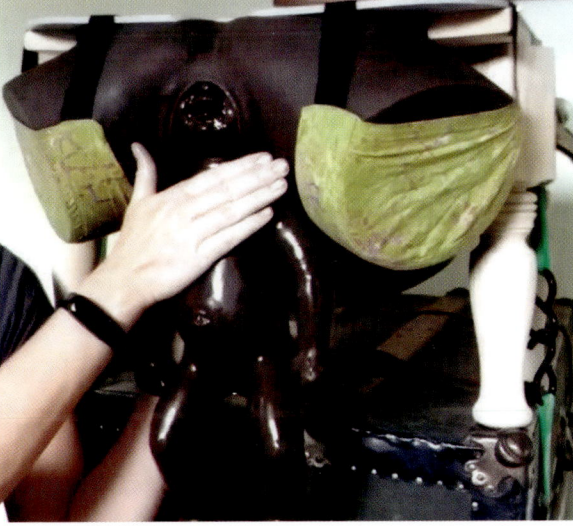

Once I can see the nose, I switch over to a flat hand shoulder press. (You could also continue doing the MSV until the head emerges.)

Hyperextended head in the pelvic inlet (rare)

One rare situation is a hyperextended head that gets stuck in the pelvic inlet between the sacral promontory and the pubic bone. The chin or the face is stuck on the sacral promontory, and the back of the baby's head is stuck on top of the pubic bone. The arms may be raised or crossed in combination with a hyperextended head—for example, see the illustration, 2nd from the left, by Gail Tully (2016 Amsterdam Breech Conference).

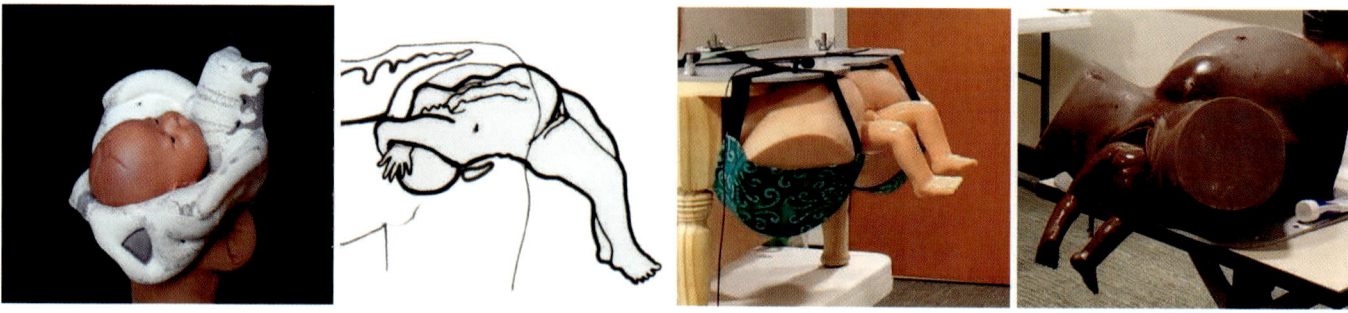

Inlet entrapment typically occurs with a constellation of 3 events:
1) The baby will rump and descend direct sacrum anterior.
2) The baby will be arrested quite high in the pelvis—the umbilicus may not even be visible. The arms will not be out at this point. No further progress will occur.
3) The baby is likely already compromised (and it is possible that pre-existing compromise led to the hyperextension in the first place).

What would you do in this situation? Flexion cannot fix this problem because the head is already stuck between the sacral promontory and the pubic rami. Traction cannot fix this problem either; pulling on the baby will just make the impaction worse. The solution involves 2 people working in tandem to disimpact significantly, flexing the baby's head against fundal counterpressure, then dropping the head into the oblique of the pelvis until the baby is low enough for an extraction maneuver (Løvset). Dr. Hayes will describe this in more detail in his lesson on maneuvers.

This G6P4 birth below, attended by a team of two midwives and an obstetrician in New Zealand, had a baby with an inlet entrapment. The birth began with a cord presenting in advance of the complete breech with dropped feet. The baby descended SA to the umbilicus and would not descend further.

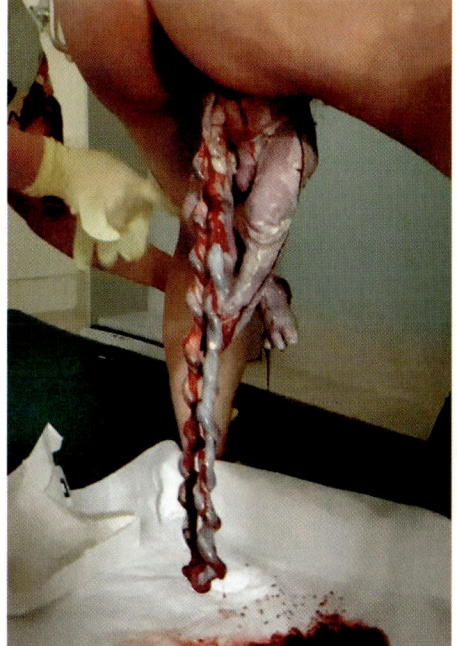

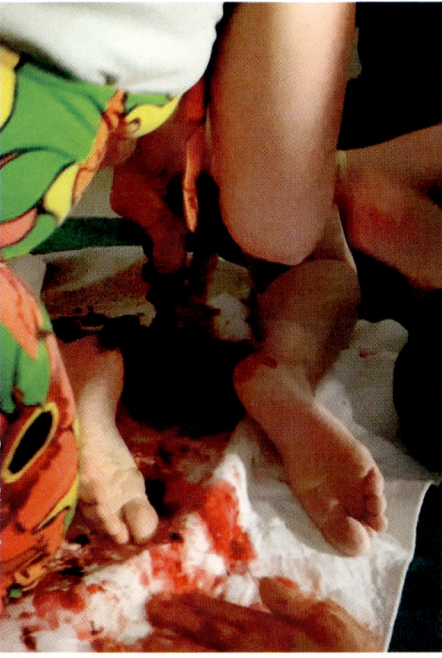

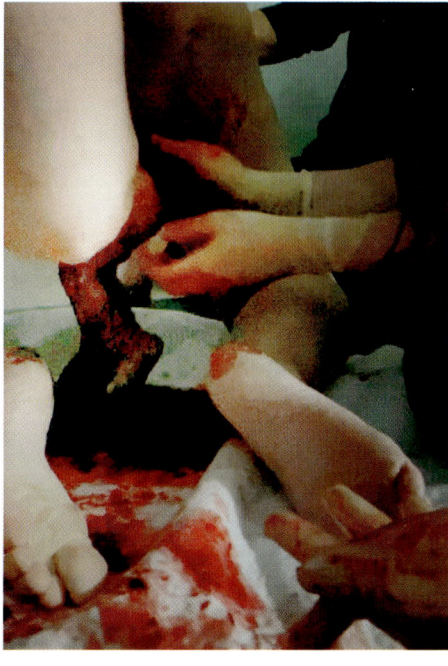

Baby remained stuck SA and high, despite vigorous pushing and position changes. Tummy crunches were absent.

After some rotational maneuvers, baby was LST but still very high.

Another Side to Side brought baby RST.

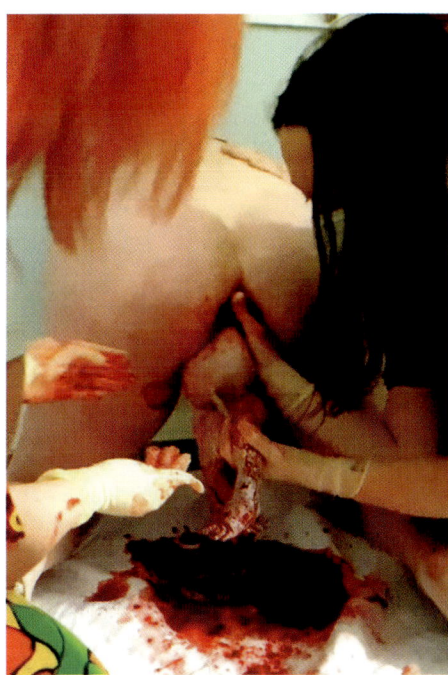

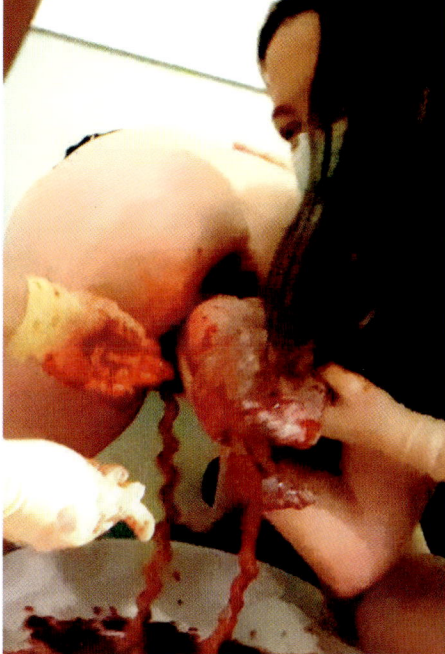

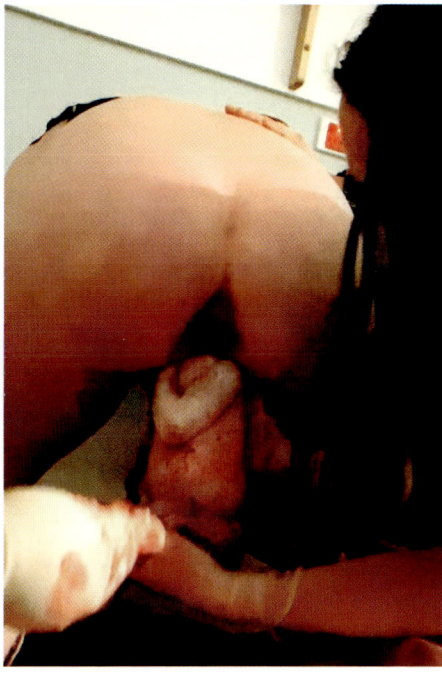

Obtetrician first tried to release posterior arm. Baby is now RSO.

Next, she tried for the anterior arm and was successful. Baby is now SA.

As soon as the anterior arm released, the posterior arm and head followed. During this arm release, the baby rotated back to RST and was born in that orientation.

The midwives performed both Front to Back and Side to Side maneuvers, reporting that the arms were impossible to reach. Finally, another partial Side to Side maneuver (180° rotation only) helped the baby descend, and the team swept down the anterior arm. The posterior arm and head were born seconds later. Interestingly, the head was born facing transverse!

In this birth, disimpacting and rotating the baby off the obstruction ultimately helped the baby descend, but it took several attempts. Although these maneuvers were designed for arm entrapment with a baby much lower in the pelvis, they ended up being effective in this situation. The baby required a few hours of NICU support (CPAP) but was released the following morning with no further complications. The birth took 5 ½ minutes from the bitrochanteric diameter and 9 ½ minutes from the first appearance of the cord to birth. The baby was 3rd centile (2657 g), smaller than anticipated based on growth scans.

If this situation occurs, it will likely not be easy and will require quick thinking, prompt action, and steady hands.

Cervical head entrapment (rare)

Cervical head entrapment is extremely rare in a normally grown full-term baby. It is more likely to occur in extremely premature or asymmetrically growth restricted babies because they have a large discrepancy between the thorax and the head. One option is to perform Duhrssen's incisions at 2 & 10 o'clock, if you are in a hospital facility and have been properly trained. Another option is to stretch the cervix up over the head. Work your fingers underneath the cervix and position them as if you are doing a MSV. Use a rocking motion to help the head work through the cervix. Anticipate that this will be extremely difficult and require maximum force to stretch and open the cervix.

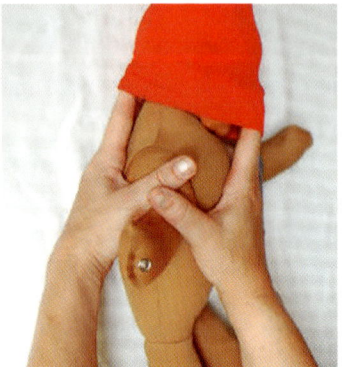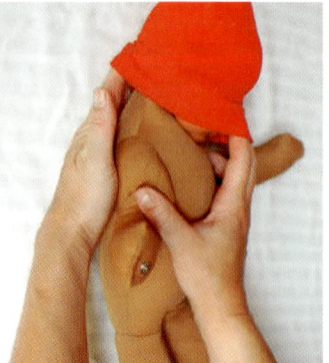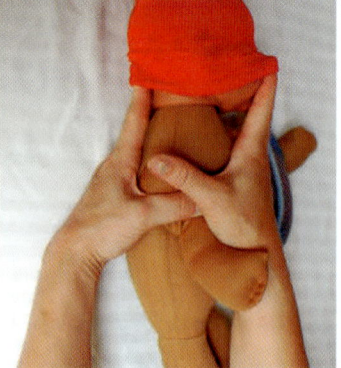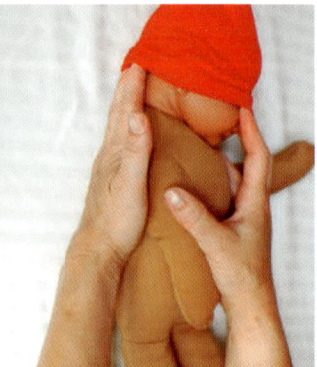

Be creative

You may need to combine more than one technique. We debriefed a birth in which a two-handed shoulder press did not free the baby's head. The midwife then did a one-handed shoulder press, and with her other hand she reached up behind the baby's occiput and pushed upwards to flex the head down. The combination of flexing the occiput and doing a shoulder press helped the baby's head release, whereas earlier efforts doing just the shoulder press had not been effective. You need to innovate, be creative, and adapt to your situations.

6d: Sacrum posterior rotation

Sometimes babies will emerge or rotate sacrum posterior (SP). Because this is so rare, we do not have good data on what the best strategy is: allow the baby to descend and wait to see what happens or correct the malrotation by disimpacting and rotating as soon as you see it happening. The baby normally descends in one of the transverse gutters in the pelvis, and it takes something very unusual to make the baby want to rotate towards the sacral promontory rather than away from it. Maternal anatomy may play a role in some cases. The majority of sacrum posterior rotations are probably likely due to a lower extremity impingement. It may be more common in incomplete or complete presentations as opposed to frank presentations.

Correcting a sacrum posterior rotation

There is little published data on the proper management of sacrum posterior presentation. Anecdotally speaking, many of them will resolve on their own, and they're amazing things to see. From my clinical experience and from other people's clinical experience, if you recognize SP rotation once rumping is occurring and you see the baby start to rotate in the wrong direction, you could try grabbing the baby by the pelvic girdle, elevating, and rotating slightly past direct transverse towards sacrum anterior to give the baby a nudge to go in the right direction.

If that is unsuccessful, I would let the baby rotate where it wants to go and see what happens. There are videos that show babies going posterior and then spontaneously rotating 270° all the way around to get to sacrum anterior. If that's what it takes for the baby to successfully navigate the sacral curve and make its way out of the pelvis, then my tendency would be to respect that—as long as descent is still occurring.

If descent is not occurring during the contraction, then here is when you can apply fundal pressure as a diagnostic tool. This will show you which direction the baby wants to rotate, and then you help it go that way. Does it matter which way it goes? It does, because if you don't know where the baby came from and which way it wants to go, and then you won't have a good idea which way the head is facing. If you've got a baby with the head facing one direction and you try to rotate the body the other direction, you may be putting unnecessary and dangerous amounts of torque on that baby's neck.

When you do the rotation, you grasp the pelvic girdle, elevate, and rotate just past sacrum transverse. If you have a neurologically intact, vigorous baby, rotate just past sacrum transverse and then ask mom to push. See if you get proper rotation and descent with that push, or even use fundal pressure again as a diagnostic tool. Again, if there's adequate descent, avoid traction.

Pay close attention to which way the baby starts rumping.
>   RST = right sacrum transverse = baby's spine facing the mother's right leg
>   LST = left sacrum transverse = baby's spine facing the mother's left leg
This will tell you which way to rotate back if you encounter this situation.

The birth below happened to a midwife before she took our training. It was her very first breech birth, and she didn't know it was breech until the rump came out. She had three seconds to prepare for a breech birth! Then the baby started rotating towards sacrum posterior, which is very unusual. This midwife was able to sweep down the arms one after another once she saw the baby was going towards sacrum posterior. As soon as the arms were both out, the baby rotated back to sacrum anterior.

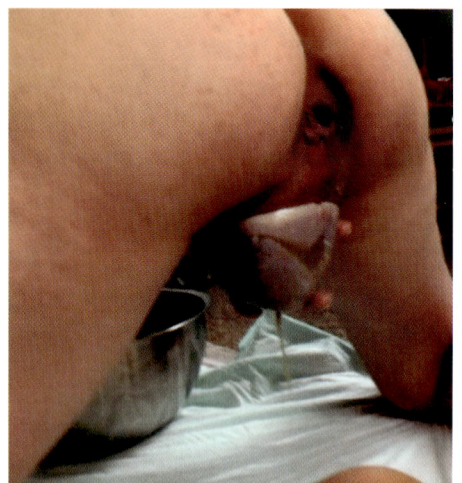 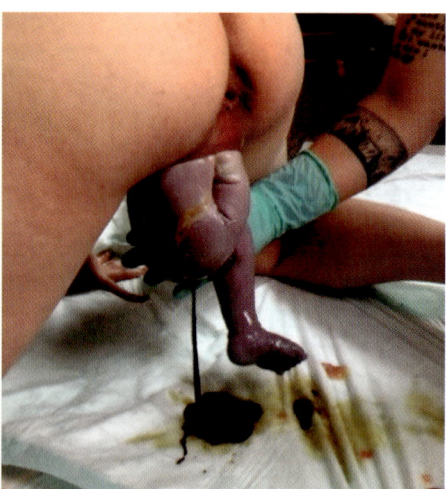 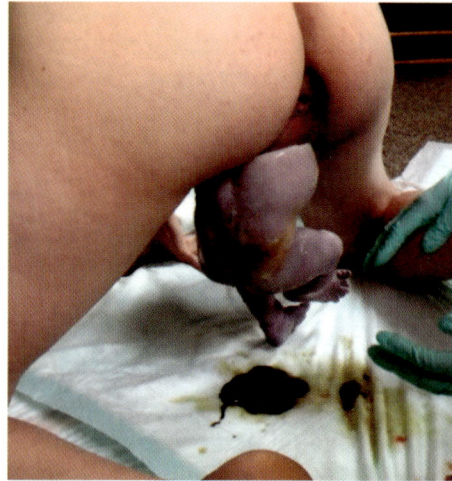

The midwife didn't realize the baby was breech until this moment! She saw what she thought was a head inside the water bag. Once the baby's foot came, she realized it wasn't a head—it was a rump!

A few seconds later, one leg was out. Notice the baby passing meconium, which is normal during a breech birth.

A few seconds later, both legs were out. Notice the baby is still facing completely transverse (LST or left sacrum transverse, with its back facing the mother's left leg).

Baby is kicking and lifting its legs up the entire time. This is very reassuring.

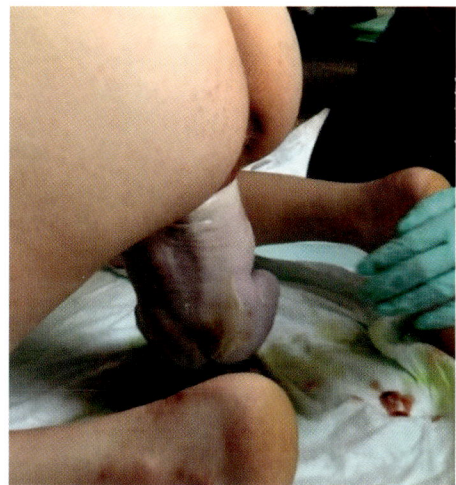

The baby started to rotate towards sacrum posterior (baby facing the mother's front). This is very unusual. Baby has good tone and is doing tummy crunches.

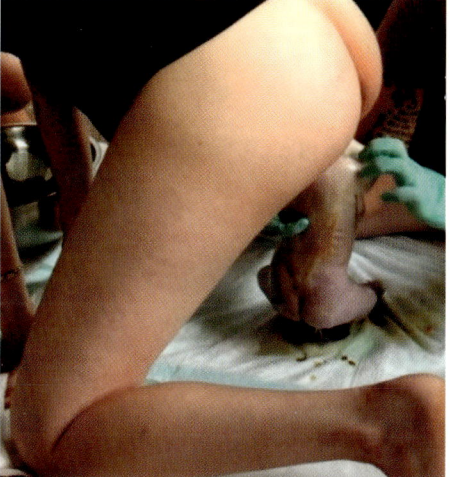

The midwife decided to release the arms. First, she gently released the posterior arm by putting her finger into the elbow and bringing the elbow down and out. She was being careful not to pull down on the baby.

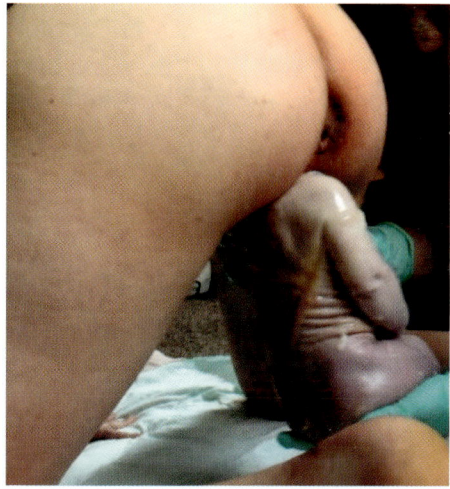

This picture shows her releasing the 2nd arm (anterior arm, or one nearest the mother's pubic bone). She was supporting the baby's bottom with her other hand.

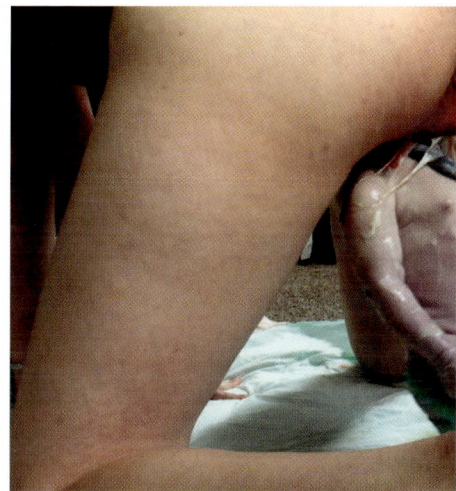

As she was releasing the anterior arm, the baby rotated back to SA. You can see the baby's left arm being released; look right behind the umbilical cord.

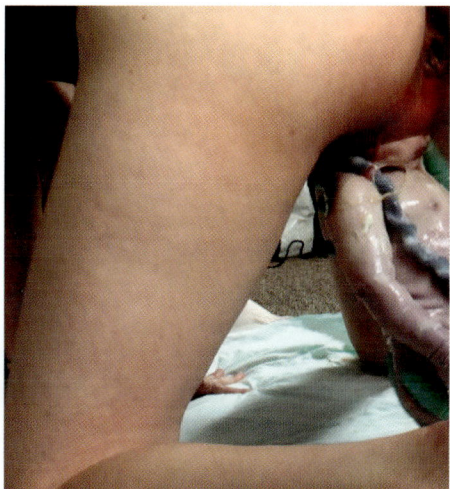

The head was already well-flexed. As soon as the arm released, the chin and mouth were already out!

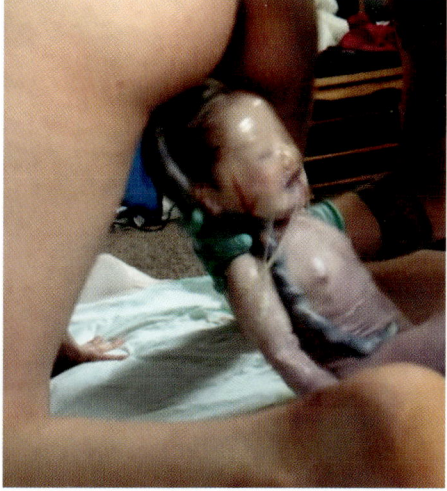

The baby's head fell out immediately after, still partly in the water bag. The baby cried immediately. Notice the full, blue umbilical cord.

Next, we show two births with sacrum posterior rotation. In the first birth, the baby rumped and descended direct SP. Note the baby's back facing the mother's back. The baby required extraction of the arms and head. In the second birth, the baby rumped and descended sacrum oblique. Once out past the umbilicus, the baby started rotating back towards sacrum transverse and beyond towards sacrum posterior. At this point, the midwife assisted by disimpacting using a shoulder grip and rotating the baby back to SA. This helped release the other arm, and the head was born with gentle assistance.

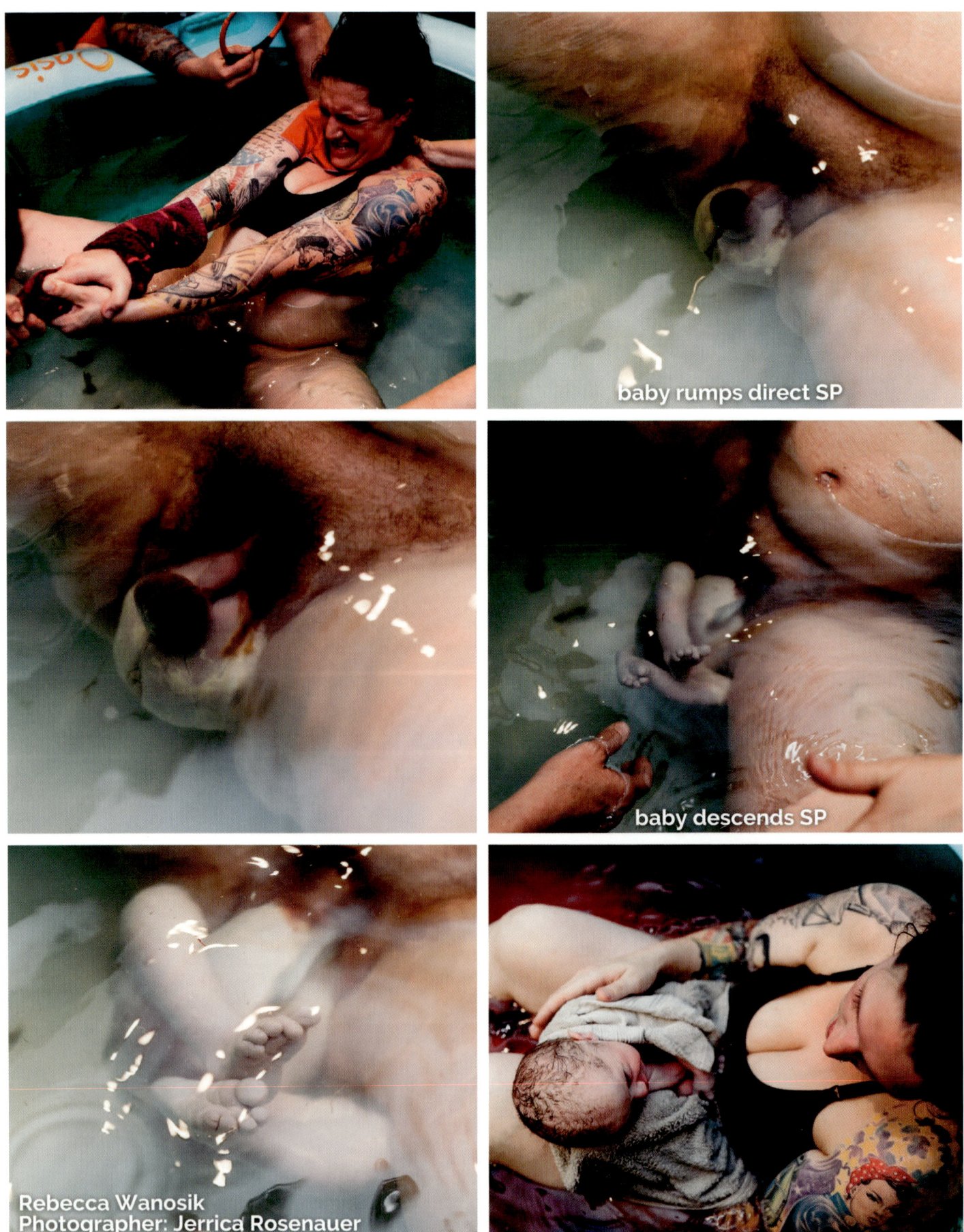

baby rumps direct SP

baby descends SP

Rebecca Wanosik
Photographer: Jerrica Rosenauer

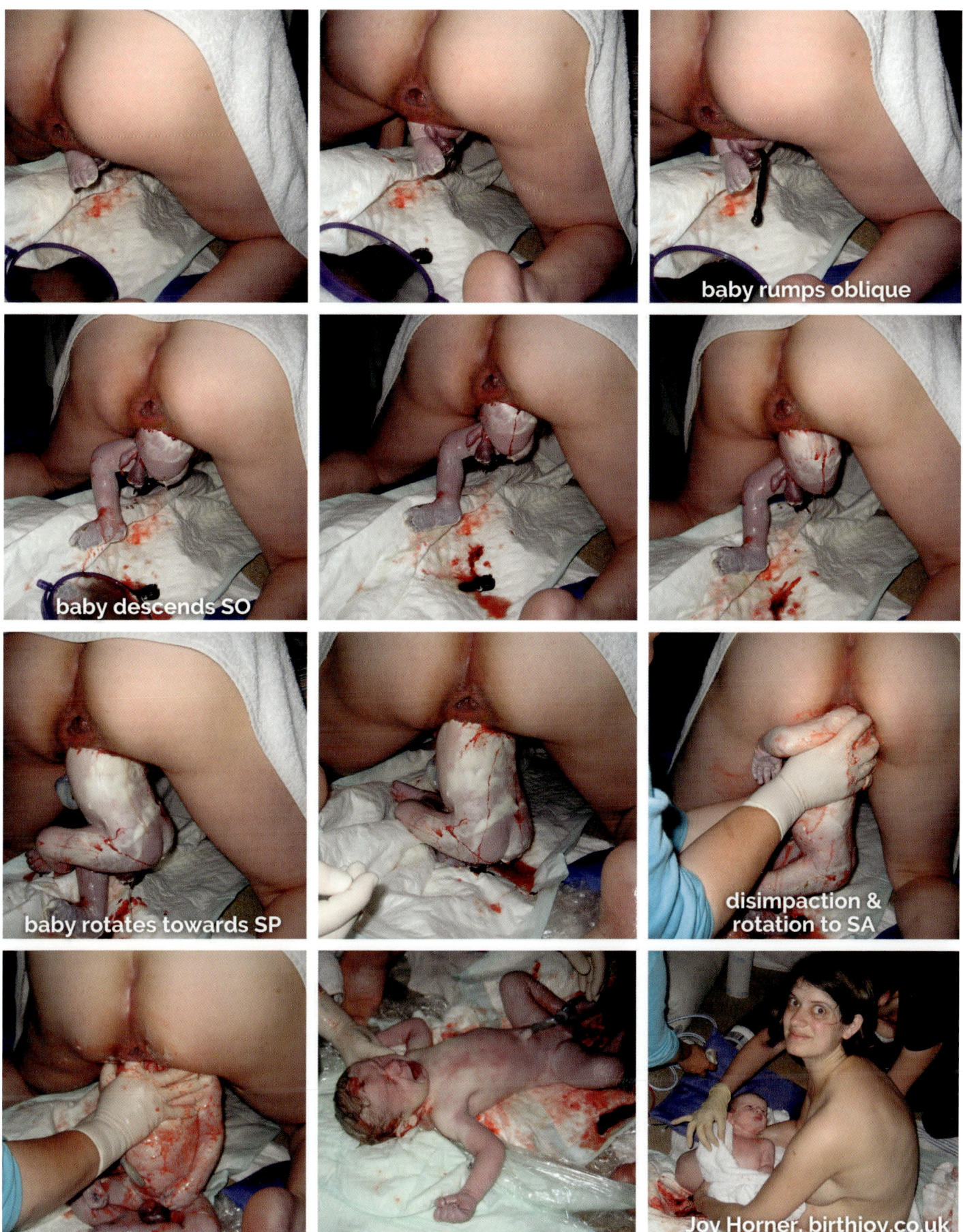

baby rumps oblique

baby descends SO

baby rotates towards SP

disimpaction & rotation to SA

Joy Horner, birthjoy.co.uk

Chin stuck on pubic bone (rare)

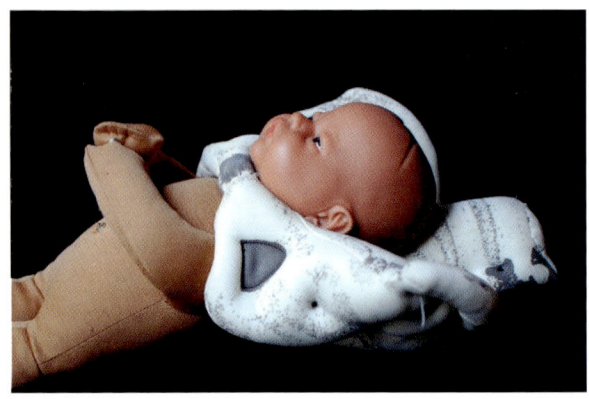

What if you have a baby that has rotated all the way to sacrum posterior (baby facing the mother's front) and gets its head deflexed, possibly with the chin stuck on the pubic bone? One strategy is to help flex the head and tuck the chin under the pubic bone. This is described in both midwifery and obstetric textbooks.

Carol Gautschi, a midwife in the USA, encountered this situation in a breech 2nd twin. The mother's abdominal tissues were loose enough for her to feel that the chin was above the pubic bone. Carol was able to grab the baby's head externally, guard the pubic bone with her other hand, and tuck the baby's head underneath the pubic bone.

Supine chin tuck

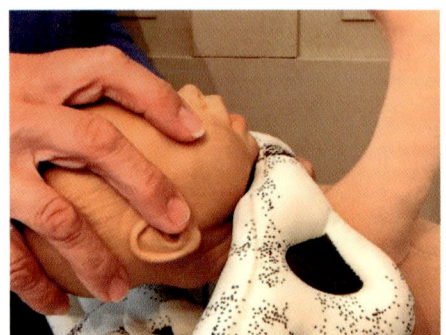 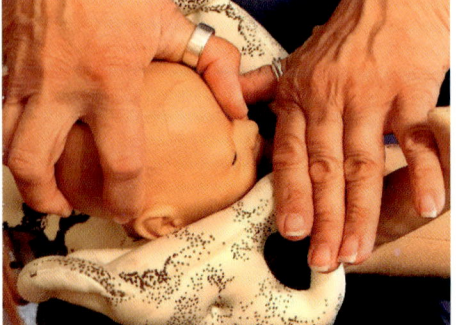 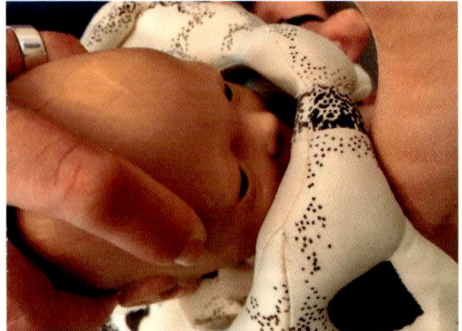

Carol Gautschi

Standing chin tuck

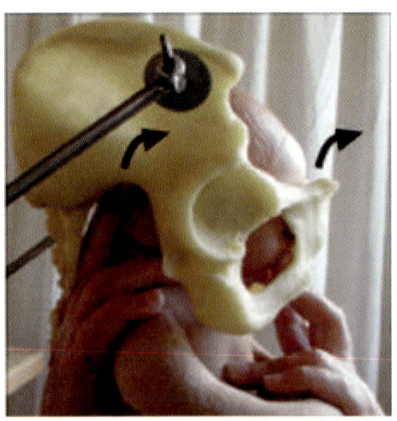

Maggie Banks, a midwife in New Zealand, describes the same situation when the mom was upright (see photo on left, from Banks 2009). She did something similar to the (MSV) Mauriceau-Smellie-Veit, but she kept the baby's spine facing towards the mother's spine (sacrum posterior). She flexed the head, brought the head underneath the pubic arch and out in the direct sacrum posterior position. There is also obstetric literature describing this same technique for supine breech births.

I have met midwives who have corrected a head facing direct SP via disimpacting and rotating back to SA. You want to be extremely careful while doing any 180° rotation, especially when the baby is already posterior and if you're not sure which way the baby started rotating in the first place. You don't want your rotation to turn into a 270° rotation by accident!

6e: Soft tissue maneuvers

Finally, let's move on to soft tissue maneuvers. You might have some births where the head is just not coming out due to soft tissue dystocia. The head might be fairly well flexed, but there is really tight skin or tissue in the way holding the head in. These soft tissue maneuvers can be used at the very end to help expedite the birth, often in combination with a shoulder press.

1. Gluteal lift

One technique is called the gluteal lift, and it's simply when you lift the mother's gluteal tissues up and out of the way with one or two hands. Sometimes it is done by itself (bottom left). Other times it is done in combination with a shoulder press (bottom right)

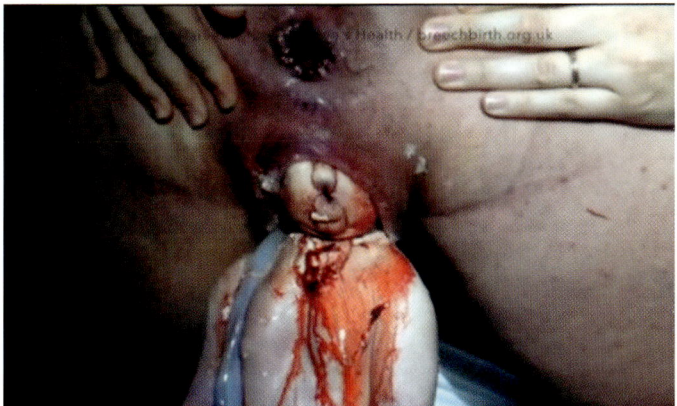 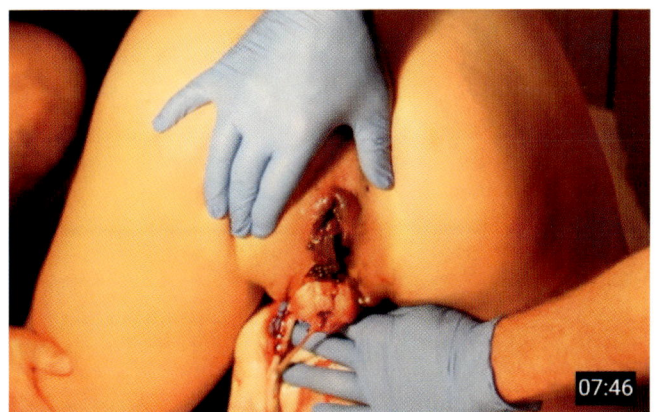

2. Perineal lift

Another technique is a perineal lift. This is where you put a few fingers under the perineum and gently lift it up and out of the way, bringing it up over the baby's face.

Mary Beliz, Birth Photographer marybelizphotos.com

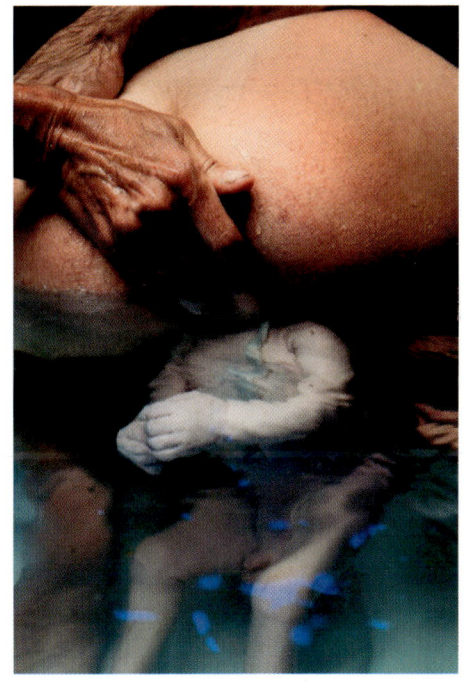

6f: Other supine maneuvers & techniques

Bracht Maneuver

The Bracht maneuver is less a maneuver and more a technique for facilitating a spontaneous supine breech birth. It recreates the normal physiological mechanism of gravity as if the woman were upright. The Bracht maneuver was first introduced in the 1930s and led to a dramatic reduction in perinatal mortality, compared to the older extraction techniques (see Plentl & Stone, 1953).

Bracht is typically initiated once the baby is born to the umbilicus and the legs have released. Keep the baby's legs splinted together with the body and guide the body around the curve of the sacrum, keeping the body as close to the maternal abdomen as possible. You are not pulling—the mother is exerting her own force via pushing, assisted if needed by fundal pressure. Continue guiding the baby as it descends.

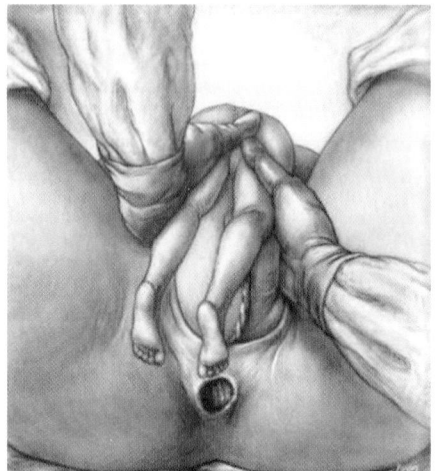 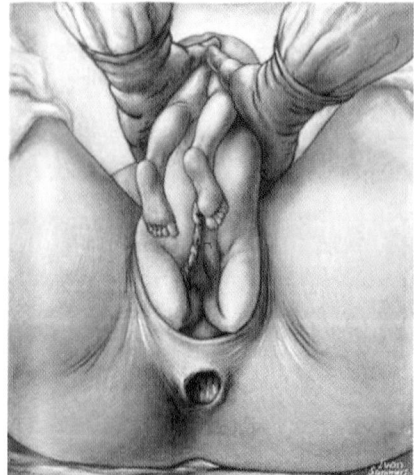 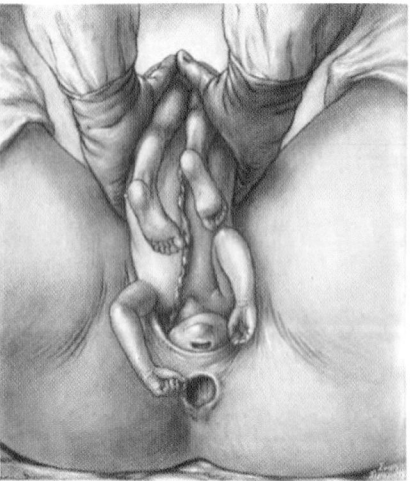

Look what happens when you turn the Bracht maneuver upside-down (or rather, right-side up!). During an upright birth, the baby does its own Bracht maneuver, thanks to gravity.

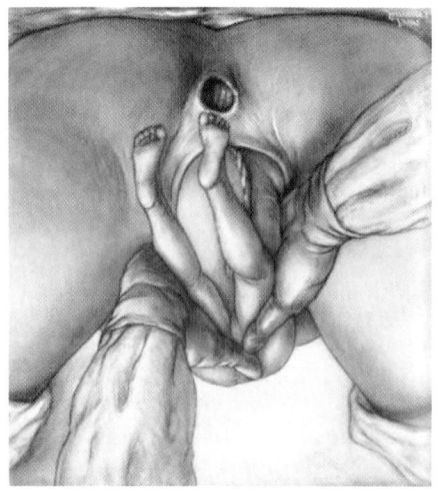 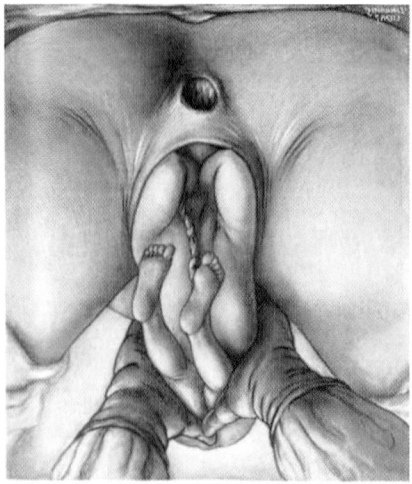 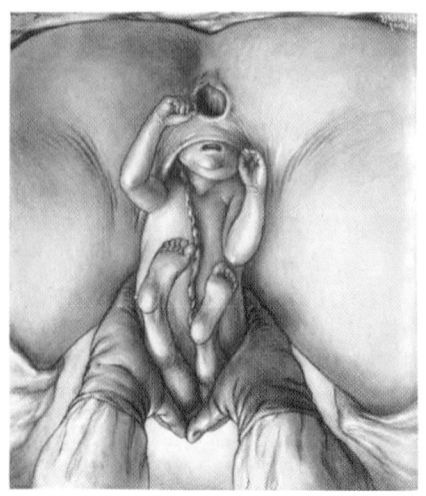

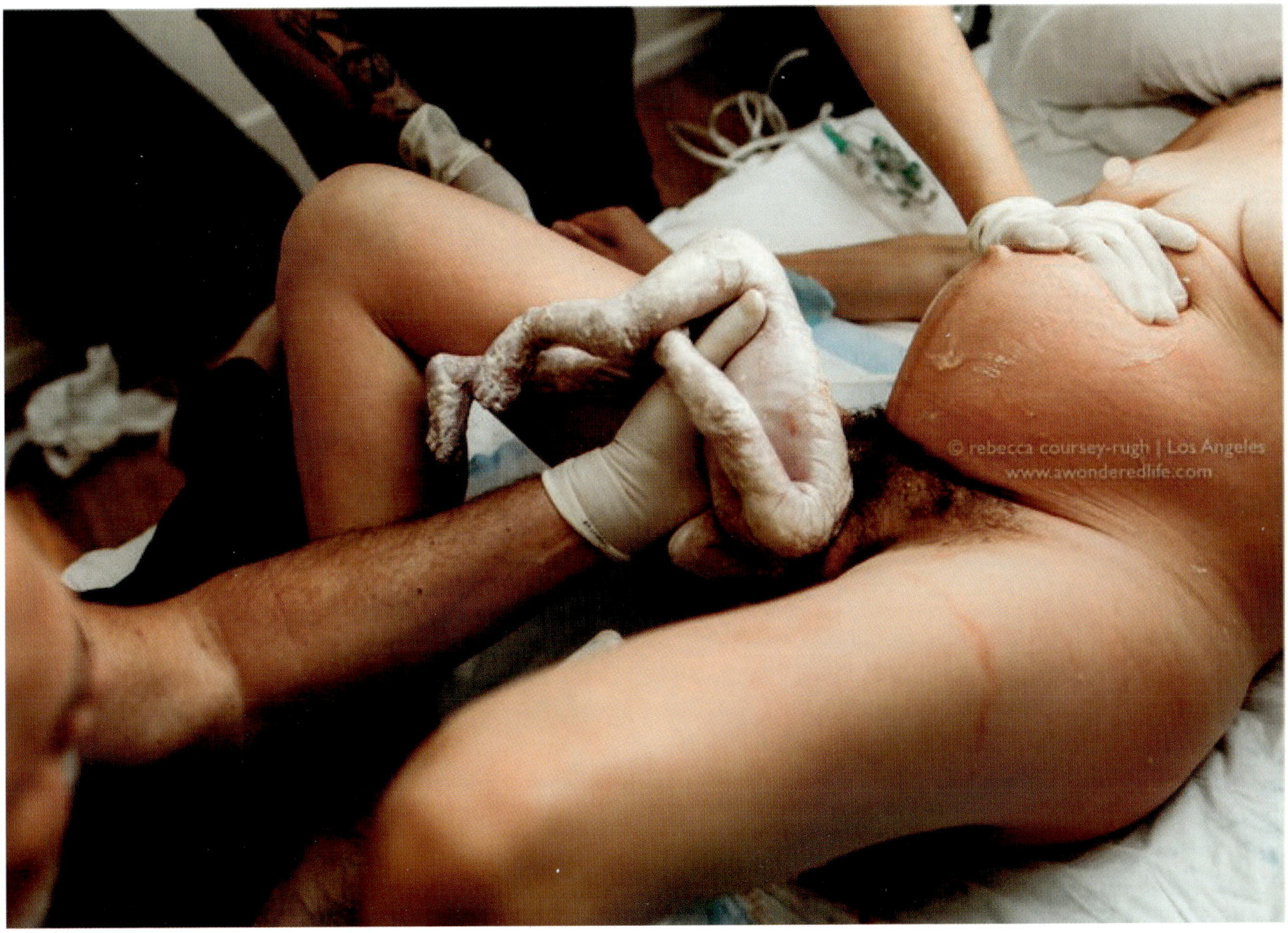

![Bracht maneuver photograph from Dr. Stuart Fischbein]

Above: This photo from Dr. Stuart Fischbein shows the Bracht maneuver. Note that an assistant is providing fundal pressure.

Right: Another picture of the Bracht maneuver. Note the baby's body staying splinted close to the maternal abdomen. The chin and mouth have passed the perineum.

Georgie Riley

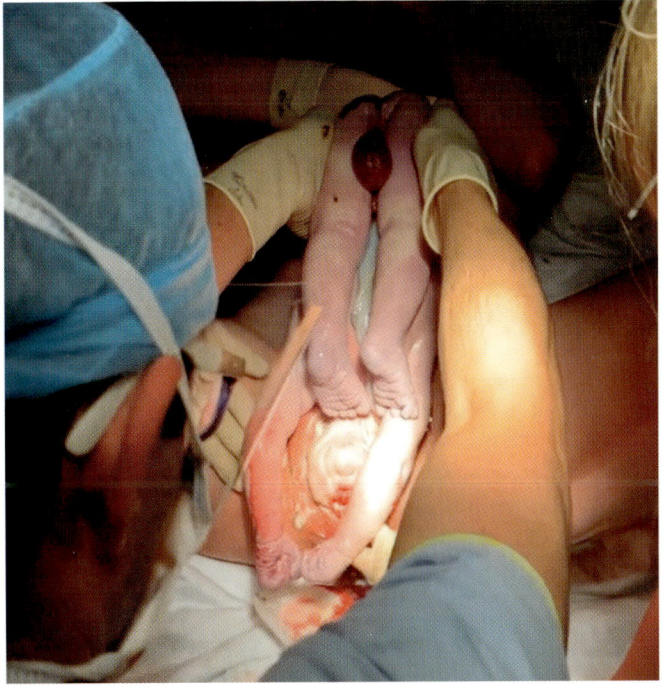

Pinard Maneuver

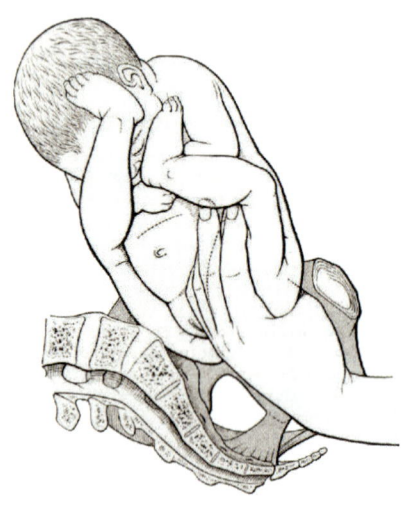

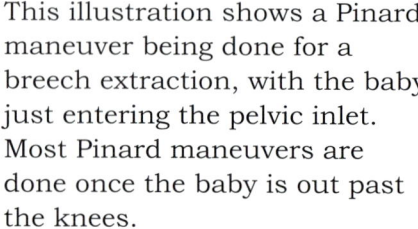

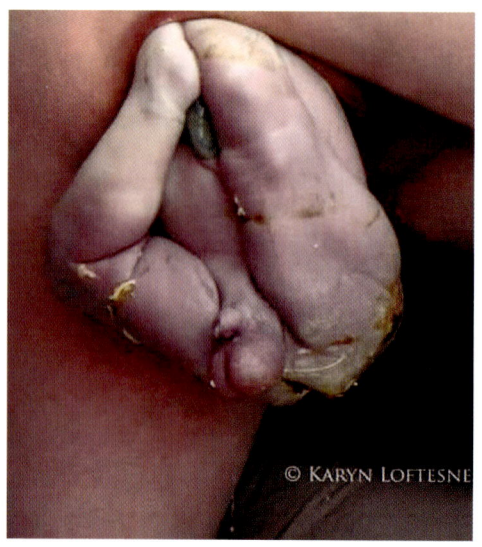

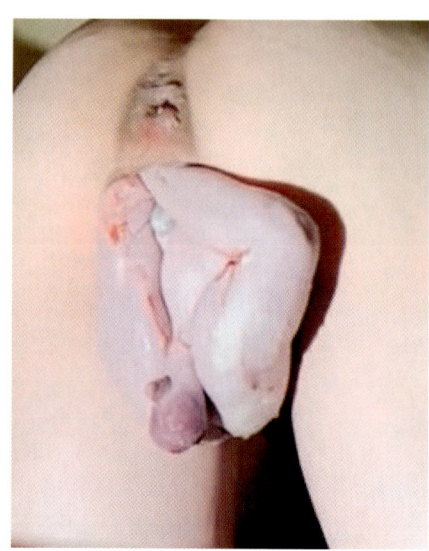

This illustration shows a Pinard maneuver being done for a breech extraction, with the baby just entering the pelvic inlet. Most Pinard maneuvers are done once the baby is out past the knees.

These babies are performing their own Pinard maneuvers! Note how they displace their knees sideways, which brings the foot into the midline and allows the foot to come down and out.

If you have a baby coming down that is frank breech and you want to do a breech extraction or expedite the birth with a maneuver and the legs are still in, you employ the Pinard maneuver. (Now that we know about fundal pressure, the Pinard maneuver is obsolete except for during full breech extractions.)

To do the Pinard maneuver, put your fingers behind the baby's knee in the popliteal fossa and push laterally (outward to the side). This bends the knee and brings the foot into the midline, where you can then sweep and deliver the foot. Then repeat on the other side.

Thoughts about the past and future of vaginal breech birth

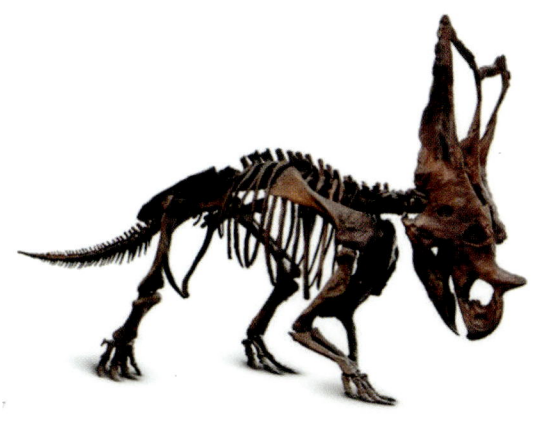

Let me share a few thoughts about the future of vaginal breech birth. Looking at how vaginal breech has been disappearing from obstetric and midwifery skill sets around the world, it can be easy to see the future of breech birth as bleak. In this future, breech birth has gone extinct. Certainly, that's one possible way of imagining the future—breech going the way of the dinosaurs.

And frankly, in most places, that is what has happened, and many people don't care otherwise. They're happy to let C-sections be the answer to breech. But maybe there's another way of looking at this near disappearance of vaginal breech birth.

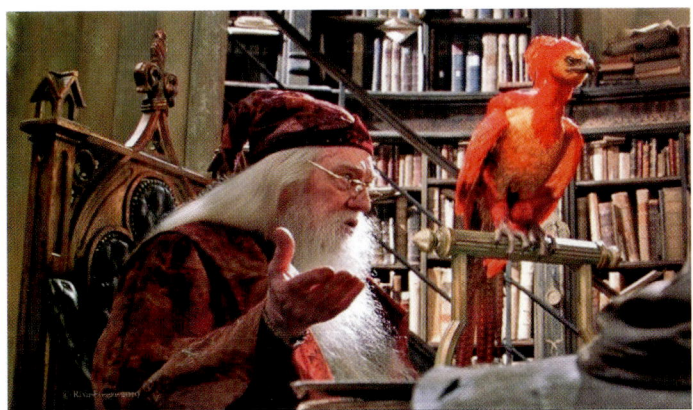

Maybe we can think of breech birth as a Phoenix rising from the ashes (as shown in this scene from *Harry Potter*). Yes, breech birth has almost entirely disappeared, but there is an opportunity for rebirth that might lead to something better.

Maybe it's a good thing. The supine, heavily medicalized and monitored births of old, using centuries-old invasive maneuvers, were not the best ways to birth breech babies. Maybe it's good that we let an entire generation of birth attendants forget how to do breech.

Perhaps this is the moment where we can reteach breech the way it should be done. We can teach breech in all its beautiful, chaotic glory where women are in a number of positions, where it's not so tightly controlled, where physiology guides the way that we do breech, and where physiological breech is the norm, not the outlier.

This is my hope. I hope that we can see this as an opportunity to move forward with excitement, with curiosity, with a desire to learn as much as we can, with a desire to be humble and to keep our skill sets alive, and with the optimism that at some point we can bring this skill back to life. Vaginal breech birth does not have to go the way of the dinosaurs.

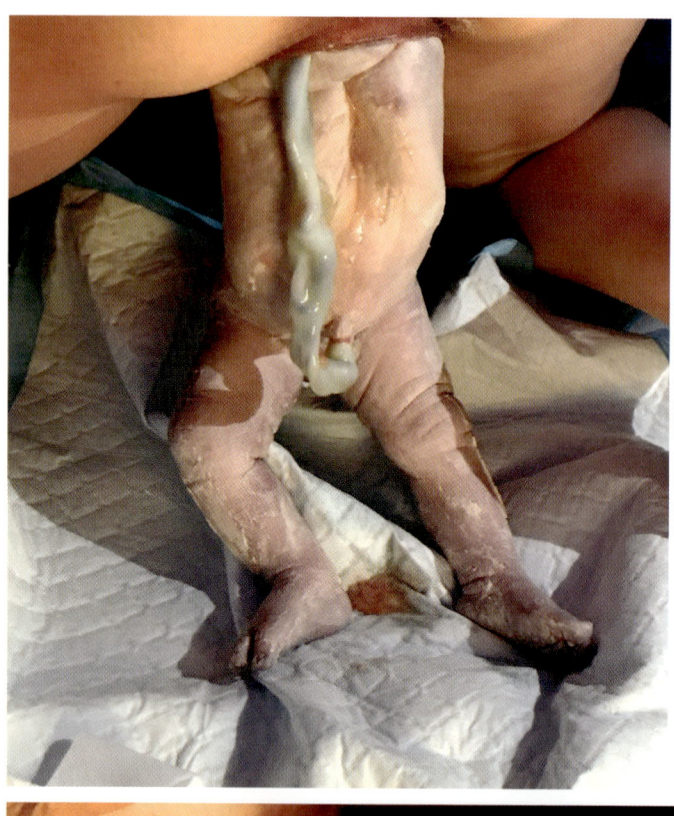
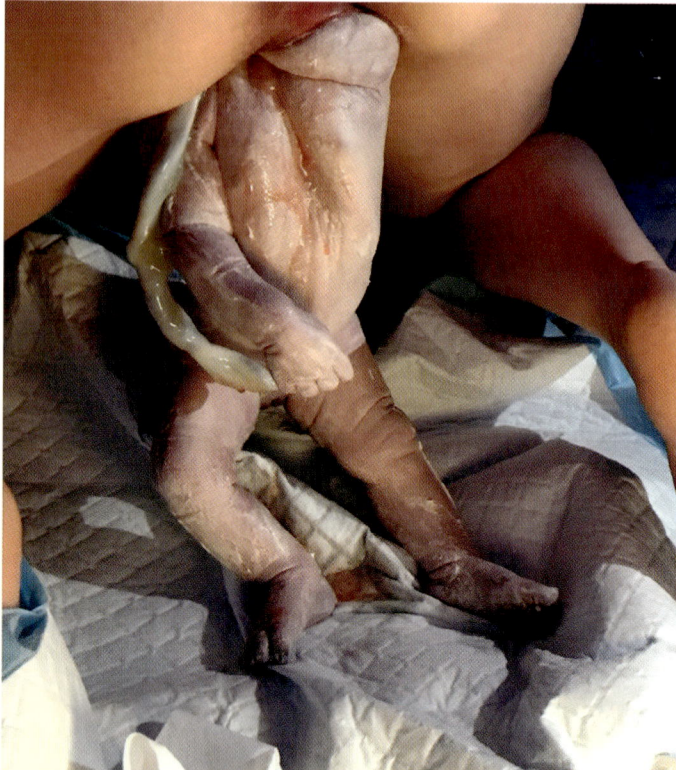
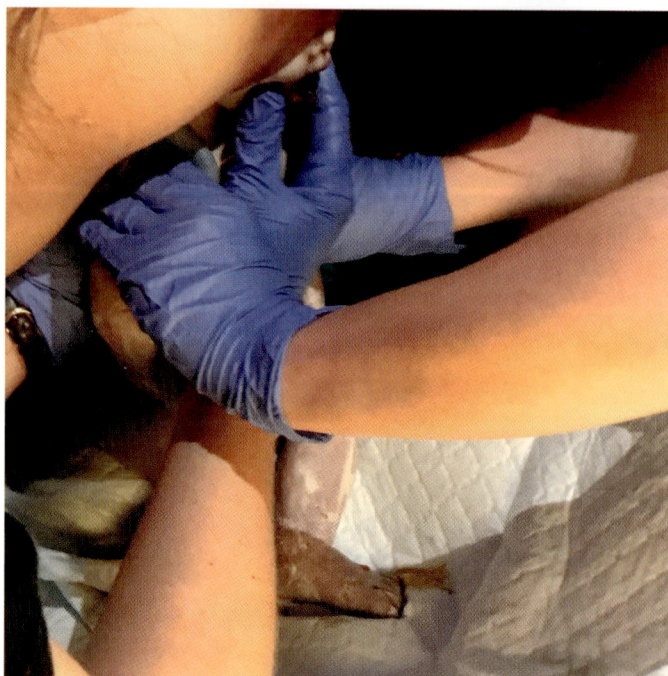
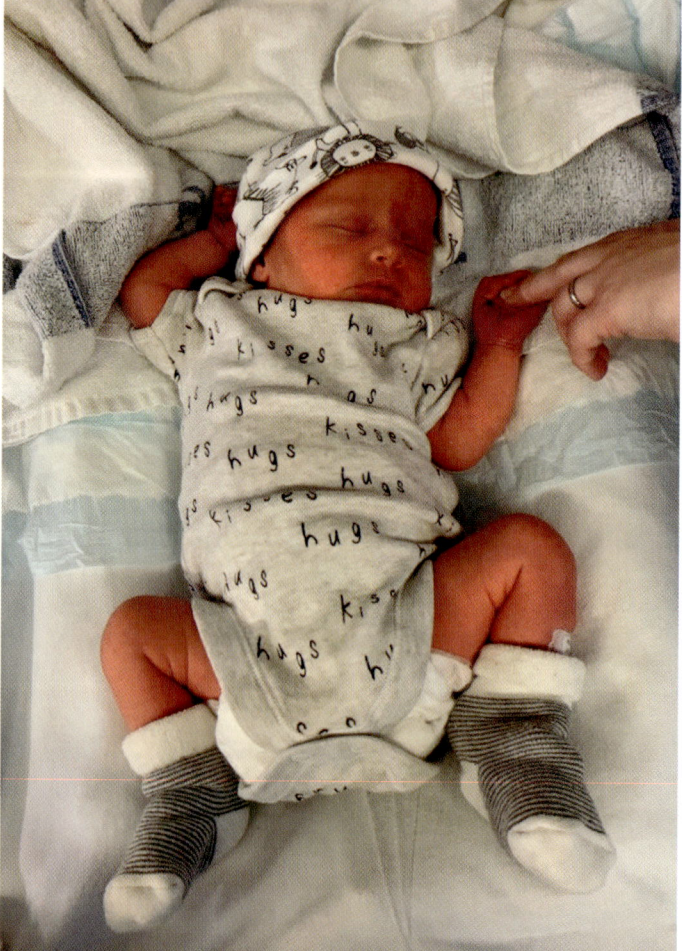

A breech birth assisted by a shoulder press
Angela Joanne Williams

Lesson 7: Nomenclature and the Risks of Various Types of Breech Presentations

By Rixa Freeze, PhD

Welcome to this lesson about breech nomenclature and the outcomes that are associated with different types of leg positions in a breech. Some parts of this lesson are very detailed. You are welcome to skim through those parts.

What is nomenclature? It means "how we name things," so I will be talking about how we name different breech presentations. By the end of this lesson, you should be convinced that it is important to properly name our breeches. It has a lot of significance for what is considered reasonably safe versus unreasonably dangerous.

We're going to start off with a few basic questions to review how you might classify and label breeches.

What is a frank breech?

A frank breech has both hips flexed and both knees fully extended, so the baby is basically folded in half. This is universally accepted in every nomenclature system.

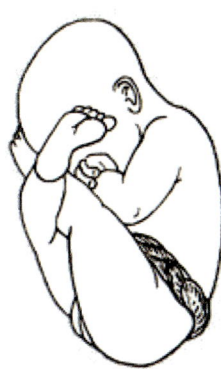

What is a complete breech?

A complete breech has both hips flexed and both knees flexed.

The feet can be above OR below the buttocks. Note that all 3 of the illustrations below, found on internet sites explaining breech presentation, show hips flexed and feet below the buttocks. All of these should be called complete breeches.

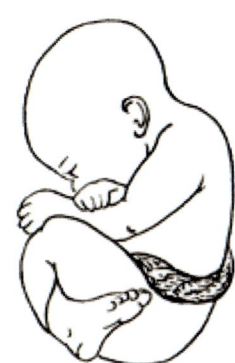

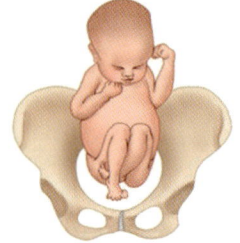 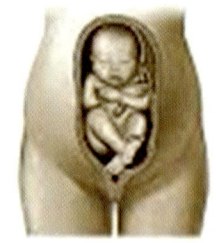 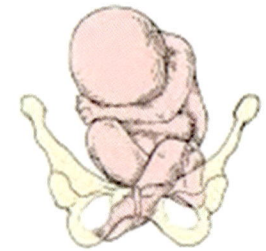

Image source unknown

Please note that many obstetric textbooks and maternity care providers mislabel some complete breeches as "footling" breeches, such as in these images above (source unknown). They see or feel a foot first and call it a footling. But that is **not** correct. The only time a breech is a footling is if one or both hips are fully extended in utero, and it is basically standing up in the uterus. We'll talk more about this later.

What is an incomplete breech?

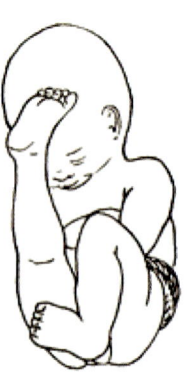

An incomplete breech is a half-frank, half-complete. One leg is fully extended up near the face (hip flexed, knee extended), whereas the other hip is also flexed, but the knee is flexed as well. This is the most common definition of an incomplete breech.

In the medical literature, "incomplete" is sometimes used as an identical term for a footling breech. And it's also as an umbrella term to mean not just a footling breech, but any footling or any kneeling breech. This becomes confusing, because you might have one article saying, "incomplete breech had this outcome" or "we did this with incomplete breech," and they might be meaning one of three different things!

As an example, here are things all labeled "incomplete" in various textbooks and websites. The circled illustration is the only correct one.

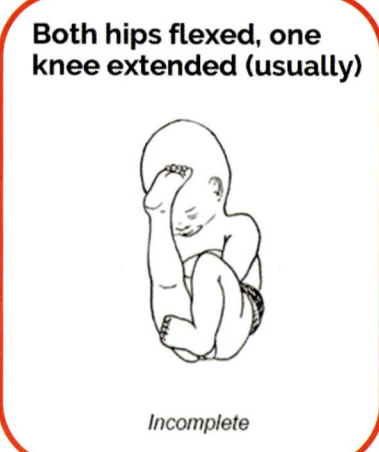

Both hips flexed, one knee extended (usually)

Incomplete

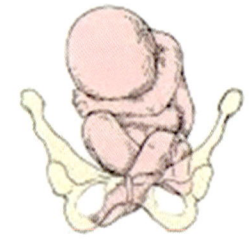

Another term for footling (sometimes)

Footling (incomplete) breech

Umbrella term for footling & kneeling (rarely)

Incomplete Breech (25%)

Footling Breech	Kneeling Breech
The baby's hip and knee joints extended on one or both sides.	The baby's hip joints are extended and knee joints are flexed on one or both sides.

What is a footling breech?

The correct definition of a footling breech is that one or both hips are fully extended, like in these illustrations. If you think of how big a full-term baby is, it is nearly impossible for it to be standing inside the uterus…which means what? It means that it's nearly impossible for a term baby to be a footling breech. Most true footlings are premature or perhaps second twins, where they have lots of room to stretch out after the first twin is born.

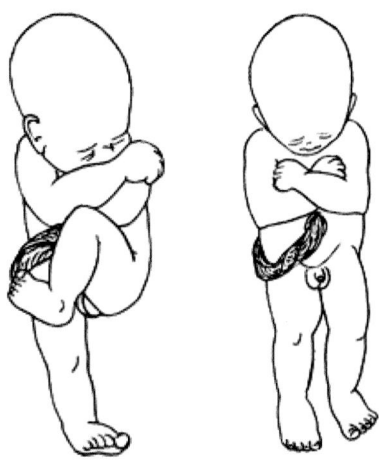

Here is a case of an exceptionally rare circumstance leading to a term baby being fully extended in utero with full hip and leg extension. This was written to me by an American Maternal Fetal Medicine specialist. He has seen this exactly once in his career. He describes what he saw:

> I had a patient recently whose baby was actually standing in the uterus. Legs extended, both feet in lower uterine segment (plus a lot of cord). I've certainly never seen that before, but it goes to show that anything is possible. This was a term baby. There was a 9 cm myoma in the lower uterine segment. The baby's body was in the fundus above the myoma, and the legs were dangling past the myoma and the feet were over the cervix. This fetal presentation probably had a lot to do with the myoma being there.

What is a kneeling breech?

A kneeling breech is where one or both knees are presenting with one or both hips fully extended. It's fairly difficult for a term baby to be kneeling. This presentation is more typical of a preterm baby. The knees are the presenting part, rather than the feet or buttocks.

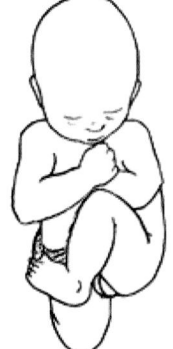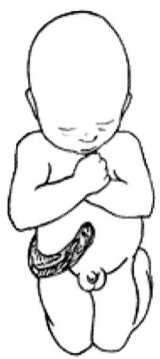

How do different countries name their breeches?

Francophone nomenclature

2 main categories in term breech literature:
- **frank** (*siège décomplété*)
- **nonfrank** (*siège complet*)

Divergence over whether *siège complet* should be translated as "complete" (PREMODA) or "nonfrank" (most other studies)

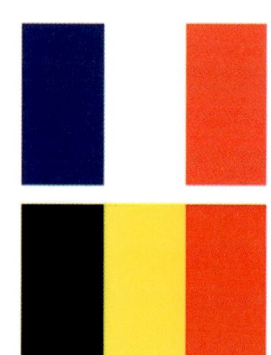

In France and other francophone countries—for a term breech specifically—there are basically two categories for breeches: frank (*siège décomplété*) and nonfrank (*siege complet*). French nomenclature runs into issues when it gets translated into English. Most studies translate *siège complet* as "nonfrank breech." However, the literal translation is "complete breech" and some studies have adopted that translation. This leads to confusion because in English, "complete breech" has a very different meaning than it does in French. This has led some studies and guidelines to mistakenly restrict incomplete and dropped foot breeches (often mislabeled as footlings) from vaginal breech birth.

Anglophone nomenclature

3-4 categories:
- frank
- complete
- footling
- incomplete

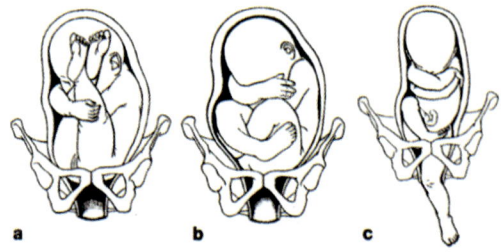

English-speaking countries typically have three or four categories of breeches: frank, complete, and footling are the most common, and sometimes incomplete is considered its own category. Sometimes incompletes are lumped in together with completes. And occasionally incompletes get lumped together with footling, which is even more confusing.

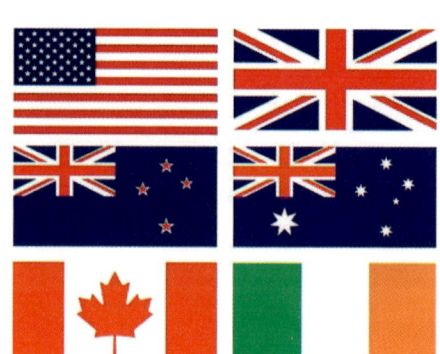

German nomenclature

German-speaking countries typically have very detailed and precise nomenclature systems, up to as many as seven different names for breeches. So, for example, this illustration below would be common in German literature. There are frank, complete, and incomplete breeches (these are all breech presentations with hip *flexion*). Then there are double and single footlings, which are considered different from each other, and even double and single kneelings, which are also considered different from footlings. Footling and kneeling breeches have hip *extension*.

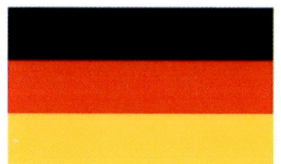

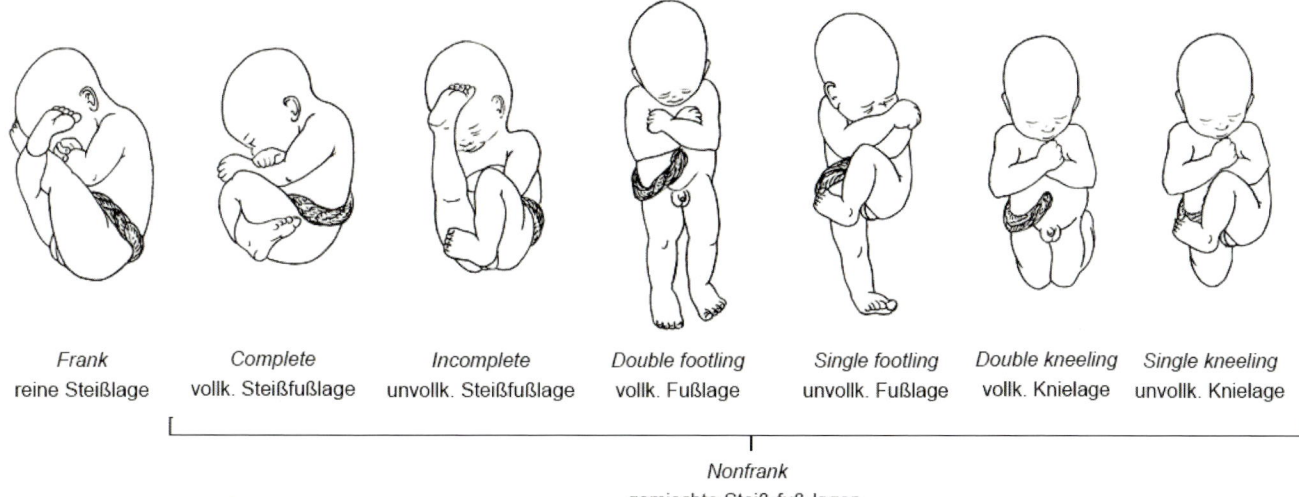

| *Frank* | *Complete* | *Incomplete* | *Double footling* | *Single footling* | *Double kneeling* | *Single kneeling* |
| reine Steißlage | vollk. Steißfußlage | unvollk. Steißfußlage | vollk. Fußlage | unvollk. Fußlage | vollk. Knielage | unvollk. Knielage |

Nonfrank
gemischte Steiß-fuß-lagen

The battle over complete vs. footling

Remember how I said that some places mislabel complete breeches and call them footlings? Let me give you one example.

TBT
"[C]omplete breech was defined as hips flexed, knees flexed, but feet not below the fetal buttocks."

SOGC
"A fetus with feet presenting but flexed hips and knees is a complete breech, therefore eligible for a TOL."

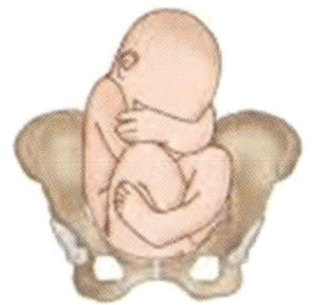

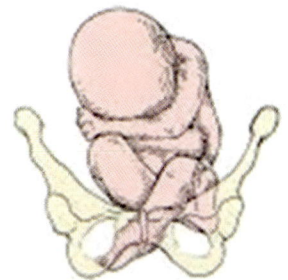

The Term Breech Trial, a study that randomly assigned 2,000 women to either vaginal birth or C-section, defined it this way: "complete breech was defined as hips flexed, knees flexed, but feet not below the fetal buttocks." Any baby that had feet below the buttocks, even if the hips & knees were flexed, was labeled "footling" and excluded from the study. On the other hand, the SOGC (the Society of Obstetricians and Gynecologists of Canada) defines it differently: "a fetus with feet presenting but flexed hips and knees is a complete breech, therefore eligible for a trial of labor."

The SOGC based their guidelines primarily on a large study from France and Belgium, called the PREMODA study. I wrote to one of the PREMODA study authors, Dr. Sophie Alexander, who I had met at a breech conference. I'm paraphrasing my questions, but I'm quoting her replies back in full.

I wrote to her about this issue. I said, "I noticed in the PREMODA study that it only listed two types of breeches possible: there were 'frank' and 'complete' and then 'unspecified' (obviously, if the medical records didn't say what type it was). But otherwise, you have two types of breeches listed as possibilities."

I then asked, "Does this mean that what we would call a footling was not included in the study, that it was excluded and sifted out? Or does this mean that 'complete' means 'nonfrank breech,' like 'anything but a frank breech'?"

She wrote back, "French and Belgian tradition accept both frank (*décomplété fesses*) and full (*complet*), NOT FOOTLING... Having said that, footling in term pregnancy is EXCEPTIONAL in my experience."

I replied, "OK, so what happened to footling breeches in the PREMODA study? If they are not accepted for planned vaginal breech birth, but they're not even listed in the PREMODA study, what's going on?"

First, she replied, "I will ask my colleagues."

Then she wrote something really fascinating. She went on to explain what she means and how they define complete versus footling breech:

> What we are taught and what we teach is that if, when you examine a lady, you feel a foot first, and it is a term baby, check with an ultrasound because mostly it will be a **complete with a foot dangling**. The idea being that the risk of the footling is that it will start descending before full dilation and get stuck, which does not happen with a complete, and only very late in the dilation (8-9 cm) with a frank. Also, we are taught, and teach, and believe that there is no way unless the lady is a giant, that a 50 cm baby can stand straight in a womb? (emphasis mine)

That made me laugh because, yes, if you think about it, there is not space in the uterus for most term babies to be fully stretched out and standing up. A term baby is going to be scrunched up, and the legs are going to be folded.

Dangling and dropped feet

We're going to talk more about this concept of a "foot dangling."

The other place I came across this concept was from a Norwegian article written in 1994 by Susanne Albrechtsen. A Norwegian obstetric colleague volunteered to translate this short article for me. Let me read you the passage that caught my attention.

> The type of breech is evaluated once labor has commenced and needs to be reevaluated later in labor as the presentation may change during the course of labor. For instance, type B and C, (as you can see here illustrated at the top), can change to type A (frank), type D (double footling), or type E (single footling). These latter two scenarios [where type B and C turn into type E or D] are called **dropped foot**. (emphasis mine)

I had never heard the phrase "dropped foot" (*fremfall av fot*) before. I wrote back to her and said, "Could you explain a little more what this 'dropped foot' thing means?"

Her reply was as follows:

> A dropped foot is when the foot drops at full dilation. But it is itself not a true foot presentation until that point and should not be perceived as one. A presenting foot is not a challenge at a point where the cervix is fully effaced over the buttock. Standing breeches are a nightmare because you have the risk of head entrapment (I had two cases with extreme prematurity in Norway and one term case in Pakistan), whereas the foot dropping in labor is no issue. (personal correspondence with Tilde Østborg, 2017)

This idea of a dropped foot this intrigued me. I wondered what I would find if I started searching through the medical literature. I wasn't looking for the term "dropped foot breech," which, until I had it translated, had never been used in English before.

A treasure hunt for dropped feet

I read through the full text of all single-center studies on term breech outcomes from 1980 to the present in PubMed. There were a lot to sift through. I read through everything in English and French and several articles in German and Spanish. I have not had all of those translated from German and Spanish, however. But I would say that I did a reasonably comprehensive review of the term breech literature.

Interestingly, I found at least 13 original research articles that describe this thing happening. Now again, they don't have a word for it, and sometimes they think that they had misdiagnosed a footling breech or missed it entirely. But when you read the circumstances of what is happening, I think you're going to be convinced that what they're describing is a dropped foot breech.

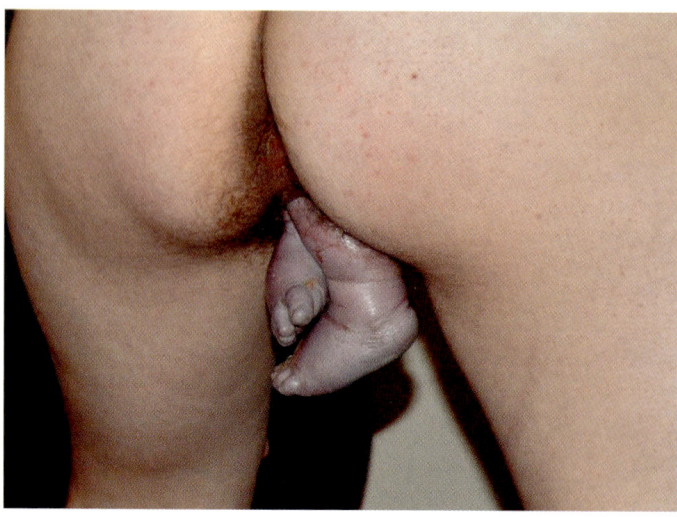 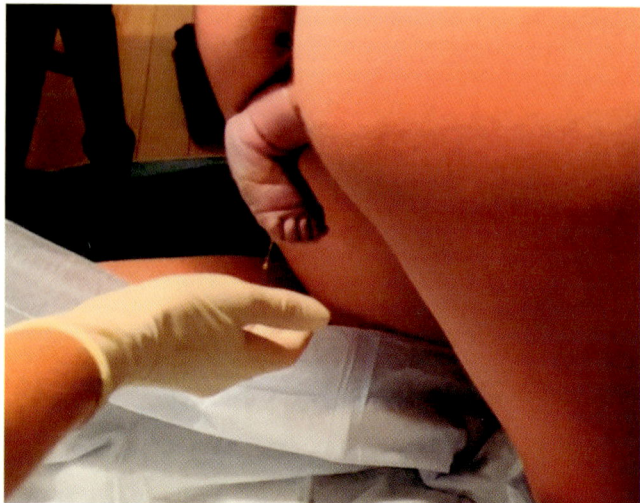

I will now discuss articles mentioning a dropped foot breech. Some describe it as missing or misdiagnosing a footling breech. This is from Bassaw 2004: "In several cases, the footling breech presentation was diagnosed first in the second stage of labor." Notice: the first time they spotted the footling was when pushing began, which means the cervix was fully open. An open cervix means that there is room for one or both feet to fall down, which is probably why they didn't diagnose a footling before that point.

Pay attention to this next statement from Schiff 1996: "Nineteen fetuses (6%), however, were delivered vaginally with footling presentation because of misdiagnosis during labor." Again, I suspect that they weren't really misdiagnosed; they probably did not drop a foot until later on in labor.

Other studies actually recognize this as a phenomenon—that the foot may drop down and that the presentation may change during labor. An article by Krause in 1997 cited 22 cases of this happening: "In 64.7% of all unplanned c-sections, the fetus began labor in an incomplete/complete breech position and converted into single/double footling breech during labor, which resulted in the move to caesarean section. The earliest possible moment of diagnostic evaluation was the complete opening of the cervix with ruptured membranes."

Note that **almost 2/3 of all the unplanned C-sections** were for this reason. Later in the article, the authors stated that they could perhaps have allowed women to keep on laboring when the "footling" was discovered. But since their policy was C-section for footlings, they went to surgery. Again, in France and Norway, this is seen as a non-issue and would not be a reason for an automatic C-section.

Which nomenclature system should you use?

With this information, let me propose a nomenclature system that I think will eliminate some of this confusion about how to label a breech. We have adopted the German way of using 7 different names. However, I think that the French nomenclature system, where you just label a term breech either frank or nonfrank, is equally reasonable. But with all the confusion we have, especially in our English-speaking world and with our intense fear of footling breeches, I don't think we're quite ready for that yet.

Breech Nomenclature

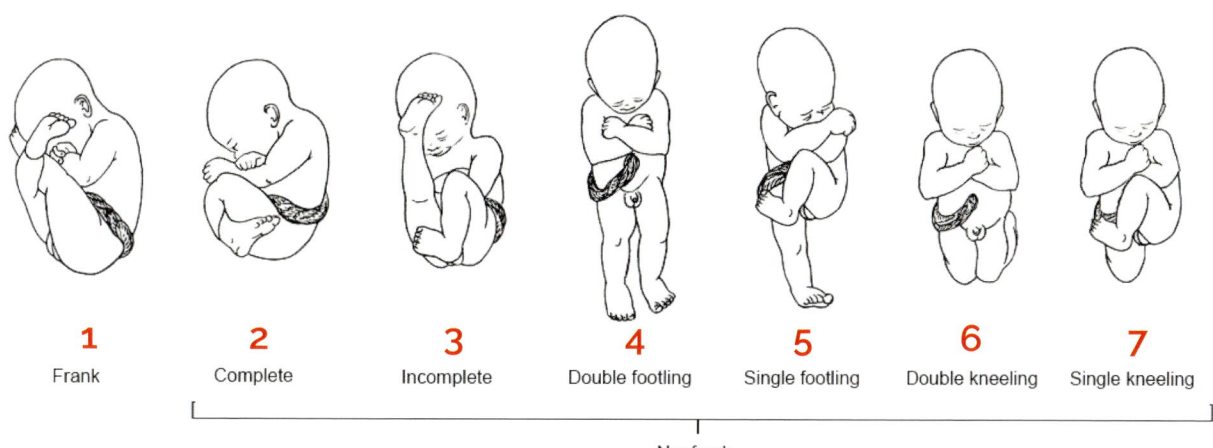

Hip flexion	Category	Type	Name	Description
Hips flexed	Frank	1	Frank	Hips flexed Knees extended
	Nonfrank	2	Complete	Hips flexed, both knees flexed. **Feet/foot may be above OR below the buttocks.**
		2+ or 2++	*(dropped foot)*	*As above; one or both feet drop down near full dilation.*
		3	Incomplete	Hips flexed, one knee extended, one knee flexed. **Foot may be above OR below buttocks.**
		3+	*(dropped foot)*	*As above; one foot drops down near full dilation*
Hips extended (usually premature)	Standing	4	Double footling	Both hips extended Both knees extended
		5	Single footling	One hip and knee extended Other hip flexed (knee flexed or extended)
		6	Double kneeling	Both hips extended Both knees flexed
		7	Single kneeling	One hip extended and knee flexed Other hip flexed (knee flexed or extended)

Our nomenclature system diagnoses breech not by the presenting part, but by **hip flexion and knee flexion**. The key question is: are the hips flexed or not? If the hips are flexed, then you're going to have a frank, a complete, or an incomplete. If the hips are extended, it will be either footling or kneeling, and the general term for those are "standing breeches" to remind us that the baby is truly standing in utero.

You could have the feet below or above the buttocks—it doesn't matter. But if the hips and knees are flexed, it is a complete breech. This nomenclature system also recognizes that true hip extension (persisting before labor, not just at the end of labor when the cervix opens up) is strongly associated with prematurity.

What if you don't have ultrasound to look at hip flexion?
It's very difficult, if not almost impossible, for a term breech baby to truly have hip extension in utero. If you don't have access to ultrasound, you can assume that a term baby will have its hips flexed.

Why do we have numbers associated with each type of breech?
Unlike words, you can't really mistranslate numbers! This ensures that, no matter which language we are speaking or translating into, we can be sure we're talking about the same thing. We would say, for example, "This was a frank breech, type 1."

What about dropped foot breeches?
This nomenclature system lets you indicate if you had a dropped foot. If you had, for example, an incomplete breech, which is type 3, and one foot dropped down during labor, then you would label it a 3+. If you had a complete with two feet dropping during labor, it would be a 2++.

Do footlings deserve their bad reputation?

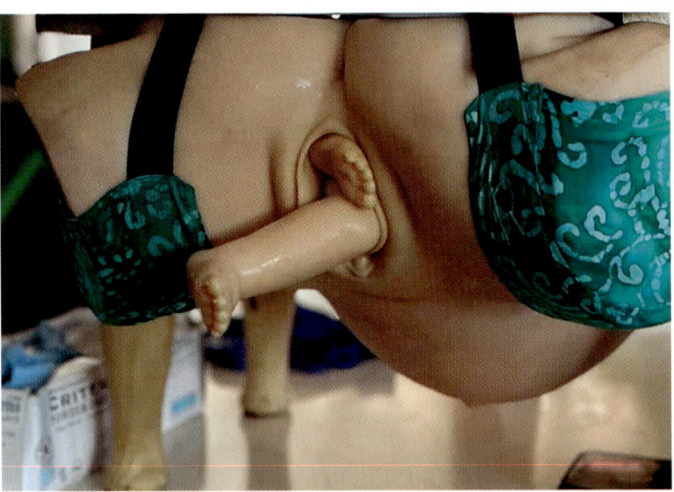

Let's now turn to what I find to be a fascinating question: Do footling breeches at term—not pre-term footlings, which is a different issue—deserve their bad reputations?

This is a surprisingly hard question to answer. I thought it would be quite easy because in the medical literature, one of the universally accepted truths is forbidding footling breeches from vaginal birth. I thought, "OK, this is a point of near consensus. Of anything in the breech literature, it's the one that almost everybody agrees on without question. So surely there must be very strong, compelling evidence for this."

That's where I started. I was shocked at how little evidence I could find for this recommendation. I started tracking the references, and then I would find the references that the first references mentioned, and on and on. I kept going backwards until I could go no further.

Think of it like digging underneath the foundation of your house. First you are at ground level, and you can't see much of your foundation. You would expect to find a solid foundation the deeper down you dig. What I found, metaphorically, is that the deeper I dug and the farther back I went in the literature, the sources got scarcer, not stronger. I realized that they would cite somebody, who would cite somebody, who at some point, maybe 5 or 6 decades ago, made a recommendation based on a study from the 1930s or the 1940s or based on general opinion. But the deeper I dug, the more I realized that there was no foundation at all.

(I had this situation happen in my garage, where one of the load-bearing walls ended up without a foundation underneath it. When we bought the house, we wondered why the garage roof was sagging…after some digging, we discovered why! If you know anything about construction, you can't leave this kind of situation alone and hope it will get better. You have to pour a new foundation to make things stable and well-supported. That is what we at Breech Without Borders are trying to do.)

Why the fear of footlings?

1. Umbilical cord prolapse

2. Head entrapment (cervical/pelvic)

3. Mechanically less efficient

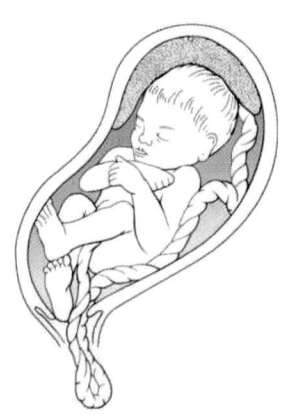 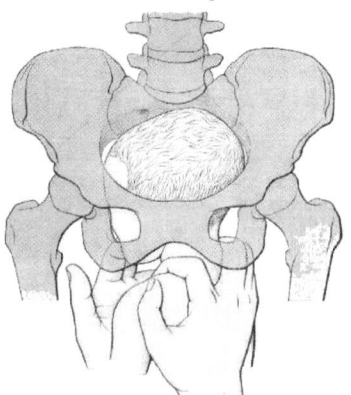 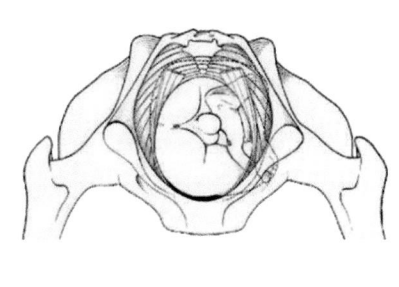

What are the reasons for not allowing a footling breech to be born vaginally, according to the medical literature? One reason is umbilical cord prolapse. Another reason is the fear of head entrapment, which is a nebulous fear because there are several kinds of head entrapment. A head can get trapped in a cervix, and that's certainly a fear and something that happens on occasion with extremely premature babies. Heads can also get trapped in the maternal pelvis, but that is not an issue with the cervix. That's due to a deflexed head not fitting properly through the bony structure of the pelvis. To add to the confusion, sometimes the literature labels a nuchal or trapped arm as a "head entrapment"—no wonder people get confused! A third reason is the belief that a footling breech is difficult to give birth to and that it's less efficient mechanically. We'll explore these three ideas and examine the evidence for all of them.

How common is a footling breech at term?

As we discussed in an earlier lesson, footling breeches are labeled inconsistently. With that in mind, studies will provide widely varying numbers as to how common footling is at term. In several recent term breech studies that I examined, the frequency ranges anywhere from 3% to over 11%. Some German textbooks state that footling breech occurs as much as 30% of the time, although they didn't specify if this meant all breeches, including preterm, or just term. And as we know in France, the term footling is often not used at all in their term studies. They just label it either frank or nonfrank breech.

Is this wide variation in the reported rate of footling breech at term due to the natural variation of babies? Or is it due to the different way these countries name their breeches? I definitely suspect that it's due to the latter reason: we're naming them differently.

1. Cord prolapse: how common and how dangerous is it?

Let's get back to the question of cord prolapse. Certainly, there is some association between footling breech and a higher rate of cord prolapse. This study by Kouam in 1980 in Germany is interesting. I had this translated with the help of a German colleague. This is the only study of its type that I have ever found. The researchers looked at all cord prolapses in their institution over a 12-year time span for both cephalic and breech babies, then classified the results by *type* of breech presentation.

Cord prolapse relative to presentation for infants > 2500 g (Kouam 1980)

Fetal presentation	%	# of births	# of cord prolapses	Rate of UCP (%)
Cephalic	96.9	19151	10	0.05
Breech	3.1	608	21	3.5
Frank breech	72.9	443	3	0.7
Nonfrank breech	27.1	165	18	10.9
- Complete	9.4	57	5	8.8
- Incomplete	7.6	46	5	10.9
- Double footling	10.0	61	5	8.2
- Single footling	1.2	7	-	0
- Kneeling	0.7	4	3	75
Total		**19759**	**31**	**0.16**

Looking at their term babies (> 2500 g), they found that, as we would expect, cephalic cord prolapse was relatively uncommon (0.05%). Cord prolapse was a little more common in breech overall. If you look at frank versus nonfrank breech, you'll see that frank breech cord prolapse was 0.7%, which was a bit more common than cephalic, but still relatively rare. Whereas for nonfrank breeches, it was 10.9% overall.

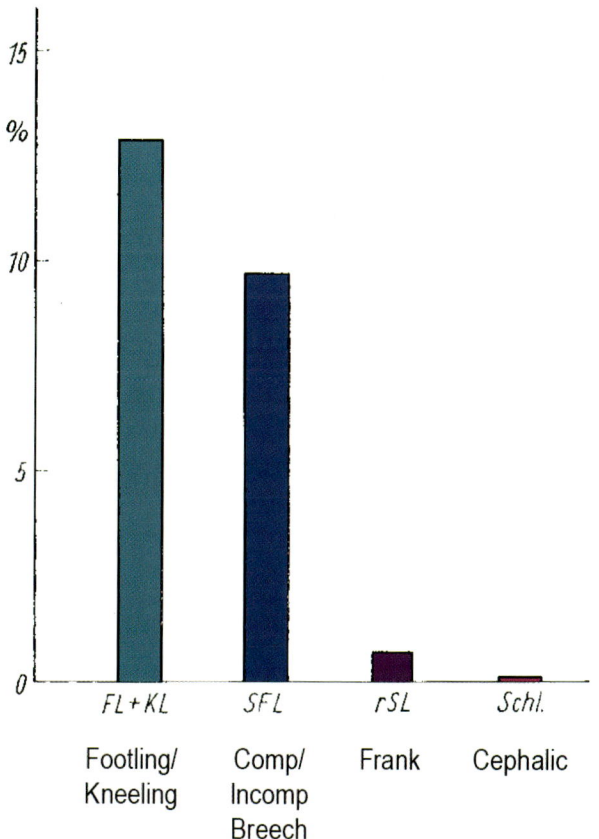

Frequency of umbilical cord prolapse,
birth weight ≥ 2500 g (n = 19,924)

When the researchers analyzed the cord prolapse rates according to type of breech, the footlings and kneelings together had rates around 13% and the completes and incompletes had rates around 9%. There were no cord prolapses in the very small number of single footlings, while 3 of the 4 kneelings had cord prolapses. But remember, we are dealing with very small numbers at this point.

In contrast, frank breech cord prolapse was much less common in this institution. With a pre-labor rupture of membranes, a cord prolapse was more likely to happen compared to a timely rupture (either spontaneous or AROM during labor).

Now here is something really interesting. The researchers tracked both Apgar scores and mortality rates after cord prolapse. They found that for frank breech and cephalic cord prolapse, the longer it took to get the baby born, the worse the Apgar scores became. There was a direct linear relationship between the diagnosis-delivery time interval and the Apgar scores. And that's exactly what probably all of us would have anticipated.

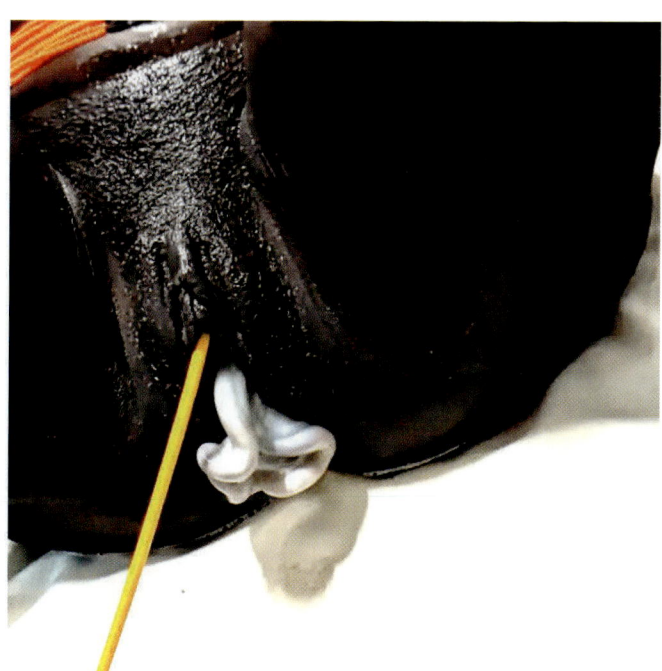

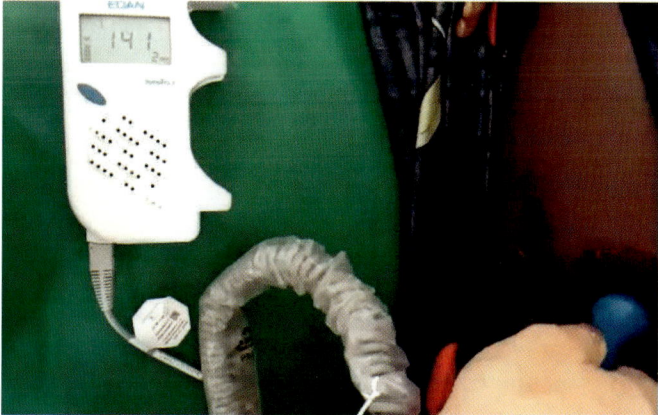

Left: Overt cord prolapse at 28 weeks gestation, nonfrank breech, primip.

Right: Heart tones remained stable throughout 17 hours of labor with cord prolapse, ending in a vaginal birth (low-resource setting).

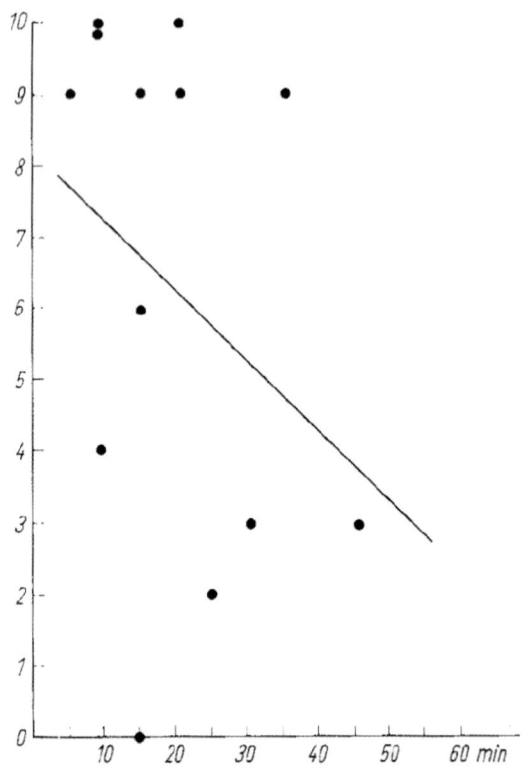

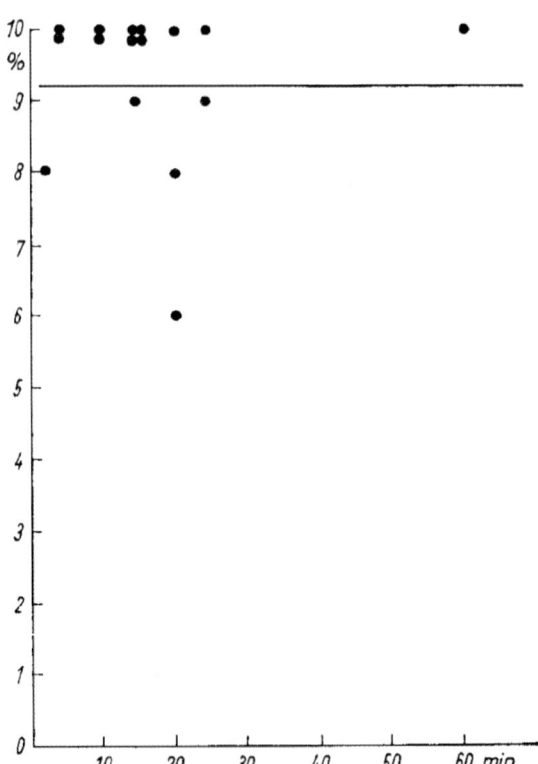

Frank breech Apgar scores depending on time to delivery: **downward slope** shows that Apgar scores get worse the more time elapses (max 45 interval from diagnosis to delivery)

Nonfrank breech Apgar scores depending on time to delivery: **horizontal line** shows that Apgar scores do not worsen with time (max 60 min interval from diagnosis to delivery)

Here is something really interesting: among the nonfrank breeches with cord prolapse, no matter how long the diagnosis-to-delivery interval was, the Apgar scores did not get any worse. (Note that the longest diagnosis-to-delivery interval was 60 minutes—they were not waiting hours after a cord prolapse.) However, Apgar scores were not time-dependent for nonfrank breech babies. But for frank or cephalic babies with cord prolapse, the Apgar scores very much depended on how long it took to get the babies delivered.

Nonfrank cord prolapse (Kouam 1980): More common but less dangerous

Mortality rate after cord prolapse
- cephalic: 30% (3/10)
- frank breech: 33% (1/3)
- nonfrank breech: 0% (0/18)

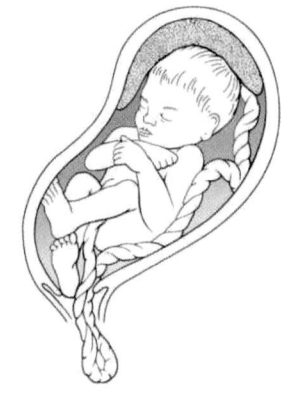

Even though the nonfrank breeches had, relatively speaking, a lot of cord prolapses, the babies did well. The Apgar scores were not time-dependent, and none of the nonfrank breeches died after cord prolapse, compared to around 1/3 the frank and cephalic babies who had cord prolapses.

The authors of this study conclude that that the risk of cord prolapse is not the same with all breeches. It depends on the type of breech. Recent data coming from France reports a cord prolapse rate of 5-6% for nonfrank breeches, which is lower than what this German clinic found. Overall, we can anticipate the rate of nonfrank cord prolapse will likely be around 6% and less than 1% for frank breeches.

Counseling points for cord prolapse

Type of breech presentation matters:
- Women with a **frank breech** should be counseled that cord prolapse is uncommon but very dangerous if it happens. The baby should be delivered immediately.
- Women with a **nonfrank breech** should be counseled that cord prolapse is relatively common but less dangerous. Labor should be closely monitored and birth should be timely—vaginally or by C-section, depending on individual circumstances.

For example, if a primip has a cord prolapse with a nonfrank breech at 4 cm, that situation would most likely end in a C-section—but a calm, un-rushed one. (In overseas locations without easy access to C-sections, this situation might very well end in a vaginal birth, especially if the baby's heart rate remains stable.) There is usually time, especially if you keep a close eye on the heart rate. In contrast, if a multip has a cord prolapse and she is already feeling pushy, it might very well be the best choice to have a vaginal birth, especially if the heart rate doesn't seem to be affected by the prolapse.

Why is cord prolapse different with nonfrank breeches?

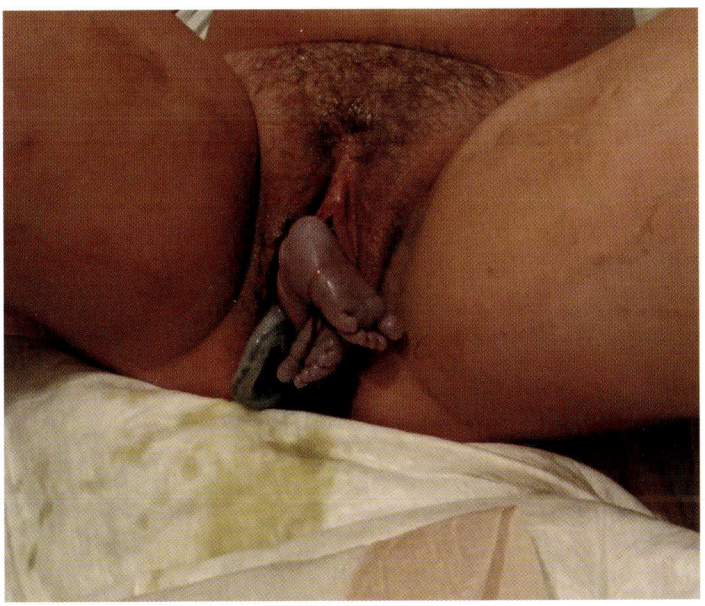

The difference in outcomes with nonfrank breeches is due to the looser fit in the lower uterine segment. A nonfrank breech has these large bent legs and large pockets of space creating room for the cord to be cushioned and protected. In contrast, a frank breech has a uniform surface all the way around. It's nearly the same as a head in that it makes a nice tight plug in the pelvis. If the cord prolapses with a frank breech, it's similar to prolapsing against a hard head; there's a higher chance for cord compression that can compromise the baby.

2. Head entrapment

Now let's talk about the second justification for being afraid of a footling breech: the fear of head entrapment. I had mentioned we have this issue with head entrapment being a couple of different things: cervical, pelvic, or even a trapped arm that gets labeled as a head entrapment.

Let's talk first about cervical head entrapment, because that's really what people are afraid of. People worry that in a footling breech, the legs and torso will slip through a partially dilated cervix, and then the cervix will clamp around the head and not allow the head to pass. This is certainly a fear that is well-founded if you have an extremely premature baby, or if you have a baby with asymmetric growth restriction, because the torso is much smaller than the head.

But is this the case in a healthy term baby? It is very difficult to answer this question because almost no research exists on this topic over the past several decades. In addition, we have already discussed how many footling breeches are mislabeled and are actually complete breeches.

From what I have found by looking through thousands of articles, cervical head entrapment in a normally developed term baby is extremely rare. It does not seem a good reason to forbid women with feet-presenting fetuses from trying to have a vaginal breech birth.

One midwife we work with, who has attended around 600 VBBs in mostly Amish communities, has only encountered cervical head entrapment twice at term. Both times happened when the mother began pushing violently and forcefully before her body was telling her to push. The mother just *wanted* to push. This caused the body to come down far before the cervix was ready.

What can we learn from this? Women should listen to their bodies and never force pushing, and birth attendants should ensure they are not encouraging women to push too early. When a woman's body is ready, it will begin pushing all on its own.

To illustrate, let's turn to France, where they don't really call term breeches footling and where they usually accept any kind of breech for vaginal breech birth. I read a study authored by Dr. Sonia Adjaoud in 2017. She analyzed outcomes of all term babies born at their hospital, both cephalic and breech. They found that when they compared planned vaginal breech birth to planned C-section to planned cephalic births, there were no increased risks for poor outcomes.

I wrote to Dr. Adjaoud and asked which types of breeches they accepted for a planned vaginal breech birth. Did it matter if it was a footling versus a complete versus a frank? She wrote back to me:

> In our study, we selected breeches without distinguishing between frank and nonfrank breech since in our hospital, the type of presentation does not affect the prognosis of the likelihood of success of a planned vaginal breech birth, nor of neonatal morbidity

and mortality. For us, we are a school with a strong tradition of vaginal breech birth that has always taught its students the techniques of vaginal breech birth. Our training in this type of delivery and a good knowledge of the mechanics leave us less afraid when we face this situation. In our practice, nonfrank breeches—whatever their nature (1 foot, 2 feet, standing)—can be born vaginally as long as they are engaged and as long as the fetal heart tones are normal (CTG is, obviously, continuous). During the expulsive efforts, either the two feet are born spontaneously, or one foot is born first. In the latter case, we do a small extraction [Pinard] by manually bringing down the second foot. Then we continue the birth with the other normal maneuvers.

(In France, the most common maneuvers are Løvset followed by Mauriceau-Smellie-Veit. Some French institutions do maneuvers routinely, not because they're necessary every time, but because they want to train their residents. Other French institutions perform those maneuvers on an as-needed basis only.)

She was also in the process of publishing another article looking at whether nonfrank breeches did any better or worse than frank breeches. She wrote to me: "Concerning the article that we are submitting, neonatal outcomes for nonfrank breeches are not any worse than for frank, except for a higher rate of in-labor cesarean section due to a higher rate of umbilical cord prolapse."

This is exactly what I was talking about earlier—that you can anticipate a higher rate of cord prolapse if you have a nonfrank breech.

3. Is one type of breech harder to birth than another?

Let's move on to this third question: Are footling breeches harder or easier to give birth to? Do they have more abnormalities in dilation or not?

Did you know that around the 1940s, footling breech was widely perceived as easier to give birth to and as less lethal than frank breech? Yes, for a time, frank breech was the scariest type of breech presentation. Today our fears are completely reversed! In 1943, this article by Moore & Steptoe stated:

> Contrary to current statements that the fetal mortality in frank breech presentation is higher than in footling presentation, we found that in primiparae the fetal mortality in the two types was almost identical, while in multiparae the mortality rate in frank breech presentation was actually lower than in footling presentation. We agree that an infant presenting by frank breech offers more difficulty during actual delivery than a footling breech, especially in primiparae, but this increase in the hazard for the infant in frank breech is compensated by the increased frequency of prolapse of the umbilical cord in footling presentations.

The authors agreed that yes, frank breeches are harder to give birth to and more dangerous in some senses, but they have a lower rate of cord prolapse. We have to balance those factors out. This should remind you that what we accept as a universal truth nowadays has not always been seen as such.

By the time we reach the 1970s and 1980s, universally frank breech is seen as the safest type of breech and footling breech is universally forbidden for a vaginal birth.

There is disagreement and lively debate about this topic. One French study by Descargues in 2001 found that a frank breech was better for dilating with fewer abnormalities: "On a mechanical level, the frank breech provides a better dilator cone. Labor in a nonfrank breech is more often complicated by PROM or PPROM, by prolapse of the foot or umbilical cord, or by abnormalities in dilation." In contrast, another French article by Dubois in 1981 found that nonfrank breeches had easier expulsive phases: "Classically, a complete/nonfrank breech was considered more favorable [than frank] because the expulsion was easier. However, it also has a higher rate of foot and cord prolapse." Nobody would argue with that last point.

A German study by Krause in 1997 measured the average length of labor and the average length of second stage for frank breeches versus completes and incompletes. Interestingly enough, they found that frank breeches, on average, took an hour longer in first stage and twice as long in second stage, compared to completes or incompletes.

Frank		**Complete/incomplete**
460 min	**Length of labor**	400 min
89 min	**Second Stage**	37 min

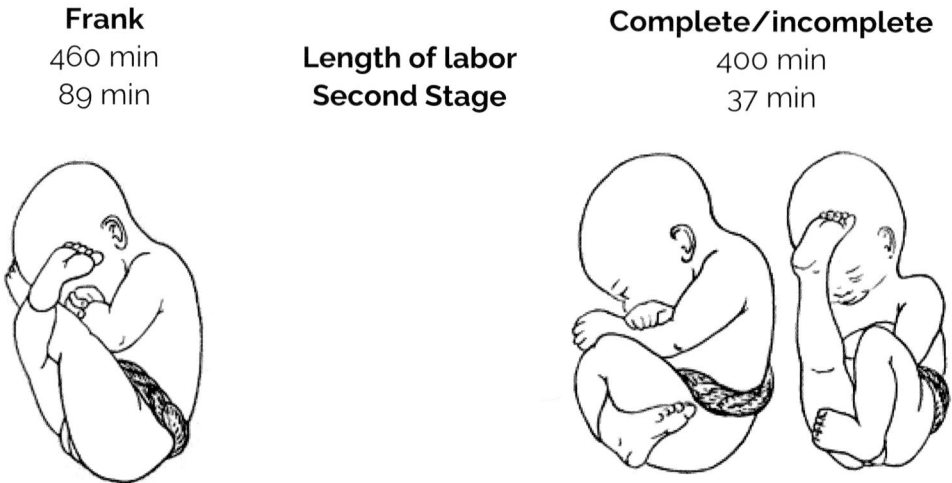

They explain it like this:

> This difference is grounded in the mechanics of birth. The presenting part of a fetus in a frank-presenting breech position is 27-28 centimeters...whereas a fetus in a complete breech position has a diameter of approximately 32-33 centimeters. Although the fetuses in a frank breech presentation occupy a smaller plane of the birth canal, they require more time to completely dilate the cervix and must negotiate a greater tissue resistance in the birth canal. For the fetus in a complete/incomplete breech position, the circumference of the presenting part is similar in size to a cephalic presentation. The greater pre-stretching makes the passage through the birth canal faster for a baby in a complete/incomplete breech possible.

They refer to this thing called the "circumference of the presenting part" or of the "dilating part" (*Geburtsmechanisch wirksamer Umfang*). Here are measurements from 3 different German textbooks.

Type of breech	Feige 2013	Mändle 2007	Stiefel 2012
Frank	28 cm	28 cm	28 cm
Complete	**33 cm**	**32 cm**	**33 cm**
Incomplete	**30 cm**	**30-32 cm**	**30 cm**
Double footling	**25 cm**	**25 cm**	**25 cm**
Single footling	27 cm	28-30 cm	27 cm
Double kneeling	**25 cm**	**25 cm**	
Single kneeling	**23-25 cm**	28 cm	

These measurements don't completely agree one with another. But notice that the largest circumferences (**in blue**) by far are completes and incompletes, while the smallest circumferences (**in red**) are double footlings and kneelings. Frank breech is not the largest by far; it's right in the middle. The Mändle textbook estimates the dilating circumference of a single footling breech to be 28-30 centimeters. That is as big as or even bigger than a frank breech!

Why is this information important? If we're scared of cervical head entrapment for footlings, with their estimated circumferences ranging from 25-30 cm, then we should be scared of frank breeches, which are not that much bigger in circumference (28 cm). This reinforces my point that a normally developing term baby is going to have a torso and a trunk that are proportionately sized to the head. Sometimes in our efforts to prevent extremely rare bad outcomes, we end up causing more harm than good (for example, forcing all women with nonfrank breeches to have C-sections due to fear of cord prolapse or head entrapment, or ALL breeches to have C-sections due to fear in general!).

Kneeling breeches

We have very little information on kneeling breeches and most of it is written in German. For example, in the German study on cord prolapse that I referenced, there were only 4 kneeling breeches in a 12-year time span. 3 of the 4 prolapsed their cords.

> High rate of cord prolapse?
> - 3 out of 4 in Kouam 1980
>
> Most evidence is in German

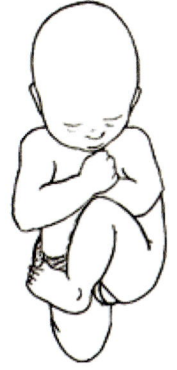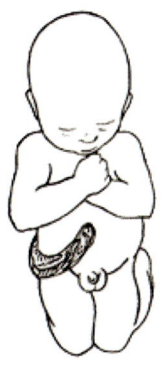

What does a kneeling breech feel like upon vaginal exam? You might get tricked and think you have a complete or a frank breech, and then you may be surprised by feeling something very strange.

What does a kneeling breech feel like upon vaginal exam?

- **Double kneeling:** "Upon vaginal exam, two sharp pointy things I couldn't identify were presenting. Felt exactly like two chicken wings."
- **Single kneeling:** "What I thought was a small butt was really a large knee! As it rumped, I kept waiting to see anus, knew it was close because we were getting lots of mec. Finally the crack I 'ass-u-med' was the anus was the crease behind the knee."

This next part are anecdotal reports from providers who have had kneeling breeches, and I want to stress very strongly that this is not systematically gathered research. When we gather anecdotal reports, we probably can expect to get the most extreme cases back. With that caveat, let's take a look.

Kneeling breech: anecdotal reports

- "undiagnosed…no cord prolapse but the baby did need extensive maneuvers and a terrible Apgar and HIE"
- "the only kneeling breech I've seen…the baby did rotate as it descended, just didn't descend fast enough…Squad was called, NRP given until squad arrived, but it never breathed"
- Undiagnosed double kneeling breech at an accredited birth center, 4-5 cm. Transfer to hospital for CS, healthy baby
- "I had a kneeling breech that I didn't recognize because I'd never heard of it at the time. Her labor progressed fine but she is one of the very few who had a deflexed head that I could only get out by using Pipers"
- [A UK provider] "has definitely supported one that was straightforward. She uses it in her breech training slides."

As you can see, some of them were born smoothly, but others had difficulties. I would be a lot more scared about a kneeling breech than I would be about a footling, due to some of these case reports coming in. But again, we have hardly any data, so don't take this as a clinical recommendation. Just take this as a word of advice based on very little information. There's something strange happening with a lot of these kneeling breeches.

Here is my hypothesis: Mostly breech birth takes part under flexion. As the baby is pushed down, the uterus is pushing on the top of the head, which then flexes the head, flexes the spine, and keeps the body nicely tucked in. There's a reason it's called the "fetal position." However, if your baby is a kneeling breech, its legs are tucked *behind* its body. If it's being squished through the birth canal, the uterus is pushing on the top of the head and flexing the head, but at the same time its legs are being forced against the back of its spine and squeezed. I think this would force spinal *extension*, rather than spinal flexion. If I bend my knees and pull my feet against my bottom, it forces my spine to arch and to extend. I can't flex my spine and round it over while simultaneously pushing my feet against my bottom. I wonder if kneeling breeches have difficulties because their bodies are being extended (arched) rather than flexed as they come through the pelvis? This is an idea that should be researched further.

Breech babies like to move their legs

We've talked a lot about properly naming breeches. But did you know that babies change their type of presentation quite frequently? In one study from the 1960s, they found that 25% of term breech babies had changed their leg positions within a 10-minute time span. And the earlier the gestation, the more the leg movement. They said: "An X-ray scan [or nowadays, an ultrasound scan] of a breech is only momentarily valid." If you send a woman in for an ultrasound because you have a suspected breech presentation, the type of breech is only valid for a few minutes!

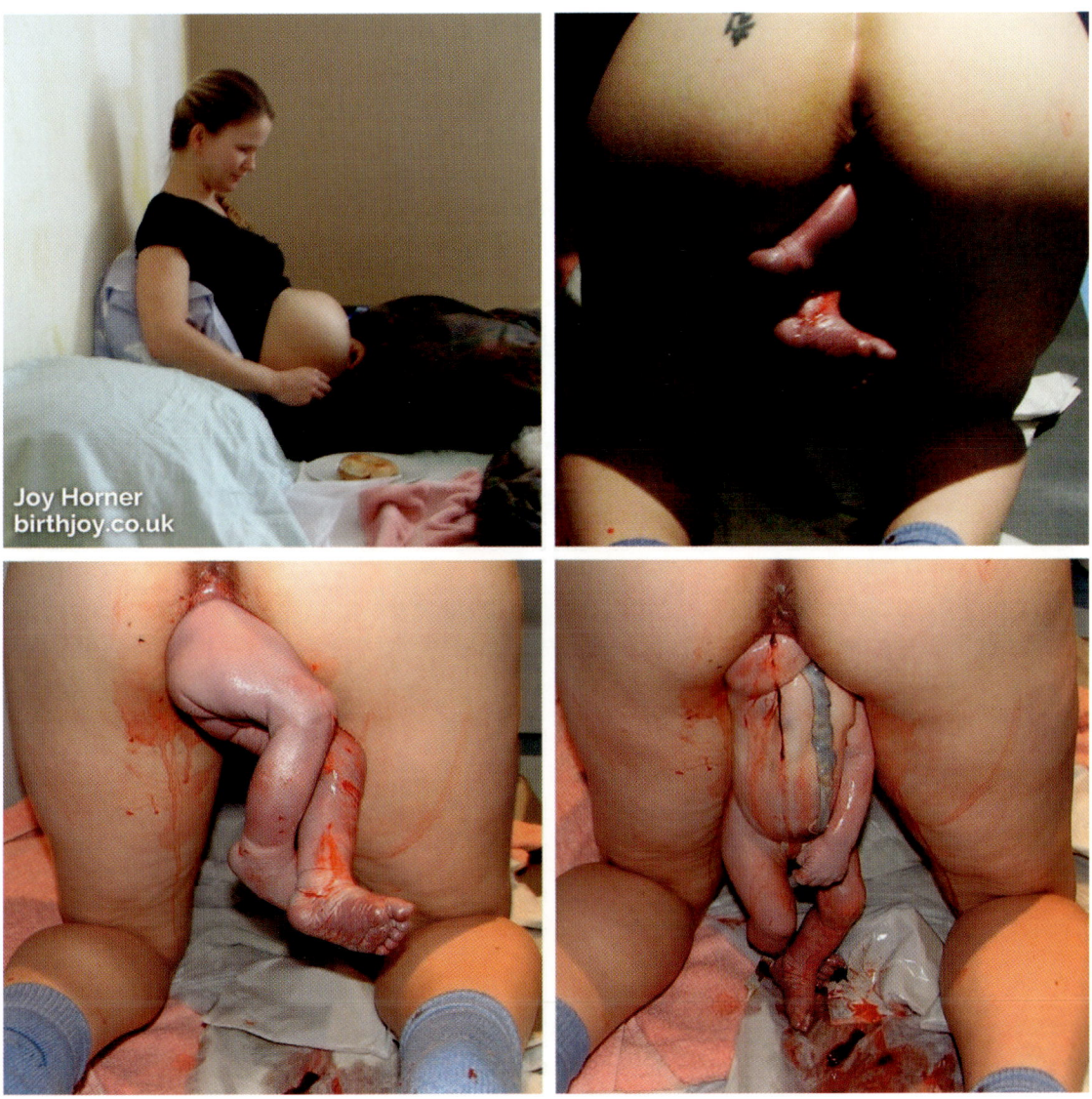

Intrapartum ECV

Although this book does not cover External Cephalic Version, I wanted you to be aware that ECV is possible during active labor; this is called "intrapartum ECV" and abbreviated as IP ECV. This may be a good option for helping women avoid surgery at the last minute. IP ECV is successful around 78% of the time. It is typically done with babies that are unengaged and/or labeled "unfavorable for vaginal birth" (which probably means "footling"). IP ECVs have been performed as late as 8 cm in published reports, usually with intact membranes. Anecdotally, I know some OBs who have done them as late as full dilation with ruptured membranes and successfully turned the baby.

Many of the IP ECVs were done in an OR, but not all. One of these studies was from an Amish birth center in LaFarge WI, so these IP ECVs did not take place in an OR. Sometimes the women had epidurals, sometimes they did not. Many of these centers would give a uterine relaxant, but not all.

This table summarizes the main studies on intrapartum ECV.

Author & year	IP ECVs Successful/ Tried (%)	Vaginal births after successful ECV (%)	Dilation	Reasons for failed ECV or failed TOL	Notes
Kaneti 2000	12/13 (92.3%)	10/12 (83.3%)	2-8 cm	Failed ECV: membranes ruptured during ECV, 8 cm Failed TOL: 1 cord presentation 1 arrest of labor	Prospective. Term footling breech. Ritodrine; regional anesthesia when possible; amniotomy after ECV. All multips (by chance). Membranes intact in all successful ECVs.
Ferguson 1985	11/15 (73.3%)	10/11 (90.9%)	1-8 cm	Failed TOL: arrest of labor in primip. All multips had successful versions & TOLs.	Participants "not good candidates" for VBB. Tocolysis. All women had intact membranes. 6 primips, 9 multips. 3 had epidurals.
Belfort 1993	1/1 (case report)	1/1	5 cm/ 70% eff.		Multip w/ unengaged complete breech, feet presenting. IV nitroglycerin; amniotomy & oxytocin to restart labor.
Leung 1999	2/5 (40%)	2/2 (100%)			Attempted on 5 out of 28 undiagnosed breeches
Deline 2012	3/?	3/3 (100%)			Amish birth center; IP ECV for nonfrank breech presentation

Conclusion

What are some takeaway points from this lesson? I hope that you will come away knowing how to properly name a breech presentation. You should now know the risks of frank versus nonfrank breech, especially relating to cord prolapse. They have mostly similar outcomes, except for a higher rate of cord prolapse in nonfrank breeches. But nonfrank breeches with cord prolapse tend to do quite well; it's more common, but less dangerous.

I think we can safely say that a true footling breech at term is nearly impossible. We should start using the phrase "dropped foot breech" to describe a complete or incomplete that drops a foot down during labor. I think we should be cautious of kneeling breeches. We don't have a lot of information, but based on what I've seen, I'd be wary with them. Intrapartum ECV is something worth exploring and might be one way of helping bring down the C-section rate in places where women cannot access vaginal breech birth with a skilled provider.

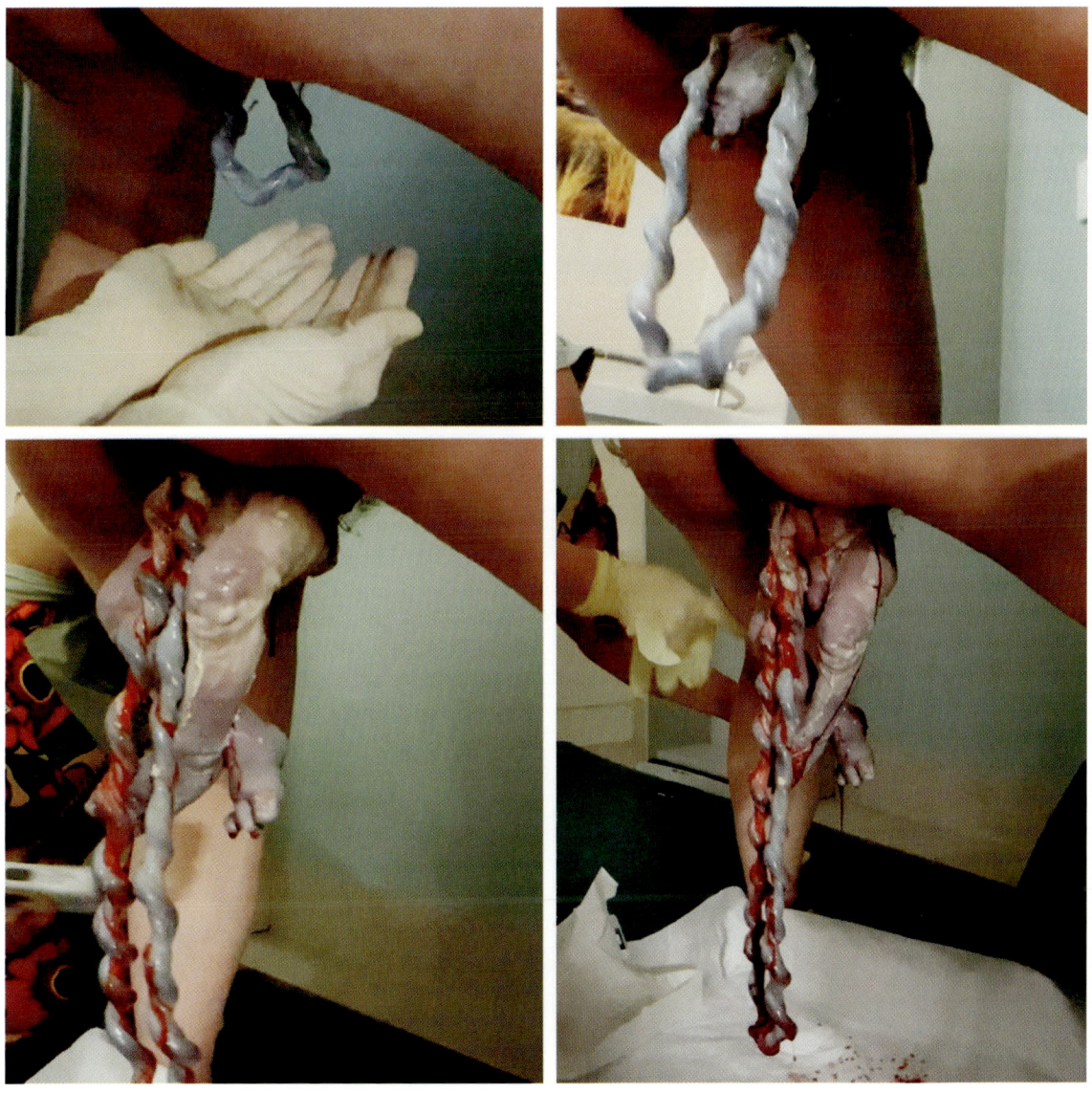

Complete breech with dropped feet and cord prolapse

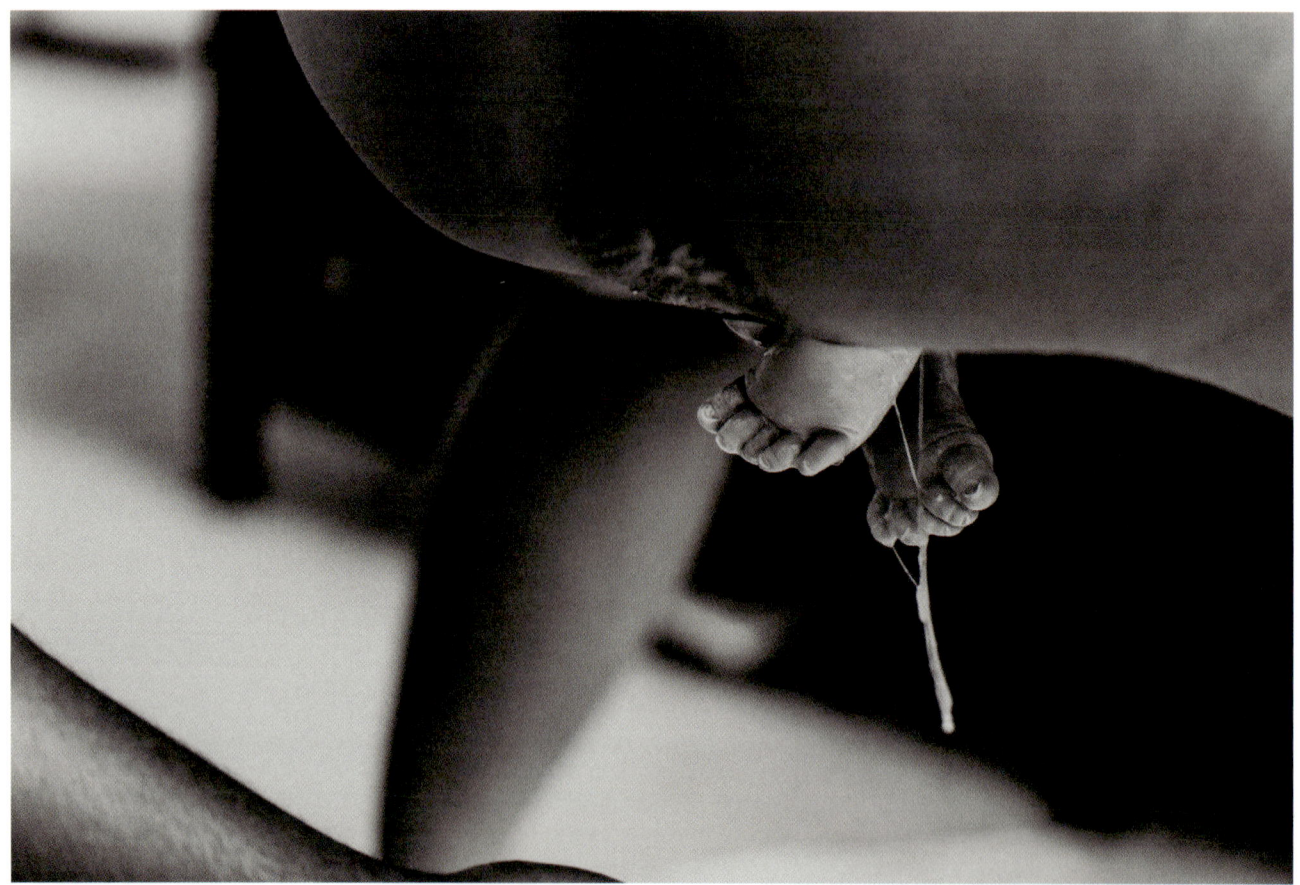

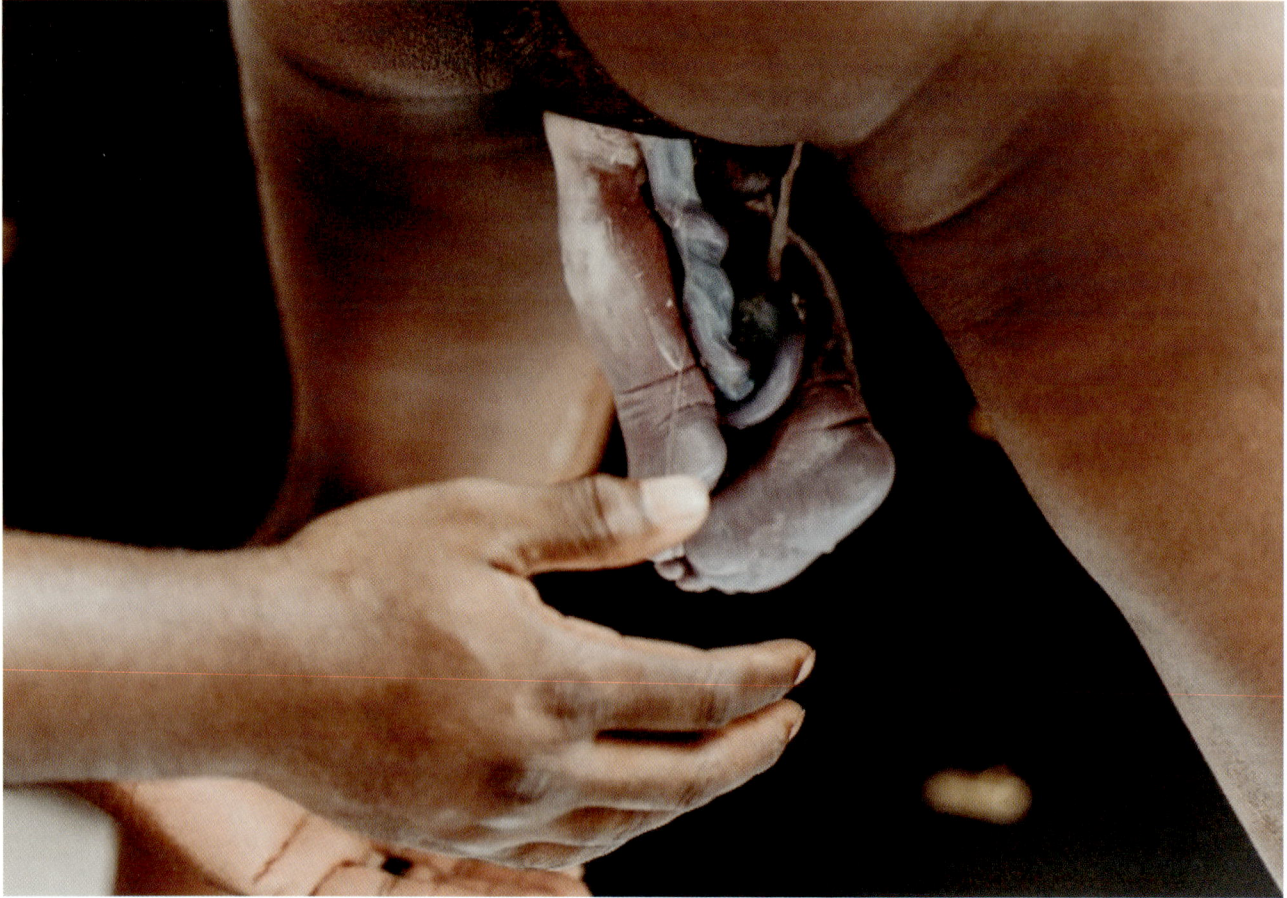

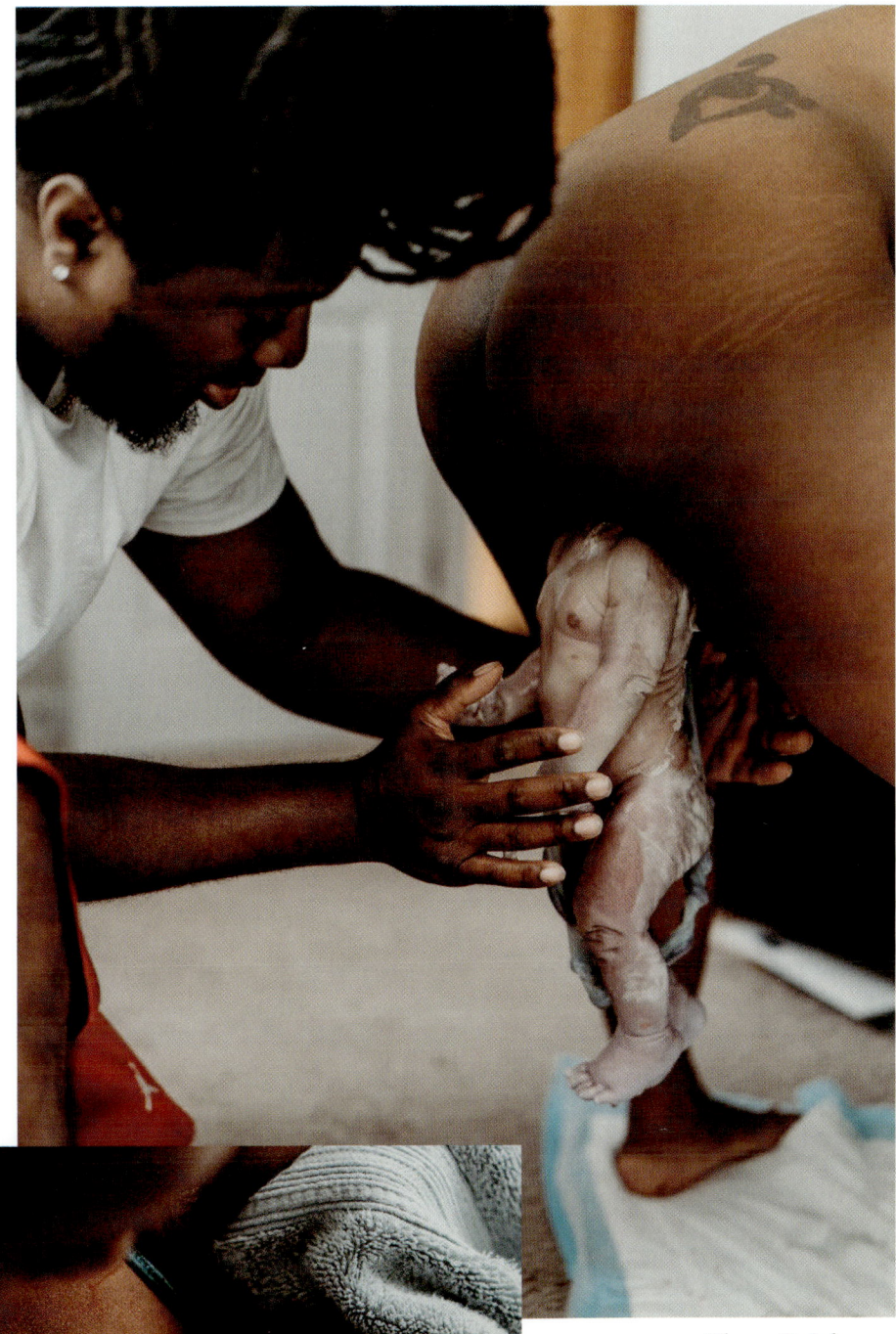

Kiana N Johnson
Baby caught by father

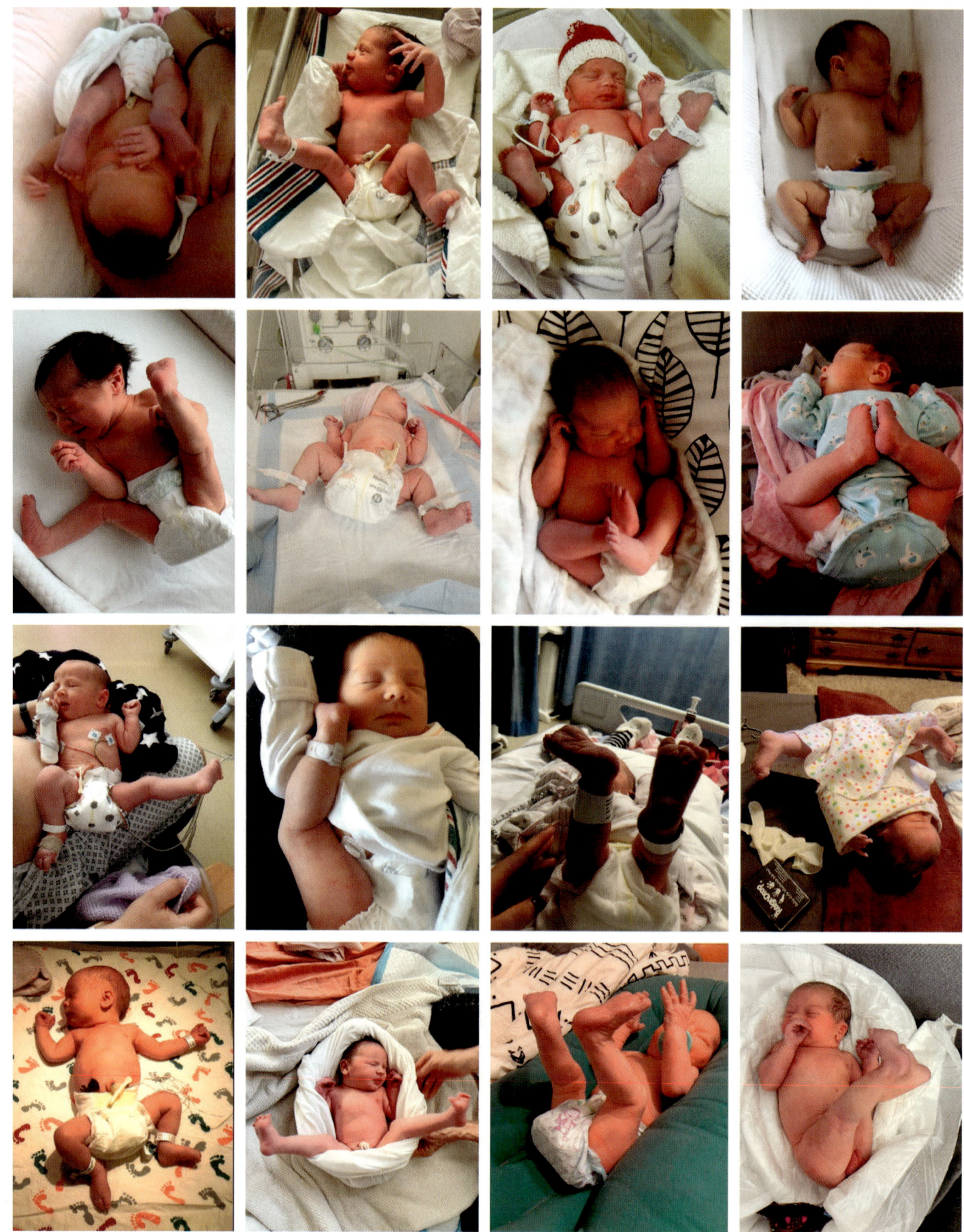

Lesson 8: Normal Breech Birth
Clinical Aspects of Physiological Vaginal Breech Birth, Part 1

By David Hayes, MD

Welcome to Clinical Aspects of Physiological Vaginal Breech Birth. In four lessons, we're going to focus on how to clinically manage a vaginal breech birth.

- What are the mechanisms of normal vaginal breech birth?
- What factors predict poor outcomes (selection/exclusion criteria)?
- How do you recognize deviations from normal mechanisms?
- How is breech labor managed? Different from cephalic?
- When is it appropriate to intervene in a birth?
- What maneuvers do you use to correct deviations from normal mechanisms or expedite the birth?

In this first lesson, we will dissect the normal mechanisms of vaginal breech birth.

Mechanisms

- **Engagement**—Sacrum Transverse
- Widest fetal dimension aligns with widest pelvis dimension
- **Descent**: Remains transverse until the fetal rump reaches the vaginal introitus
- Unlike cephalic mechanisms, there is no rotation between engagement and "rumping," only lateral flexion.
- The anterior buttock presents first.
- As the rump approaches the introitus, expect meconium.
- **Rumping = birth of the bitrochanteric diameter (widest part of the fetal hips)**

Typically, in vaginal breech birth, women are not lying flat on their backs in the bed with monitors strapped to them. They are generally upright or on hands & knees or all fours. Those positions tend to be preferred and we have good evidence for using those upright positions. That is what you're going to be seeing as a practitioner of physiological vaginal breech birth, which means you're going to be facing the mama from the back. You'll get used to seeing that position.

Engagement

The baby engages like a head-down baby engages. It finds its way into a nice snug fit in the pelvic inlet, and it does so in a very particular manner. It either is going to be right sacrum transverse or left sacrum transverse. The widest diameter of the baby naturally rotates to fit the widest diameter of the pelvis. As you can see in this doll & pelvis below, the widest part of the baby is from its front to back, so it likes to enter facing transverse (sideways).

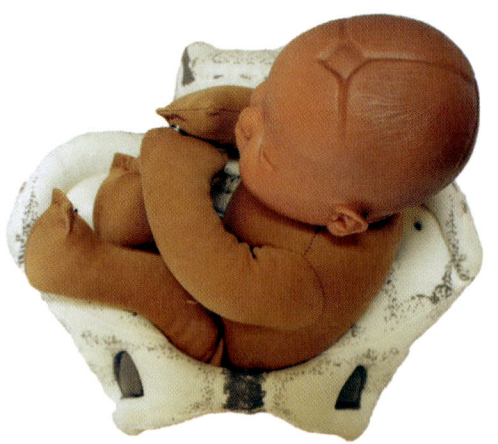 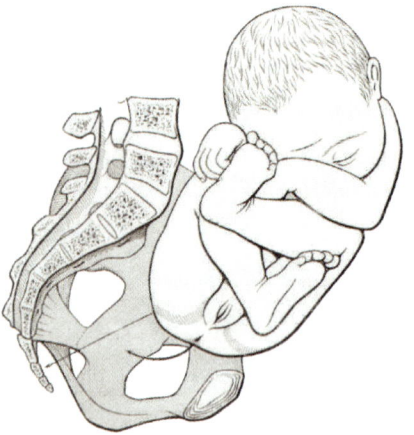 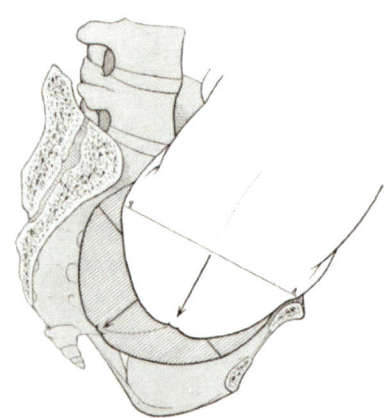

It's not overly complicated. It's a mechanism that has evolved and works very nicely. You can expect in almost every instance that your baby will engage and enter the pelvis either right or left sacrum transverse (RST or LST). My personal experience with LST babies is no different than with RST babies. In fact, they are somewhat fewer, but they have gone extremely smoothly.

In cephalic birth, the baby's head enters the pelvis. It flexes, it internally rotates, it extends, and then it externally rotates as it navigates through the pelvis. In breech presentations, that does not happen. Descent is much simpler. The baby enters the pelvis transverse to one side or the other. The baby then proceeds to descend directly through the pelvis with no rotation whatsoever. It does have a little bit of lateral flexion so that it can follow the sacral curve, but there is no rotation until the baby's rump gets on the perineum, which we call "rumping."

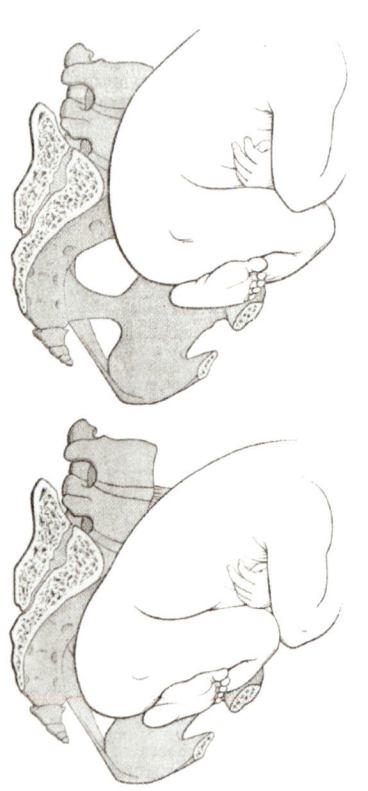

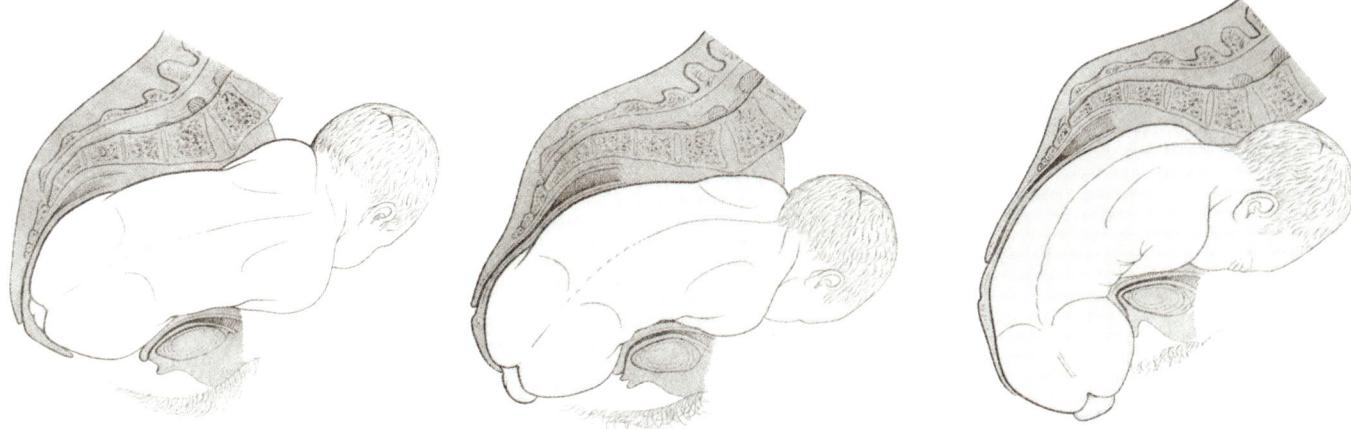

Technically, rumping is the birth of the bitrochanteric diameter, not just the first appearance of the buttocks on the perineum. But up until that point, you expect to see the baby descending transverse with absolutely no rotation. That is completely normal. You also might expect to see copious quantities of meconium as that baby's butt does a lateral flexion and starts being squeezed through the pelvic outlet. That is also perfectly normal.

Here are some pictures of the anal cleft starting to peek through the perineum. You will always see the anterior buttock first due to the lateral flexion through the curve of the sacrum.

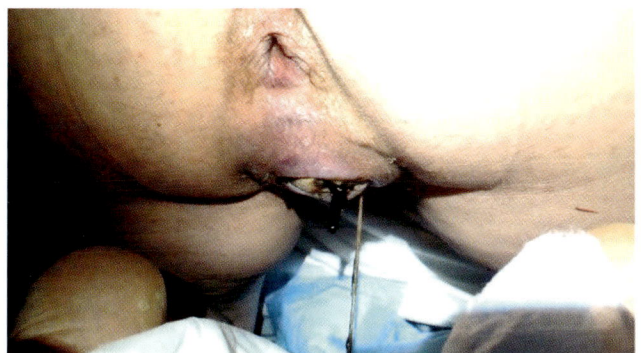
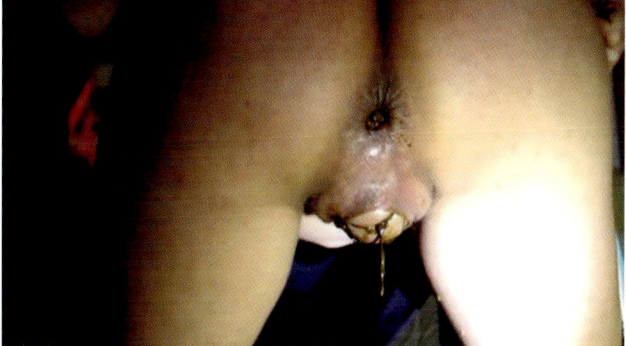

Rotation and descent

- Rotation to sacrum anterior and descent to the chest normally complete in one contraction
- The point at which the umbilicus passes through the introitus is the point at which the cord can become compromised.
- Timing is now important
- **Clinical tip:** Have an assistant keep accurate time once "rumping" is firmly established.
- **What fetal event drives rotation?**

During that first contraction after rumping and during descent and rotation, the umbilicus is exposed for the first time. The umbilical cord is still attached to the placenta inside and is going through the perineum or between the perineum and the baby's body. The potential for compromise of the cord increases. Timing is fairly important at this stage of the game. A normal undisturbed vaginal breech birth after rumping typically takes on the average of 2 to 5 minutes. In a primip, it may take 7 to 8 to 10 minutes. But usually, it's a fairly quick process. Obviously, there is concern if there is potential for the cord to be compromised.

As a **clinical tip**, I recommend that you have a person available whose only job is to start a stopwatch and be able to give you, as the attendant, an accurate account of how much time has elapsed since rumping occurred.

What fetal event drives rotation? The baby has entered the pelvis with its widest diameter fitting the widest diameter of the pelvis. It has descended without any rotation. And now all of a sudden, as the rump gets to the perineum, it begins to rotate as it further descends.

What causes that to happen? The answer, of course, is that when the shoulders reach the pelvic inlet, they are now the widest presenting part of the fetus to the pelvis. The pelvic anatomy encourages them to rotate so that the widest part of the baby is engaged in the widest part of the pelvis, the transverse diameter. This is also the point where frank and complete breech presentations diverge somewhat. In a frank presentation, descent brings the shoulders to the pelvic inlet, which we've already mentioned. The sacrum anterior position lines the shoulders up with the transverse diameter of the pelvic inlet. You can see all of this happen.

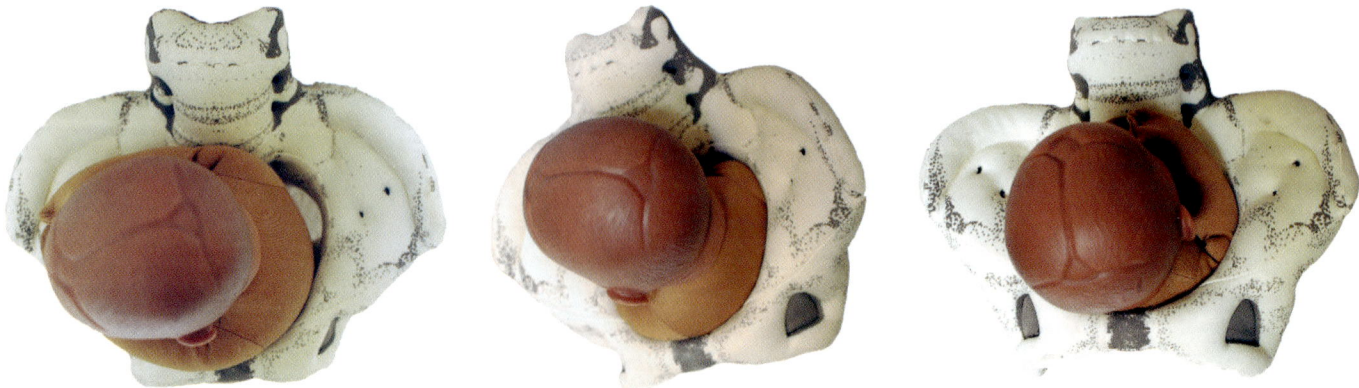

Rotation and descent: Frank

- Descent brings the shoulders to the pelvic inlet and rotation allows them to enter
- Sacrum anterior position lines the shoulders up with the transverse diameter of the pelvic inlet
- The beauty of VBB is that the baby is right in front of your eyes. You can see the mechanism in action!
- **What causes the baby to rotate to sacrum anterior?**

Why does the baby rotate to sacrum anterior and not, for example, sacrum posterior? We know that it rotates away from transverse because the baby's shoulders are the widest diameter and they're going to fit into the transverse portion of the pelvic inlet. But why does it almost always go sacrum anterior, instead of rotating sacrum posterior? The answer, of course, again is the pelvic anatomy. The baby is in either the right or the left gutter of the pelvis; it doesn't matter which one.

The baby is in a transverse presentation coming down through the pelvis, and once the shoulders reach the inlet, it wants to rotate. It has the option of rotating towards the pubic bone—which is a nice, smooth, open space—or towards the sacral promontory, which is a massive chunk of spine. So of course, when the baby wants to rotate, it's going to rotate in the direction that has the least resistance, which is *away* from the sacral promontory. That is why the baby rotates to sacrum anterior.

Note the protruding sacral promontory in the pelvic inlet in these illustrations below.

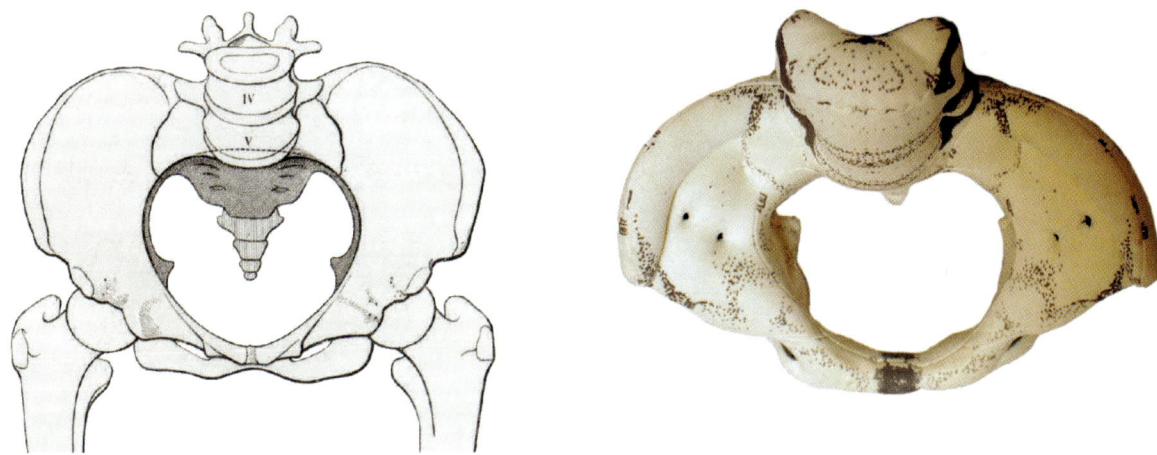

Your vantage point is usually behind the mother. You will see the baby rump sideways and then turn to face you.

If the mother is on a birth stool or supine, your vantage point will be from the front of the mother. In the picture below left (birth stool), we see a complete breech that has partially rotated to SO (sacrum oblique). On the picture on below right (supine), we see full rotation to SA; the baby's back is facing the mother's front.

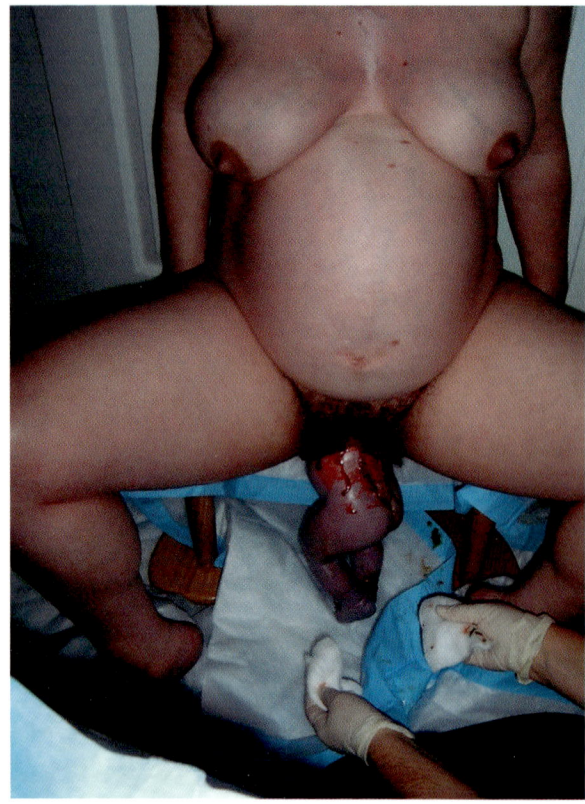

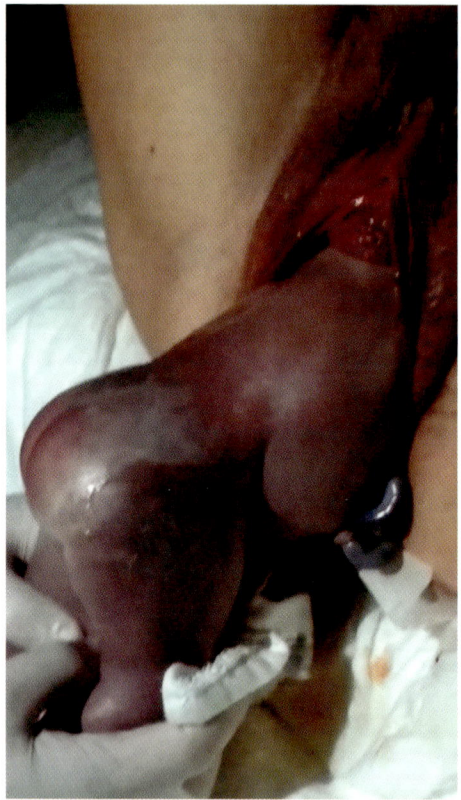

Charity Pitcher-Cooper, Photographer: Heidi Petty,
Midwife: Marilee Pinkleton

Eirini

We will follow several births in this lesson. Example 1 below is a primip and the first physiological breech birth I attended, assisted by Shawn Walker of the UK. Example 2 is a second-time mother who stood up during the pushing stage. She was quite tall, and I worried about dropping her baby, since it was very far to the floor!

Example 1: Rumping and rotation

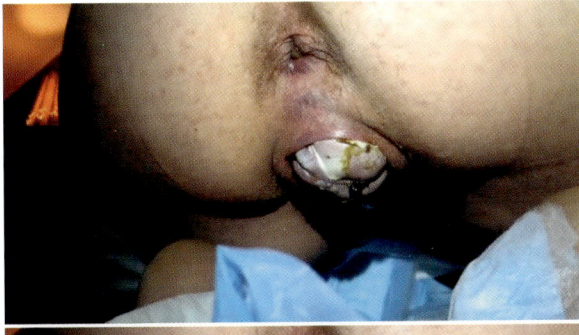

This series of photos comes from a mother who was a primip and one of my first physiological breeches.

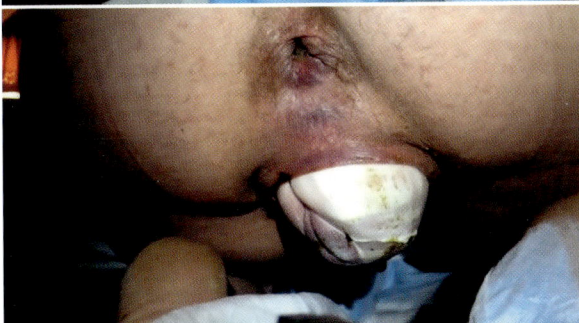

Notice the bitrochanteric diameter just came out.

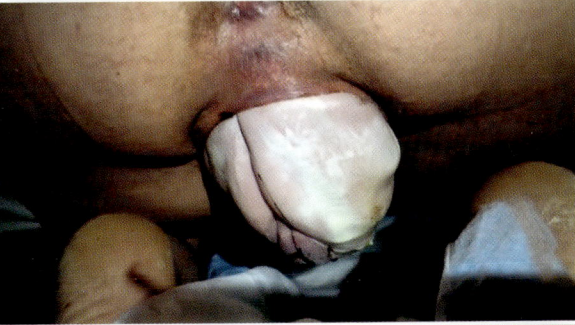

Rotation is happening beautifully.

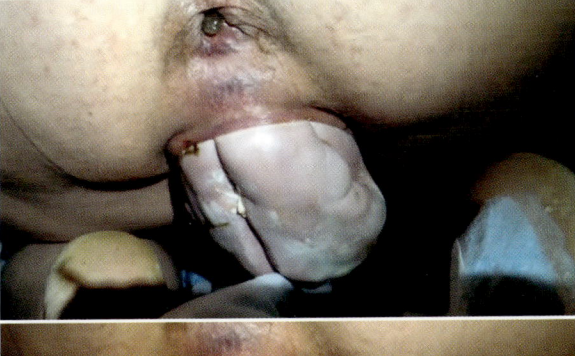

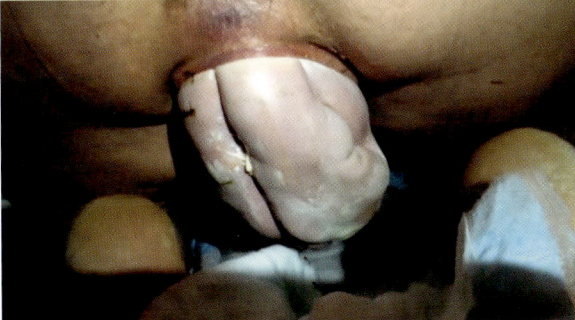

And there we have a perfectly normal rotation to sacrum anterior.

Example 2: Rumping and rotation

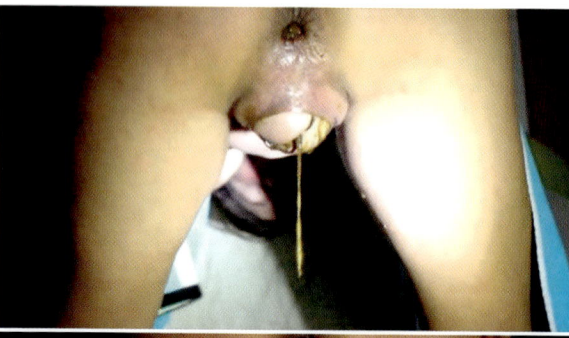

The baby is rotating to left sacrum anterior and presenting its front to the observer. This is the mother's 2nd baby.

The mother is completely bent over looking at her rumping baby; you can see her face between her legs.

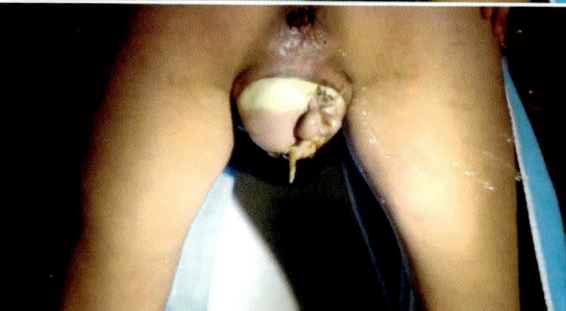

Descent is going beautifully.

(And yes, the baby peed on me!)

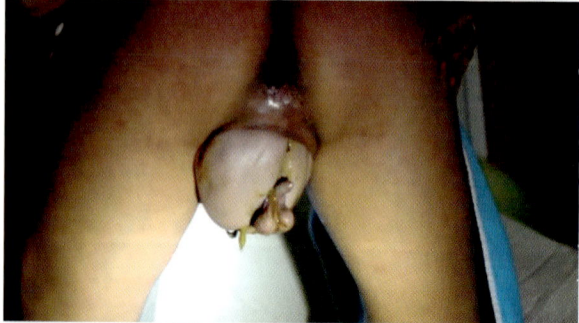

The mom is doing little standing squats. None of this is coached. She is doing it on her own, responding to what she feels.

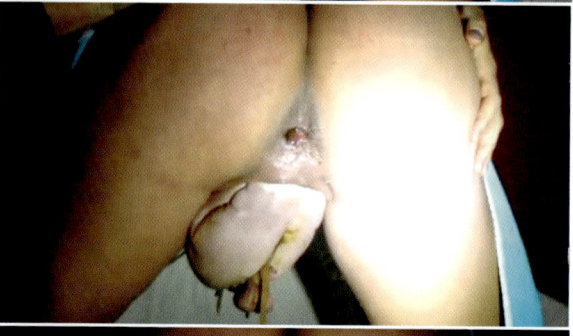

Notice the baby is still asymmetric and jammed against the mother's left thigh.

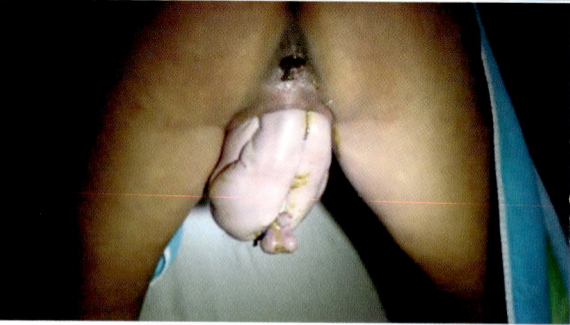

Waiting for the baby to finish its rotation.

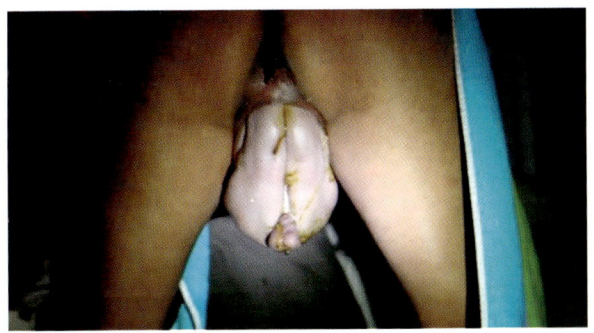

Now the baby is very symmetric, which indicates that there is nothing hanging the baby up in there. If the baby gets caught on something, it tends to want to lean to one side or the other. When it comes down symmetrically hangs straight like that, that's a very good sign that that there's not an obstruction in its labor.

That's a nice illustration of how this is a cooperative dance between the baby and the mom.

Rotation and descent: Complete

- Just as in frank presentation, descent brings the shoulders to the pelvic inlet and rotation allows them to enter
- However, often in complete presentations, the lower extremities interfere with rotation
- If descent continues normally, the deviation of rotation in a complete breech is normal and expected

Moving on to complete presentations: just as with frank breeches, the same mechanism starts to play out. That is, the shoulders reach the pelvic inlet and there's an impetus for the shoulders to turn so that the widest diameter of the baby matches up with the transverse diameter of the pelvis. However, instead of having a frank breech and a smooth cone-shaped presenting dilating part, with the complete breech, you have two large legs folded up inside the pelvis. Those legs can and often do interfere with rotation. **The key issue here is whether or not descent continues**. If rotation is interfered with and there is continuing descent, that means the baby's shoulders—which are flexible and compressible—have entered the pelvis in the orientation where the rotation was arrested.

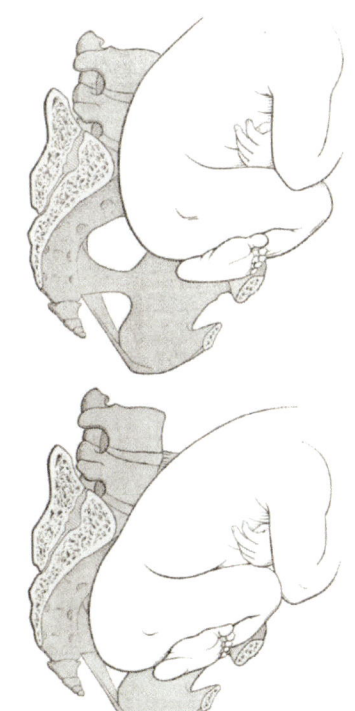

In these two illustrations on the right, you can see how the folded-up legs of a complete breech have to compress to fit into the pelvis. It makes sense why those legs may sometimes lock the baby into a certain orientation. As long as descent continues, the arrest of rotation doesn't seem to interfere with the birth in any measurable way.

I'm not nearly as flexible as a newborn, but even my shoulders can compress fairly significantly from where they started at. In a newborn, the shoulders can compress to about 2/3 of their resting diameter. There is plenty of room for the shoulders to come down. And if descent is not interfered with, they will indeed come down. But that compression keeps the baby from rotating.

There is nothing else in there that is an impetus for rotation. There is the head that follows, but the head obviously swivels on its own axis, so it's not going to be pushing the body to rotate back. So that is a distinct difference between frank and complete breeches.

Example 3: Arrested rotation with continued descent

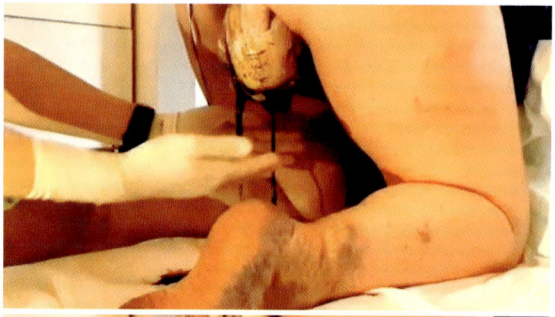

You see the breech coming down. If you look at the midwife's posterior hand, there is one foot out just below the baby's buttocks. This is obviously a complete breech.

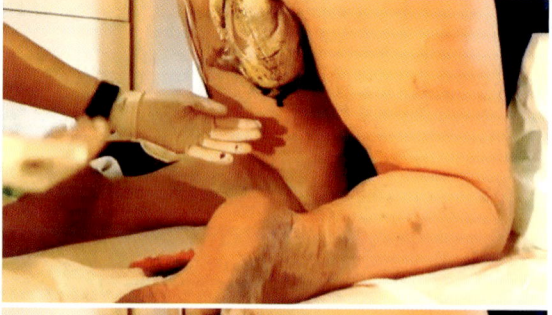

The baby appears to be trying to rotate. The legs are trying to come out

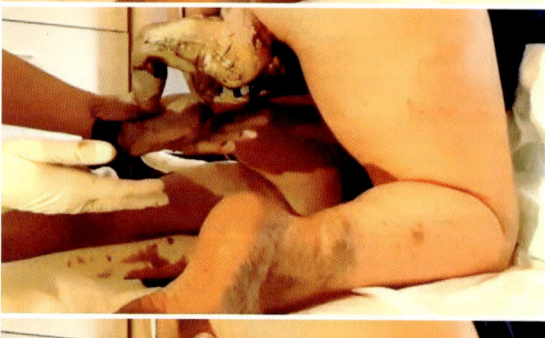

You see the legs come out now. The midwife is trying very hard not to interfere with the birth. She's doing a pretty good job. The baby continues to come down very nicely. The baby does a tummy crunch, which indicates that it's vigorous and trying to maintain its head flexion and tummy flexion.

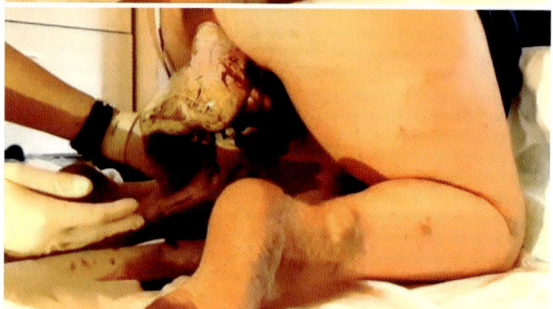

But you also notice that the baby has not rotated. It actually tried to rotate a little bit and went back, so it ended up directly transverse. But as long as it's descending, that's okay. And that is to be expected in complete breech births.

Example 4: Grand multip (baby #7)

This birth took 1 minute from rumping to birth! Notice how the baby rumped RST, descended transvers/oblique e, and only rotated to SA at the very last moment.

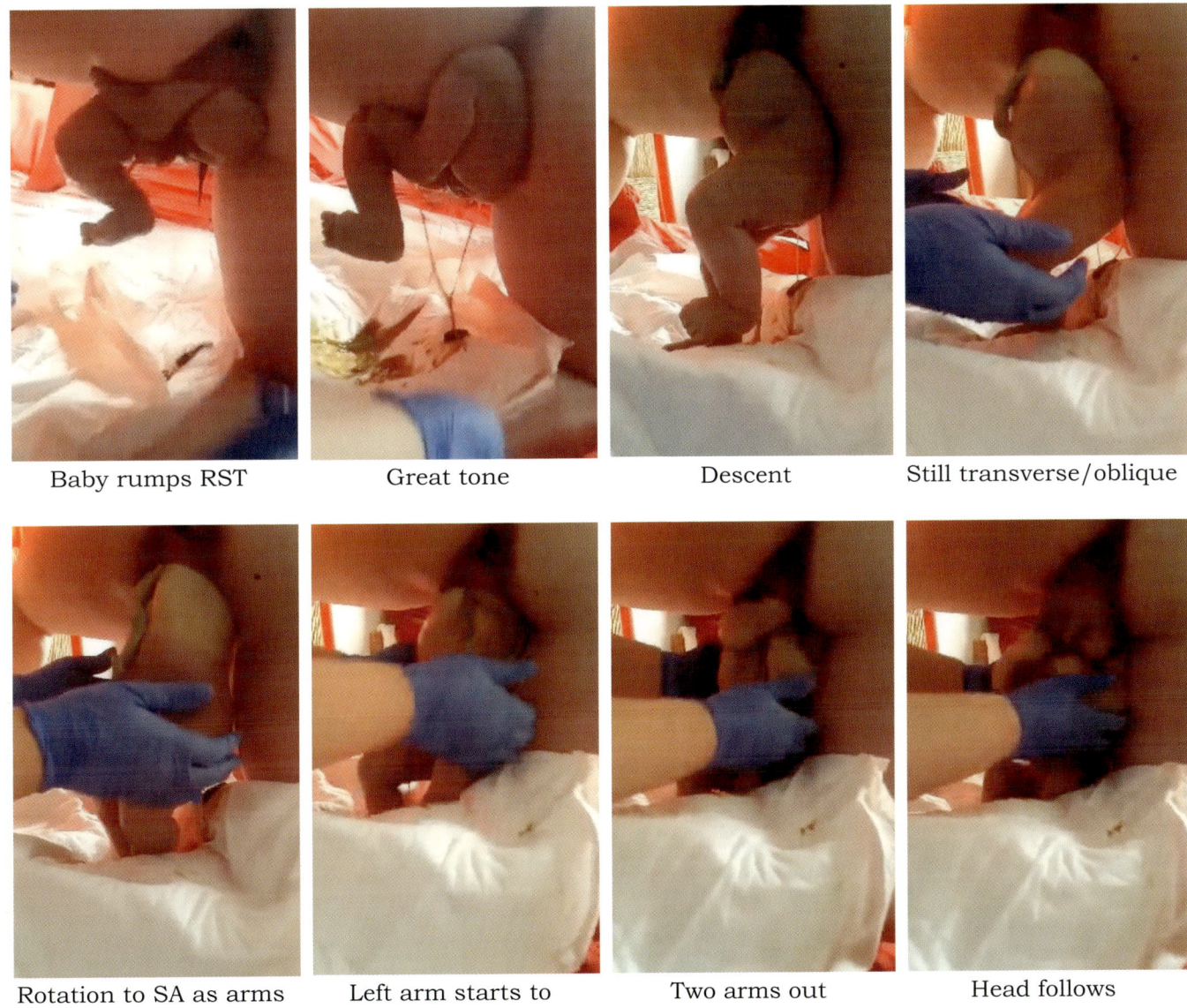

| Baby rumps RST | Great tone | Descent | Still transverse/oblique |

| Rotation to SA as arms start to release | Left arm starts to appear | Two arms out | Head follows immediately |

Descent in incomplete breeches

Incomplete breeches are relatively rare, and they tend to be more difficult births. An incomplete breech is functionally like an asynclitic head. The body is asynclitic, and the center of rotation goes up through one leg, rather than the center of the body. The leg, thigh, and one buttock are trying to come out, and they get centered on the vaginal introitus and take all the available space. The other buttock and leg are up high and get pushed up and off to the side. In that circumstance, the rump has a harder time getting to the perineum. I tend to leave them be. It can be difficult to watch as the leg may descend and then recede significantly as the baby figures out how to navigate the pelvis. Fundal pressure can help if the baby is showing signs of compromise (see Lesson 10). In this birth below (Example 5), the baby had to descend 3 times before finally making its way out.

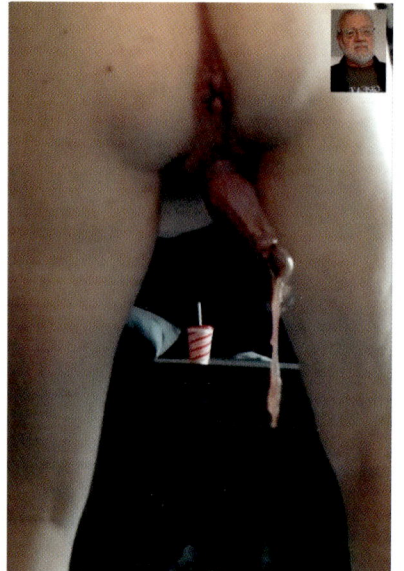
Leg out to the knee

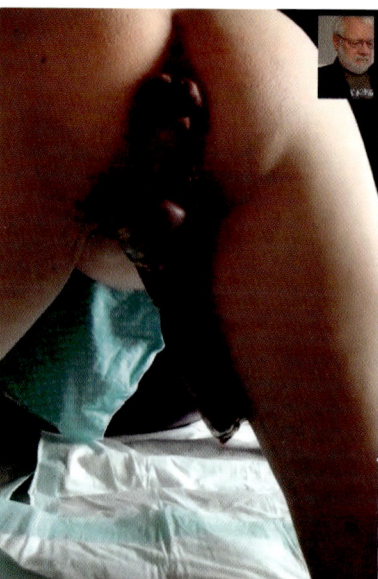
Leg out to upper thigh

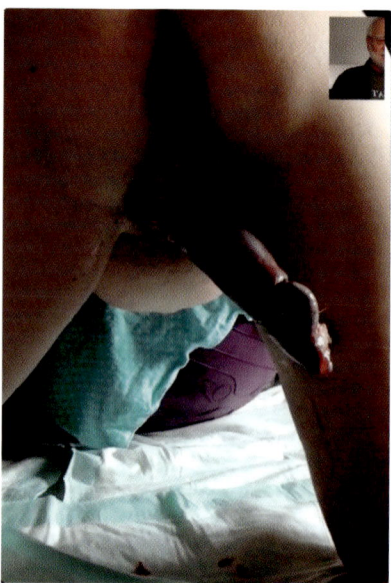
Leg goes back up to the knee

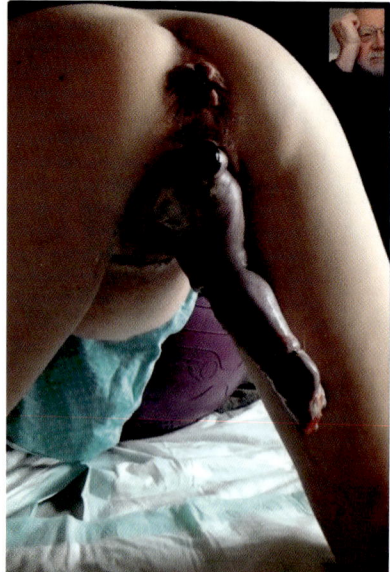
Leg out again to upper thigh

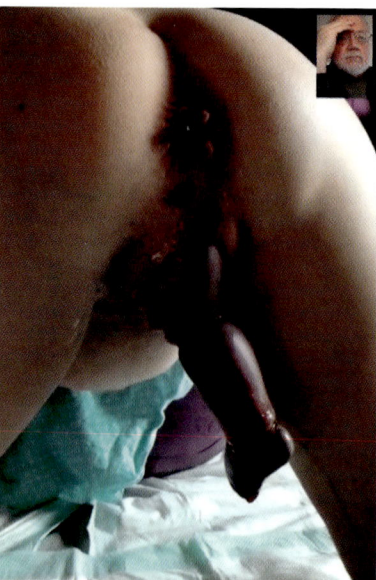
Leg goes back up to mid-thigh

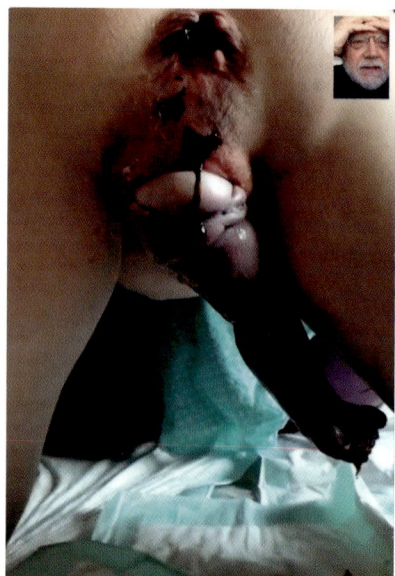
Baby finally rumps LST; quick descent to nipples

Birth of the legs: Frank

- With further descent, the legs are born simultaneously
- When the legs deliver, the chest and umbilical cord are exposed
- By the time the cord is exposed, it has already passed through the perineum at some undetermined point.
- Look for cleavage! Chest cleavage may provide protection from cord compression
- **What is the position of the head now?**

With further descent, the legs are born simultaneously. Once those legs are born, it exposes the umbilical cord, which is easily available as a measure for fetal well-being. It also exposes the chest, allowing you to easily listen to the baby's heart rate directly. In a frank breech baby, those shoulders are also compressed. The baby has rotated to the sacrum anterior position in a frank breech.

Descent of the shoulders: Frank

- Shoulders are now nearing the pelvic outlet. Unlike cephalic birth, they will not rotate. They will deliver with the trunk still facing SA (sacrum anterior)
- Shoulders are flexible. They can decrease to less than 2/3 of their resting diameter.

As they come down, the shoulders—instead of rotating to an anterior-posterior orientation, with one shoulder anterior and the other shoulder posterior, as they would in a cephalic birth—they maintain their side-to-side orientation in the pelvis, which means they get compressed. That compression creates cleavage or what is also called a chest crease. The umbilical cord usually runs through that crease and up and over the shoulder.

There are two things about that chest crease that are important. First, it tells you that the baby's arms are free and they're still above the perineum. You don't see the arms, but if there is cleavage, the baby's arms must be free. Why? If the baby's arms are stuck or extended, then that will affect the ability of the shoulders to produce that cleavage. A chest crease is an indication that the arms are free and not caught.

Second, the chest crease provides a protective channel for the umbilical cord to run through that helps to prevent the umbilical cord from being compressed as it runs back up into contact with the placenta.

What is the position of the head now? At this point, with chest cleavage visible, the head is entering the pelvic inlet.

The head is going to enter in an oblique or transverse orientation, just off from where the shoulders are already compressed in the lower pelvis. As the baby descends further through the pelvis, if the head remains properly flexed, it will rotate directly forward to an anterior-posterior (AP) position, which is the widest diameter of the pelvic outlet.

Look at this series of pictures. You can see the umbilical cord, and you see the legs come out simultaneously, which is an indication that the baby is coming straight down. The baby's body is not skewed off to one side, which means there is probably not an arm caught somewhere. Although the cord is starting to look a little flaccid, notice how well-protected it is in the chest cleavage. That's a pretty dramatic indication that the arms are not stuck.

Example 1, cont'd:

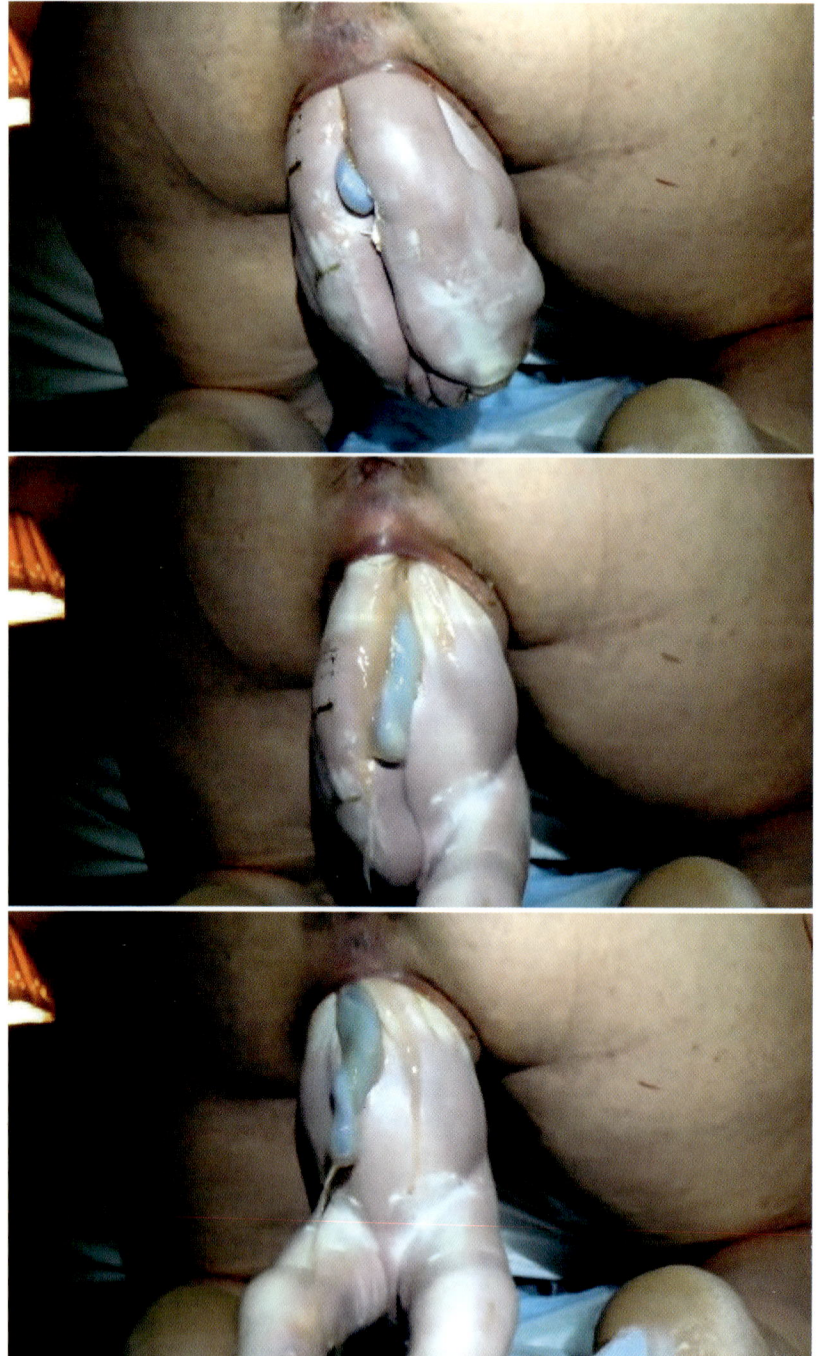

Example 2, cont'd:

Here is the other birth we have been following (mother's 2ⁿᵈ baby).

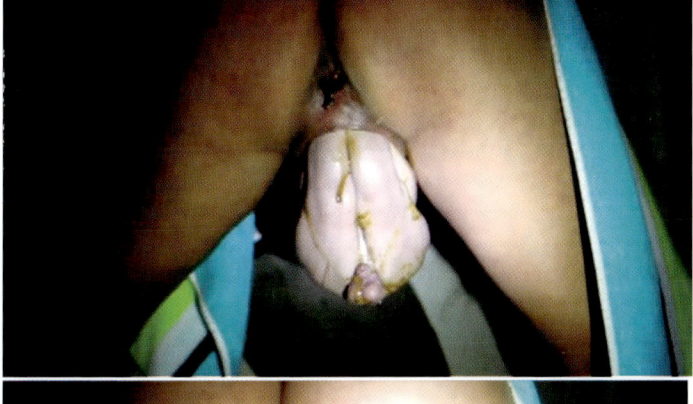

The presentation is now very symmetrical, although it had started off leaning to one side in the earlier photos.

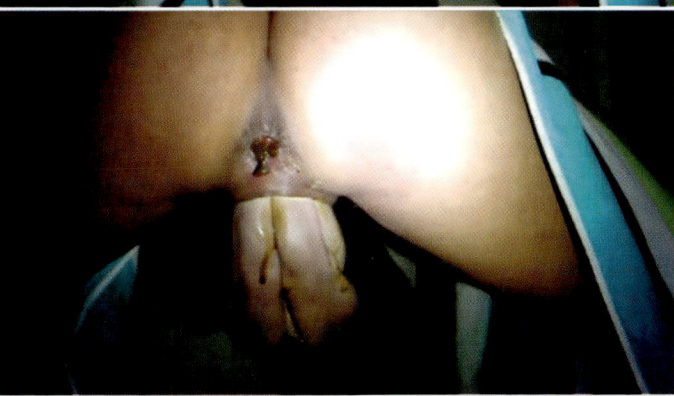

You see mom doing that deep squat. That's in response to something she feels inside. This is totally uncoached, and whatever she's doing seems to be functional. Nice, deep squat.

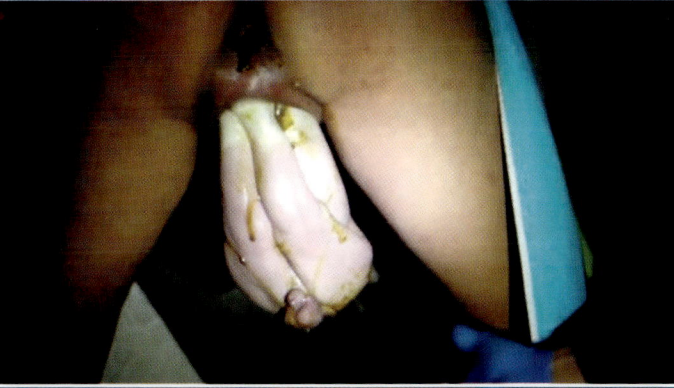

There come the legs; the heels are right behind the perineum.

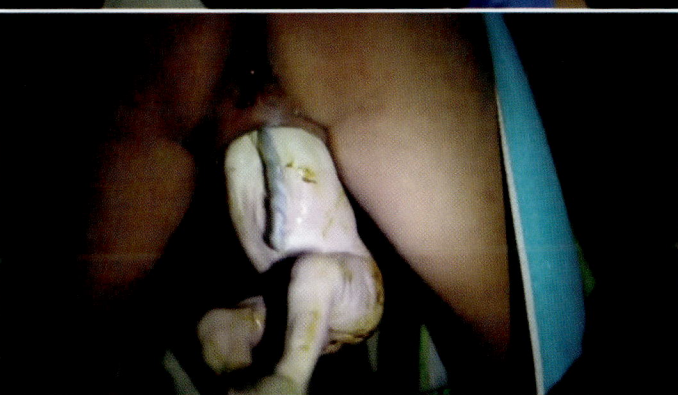

We have two legs and a nice beefy looking cord. You've got a baby with good muscle tone. The legs flexing indicate muscle tone in the trunk. All in all, it looks like a very healthy presentation

- Release of the legs exposes the lower trunk to the effects of gravity, for the first time ever! A neurologically intact baby responds to that extension by maintaining tone in all voluntary muscles and flexing its whole body
- This is commonly referred to as the "Tummy Crunch"

The shoulders are nearing the pelvic outlet. Unlike cephalic birth, as I have said before, the shoulders will not rotate anterior-posterior. They deliver transverse, still facing towards the mother's sides.

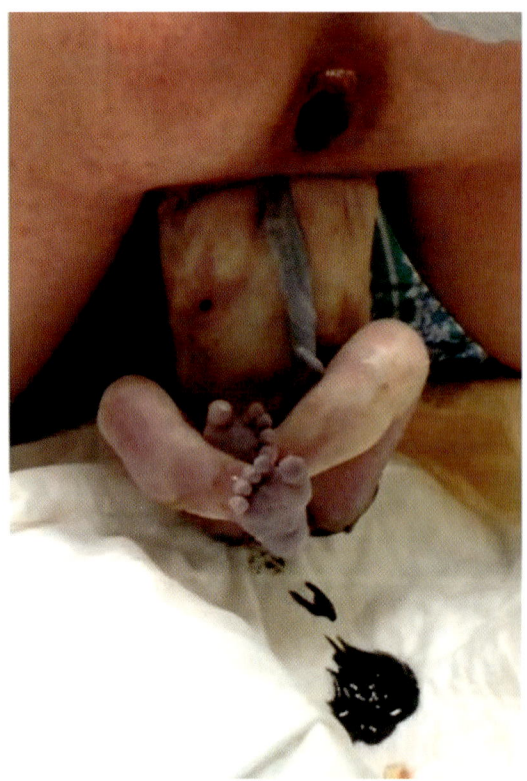

The release of the legs exposes the lower trunk to the effects of gravity, and a neurologically intact baby responds to that by trying to pull them back up into the position that it's used to them being in. Recall that flexing is euphemistically referred to as the "tummy crunch." But it's very valuable because when the baby flexes, it's a whole-body motion. That flexion helps to flex the baby's head as well. We want the baby's head as flexed as possible because that's the smallest diameter that presents to the pelvic outlet.

This brings me to another question: **Why is shoulder dystocia such a common and feared complication in cephalic births?** If the shoulders are so flexible, how is it that they get stuck fairly often in cephalic births?

The issue is not, as many people believe, the shoulders being too wide and thus getting stuck coming out. Instead, in a cephalic birth, you have the head tucked and coming, navigating the pelvis. The shoulders are in an anterior-posterior diameter. Typically, there is plenty of room posteriorly. If you're seeing this in a normal dorsal supine position and you do an exam back here, you'll find that there is plenty of room posteriorly.

The dystocia is not the width of the shoulders. **It is the uterine fundus pushing on the baby and pushing the anterior shoulder into the pubic symphysis**, because this is the only shelf that's available to catch something on inside. In the back you've got this big sacral promontory. We've already discussed this earlier. On the sides of the pelvis are muscles, which create a very smooth pathway. There is no shelf; there's nothing sticking out in the sides or back of the pelvis. In the front, however, the pubic symphysis presents an actual physical barrier that the shoulder can get caught on. That's why you may have a problem with shoulder dystocia, much more so in cephalic birth than in breech birth.

Descent of the shoulders: Complete

- Shoulders will descend and deliver in the orientation in which they entered the pelvic inlet.
- This is a normal and expected characteristic of complete breech births.

A complete breech may often have arrested rotation but with continued descent. This is normal. What causes this? Sometimes the folded-up legs of a complete breech "lock" the baby into place inside the pelvis, and the shoulders will then descend through the pelvis in the orientation in which entered the pelvis. Once the shoulders are compressed and locked into position inside the pelvis, there is no rotational force applied to them as they descend. This is why is it fairly common to see complete breech babies descend sacrum oblique or transverse. Continued descent, even without full rotation, is reassuring.

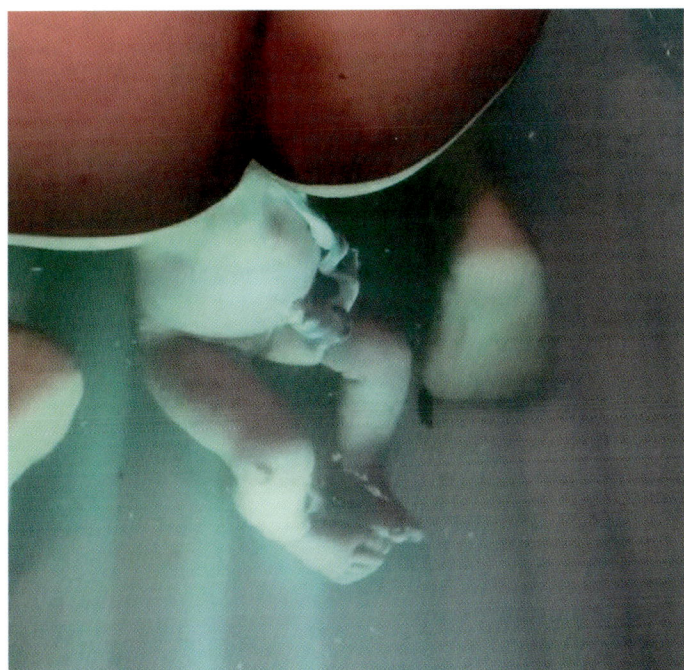 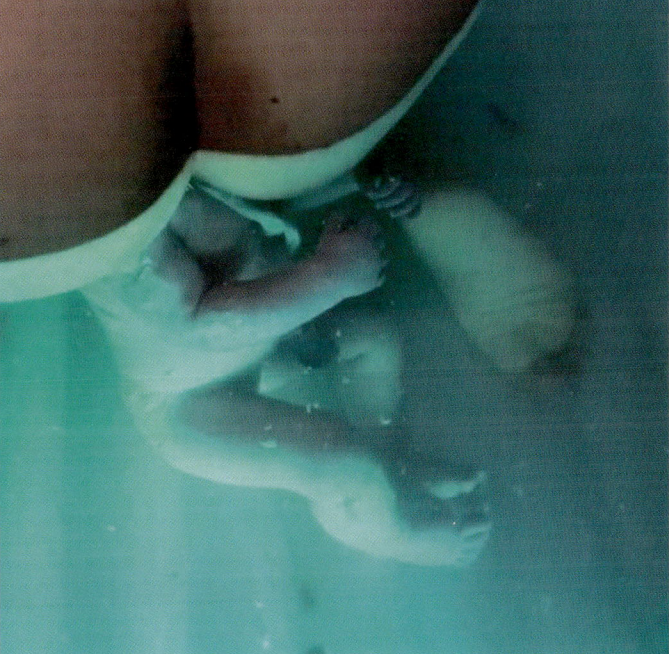

This baby descended oblique and delivered its arms in that same orientation.

Birth of the arms

- The arms are typically not born simultaneously
- There may be a slight rotation to one side as the arm on that side delivers, followed by a slight rotation toward the remaining arm, which helps it deliver
- When the arms deliver, the shoulders are out and the baby is now being supported only by its head
- The perineum may appear hollow at first, but it should soon appear full
- This indicates that the head is properly flexed

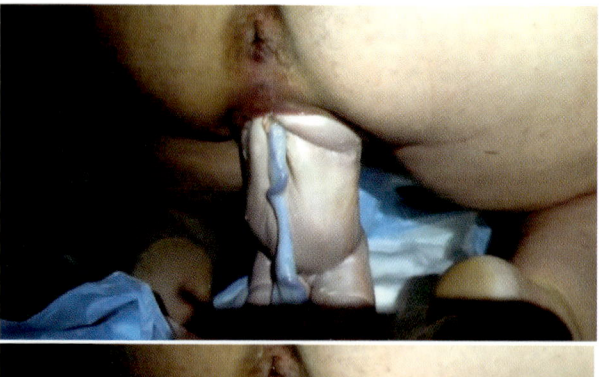

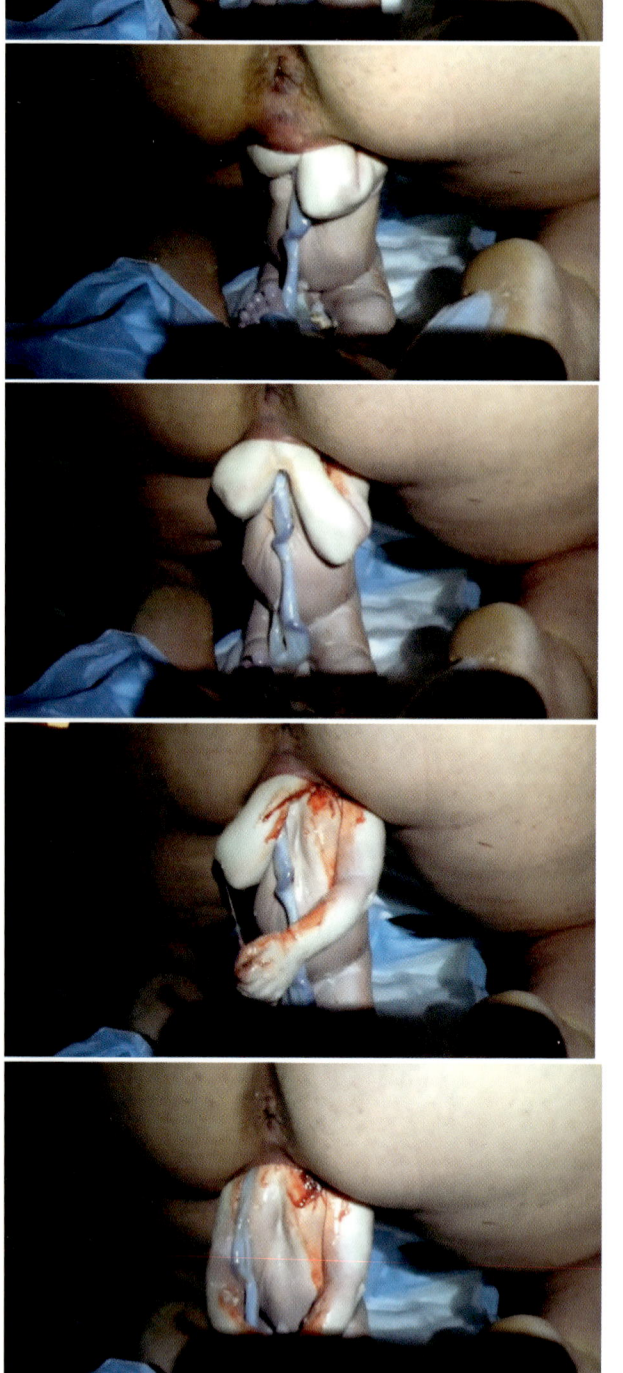

These are the 2 frank breech births we have been studying in this lesson. The baby on the left (Example 1) took several seconds to release the arms, while the baby on the right (Example 2) released both arms within about 2 seconds.

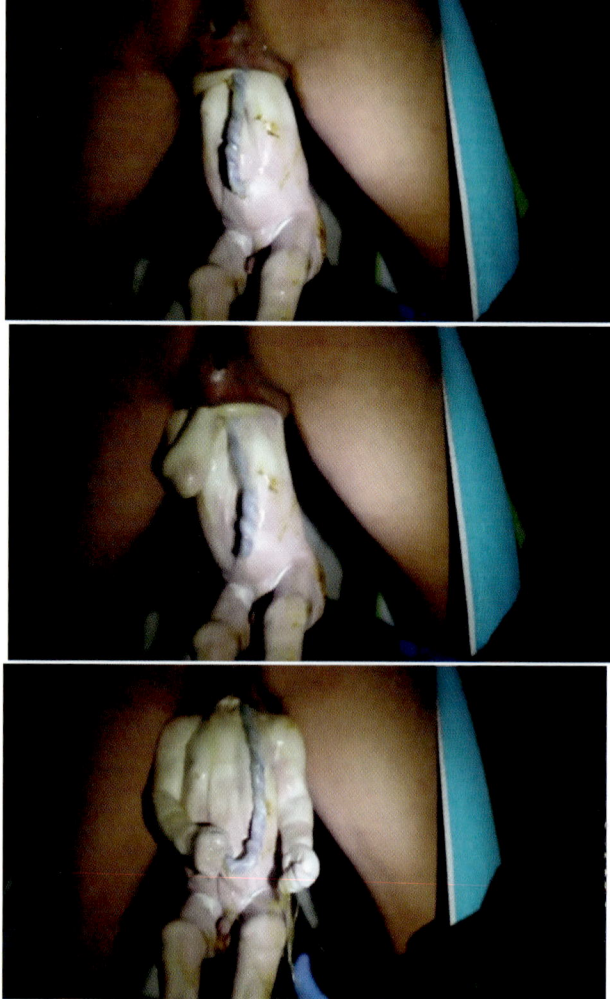

Unlike the legs, arms are not typically born simultaneously. They may be, but there's usually some wiggling and rotating of the shoulders. If the baby is vigorous, it will often pull its own arms out.

Notice that the baby on the left (above) has a deflexed head; the perineum appears hollow and deflated, and it looks as if the baby is looking upward. This baby eventually was assisted with a shoulder press and gluteal lift due to its low tone. (This was a primip birth, and typically they take a bit longer.) The baby on the right (above) already has part of the neck and chin visible behind the perineum. It was vigorous the whole time and fell out a few seconds later. (This was a 2nd-time mom.)

Example 5 cont'd (incomplete breech):

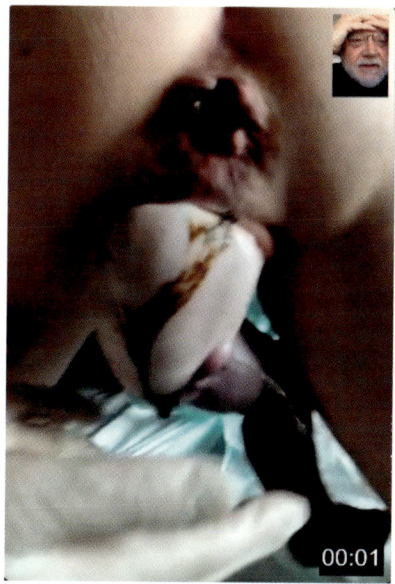
Quick descent

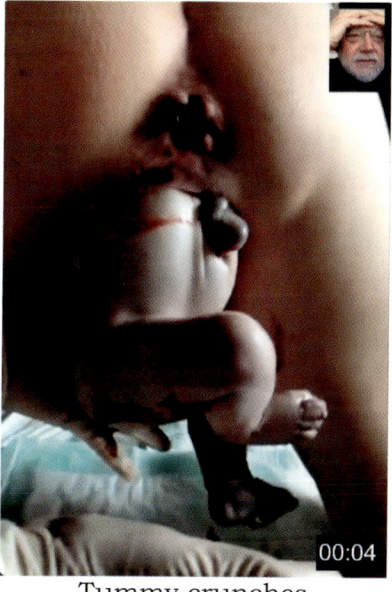
Tummy crunches

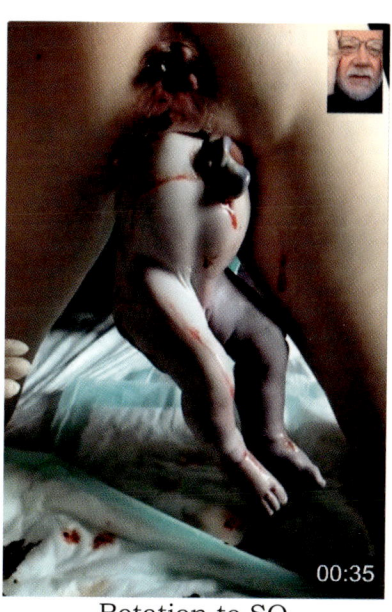
Rotation to SO

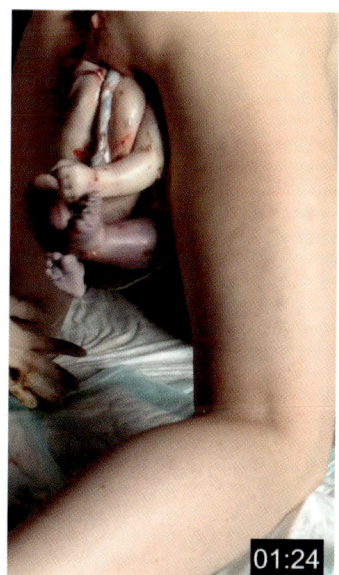
Left arm releases

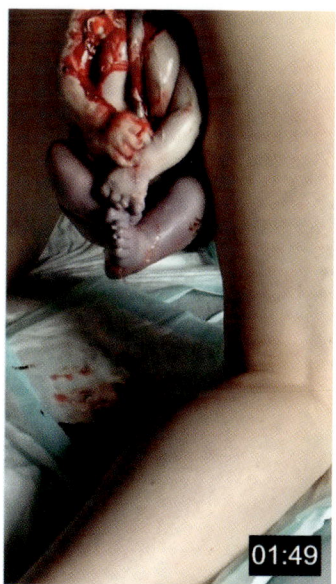
Right arm releases

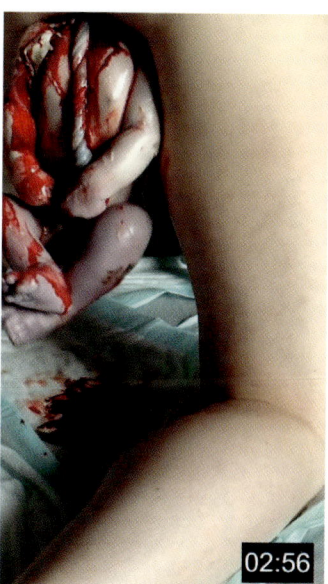
Baby facing SA

Positioning the head

- The head rotates from transverse/oblique to direct A-P as the shoulders deliver. This puts the longest diameter of the head in alignment with the widest diameter of the pelvic outlet.
- The body is now hanging by the head and again, gravity causes the head to extend.
- As before, the baby responds to this extension of its neck by flexing its entire body. Once again, the "tummy crunch" helps flex the head to present the smallest profile to the pelvic outlet.
- Mom may reflexively move backwards and "sit" on the baby. This also helps to flex the head.

Once the arms deliver, that means the shoulders are out, and typically the baby drops a little bit. At this point, when the baby drops, the baby is sacrum anterior. That has the effect of somewhat extending the baby's head. That's why those tummy crunches are so important. A tummy crunch helps the baby pull its head down and get it into the smallest possible profile in order to exit the pelvis.

If you look carefully at the perineum after the shoulders come out, it's probably going to look a little bit hollow. Then after that head flexion occurs, the baby's face comes down behind the perineum and it fills out because there is a nose and a face behind it. The pictures below are from Example 1.

Hollow	Full

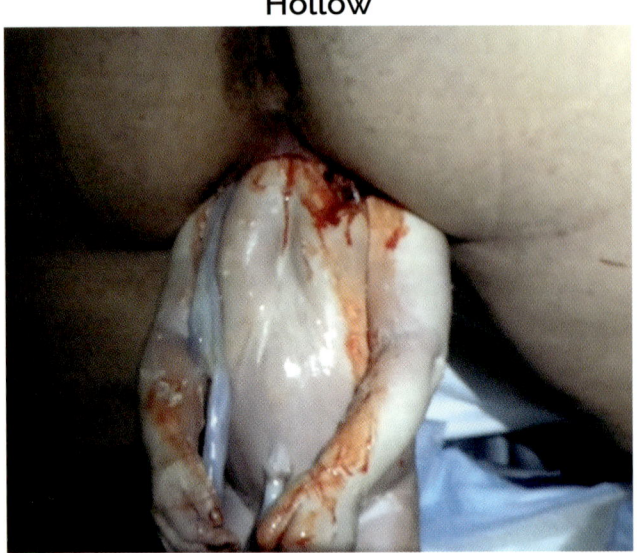 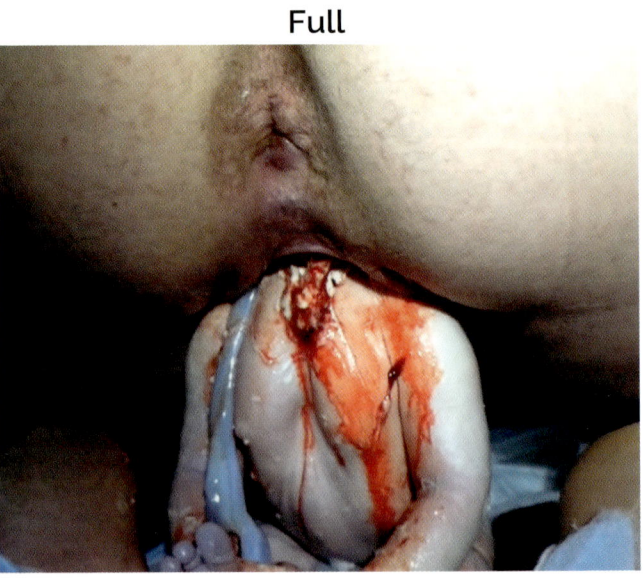

The head rotates from transverse oblique to direct AP (anterior-posterior) as the shoulders deliver. This puts the longest diameter of the head in alignment with the widest diameter of the pelvic outlet.

Head entering the pelvic inlet

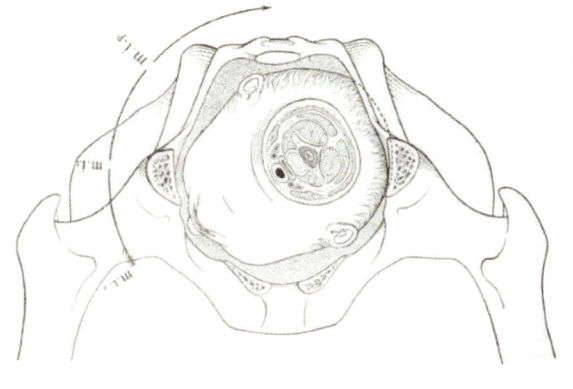

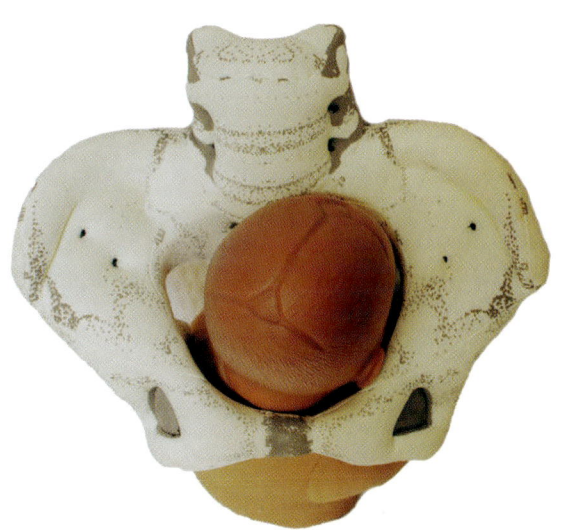

Head descends and rotates to the AP diameter in the pelvic outlet

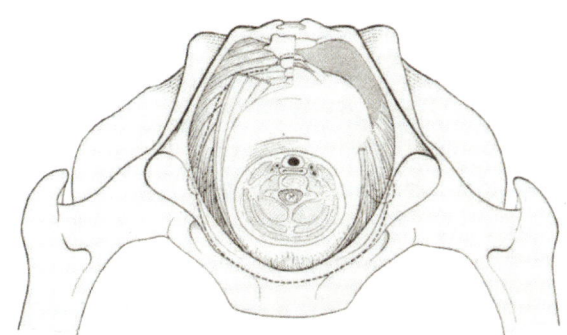

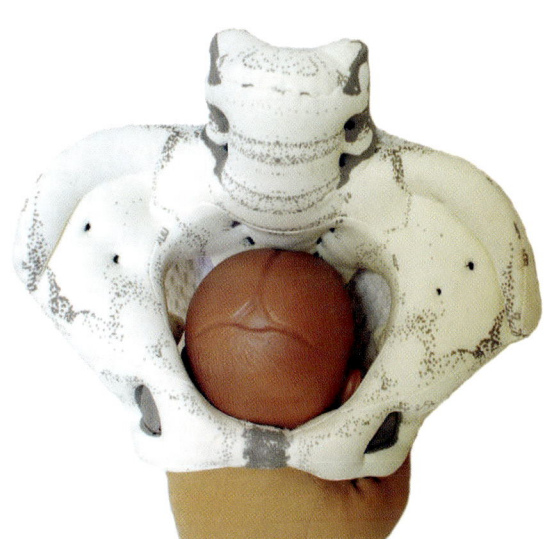

The body is now actually hanging by the head, and gravity is causing the head to extend. The baby responds to that extending of the head by flexing its body and doing a tummy crunch, which you've seen examples of. The tummy crunch, again, helps to flex the head and put the smallest diameter of the head in position to exit the pelvic outlet.

Sometimes in this situation, you will also see a mom on all fours or squatting, and her urge will be to sit down on the baby or squat down on the baby a little bit. That too helps to flex the baby's head. She feels a larger diameter that needs to be there, and by sitting on the baby, squatting on the baby a little bit, it decreases that diameter and decreases the pressure. It feels better to her and helps the baby flex its head.

The impact of flexion

Head flexion is extremely important. This illustration is from a German study. Notice figure A. The baby's head is properly flexed and that presents, on average, a 9.5 cm diameter to the pelvic outlet. That's what you want: the smallest diameter you can come up with. The head in a neutral position is up to 12.5 cm. The head in an extended position is up to 13.5 cm.

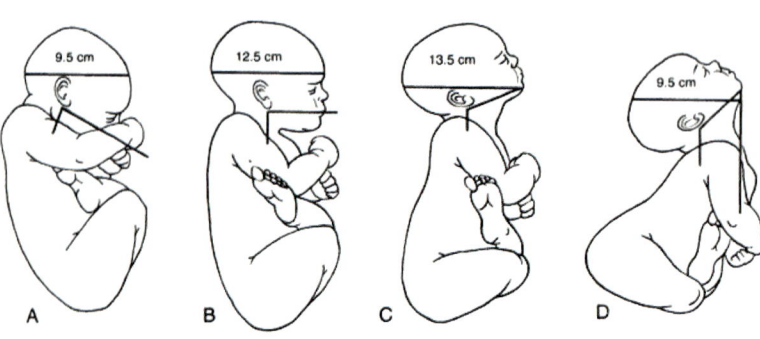

Those are the situations where you are concerned about the head becoming trapped. And fortunately, there are maneuvers to help flex that head, which we'll talk about in another lesson and which Rixa Freeze has already introduced briefly.

In figure D, the baby can also present a small diameter by being hyperextended. However, when the baby's head is hyperextended, that puts the neck at an unsafe angle relative to the head position and is worrisome for traction on the spine. It's also a position that is not normally seen in a neurologically intact baby. I would be concerned that the baby is already compromised if I encountered a hyperextended head.

Birth!

- With the head properly positioned, the perineum should now look full.
- This extension, and the "tummy crunch" that follows, helps to move the head into a properly flexed position.
- Birth of the head should follow shortly after.

In Example 2, the head flexes and releases spontaneously.

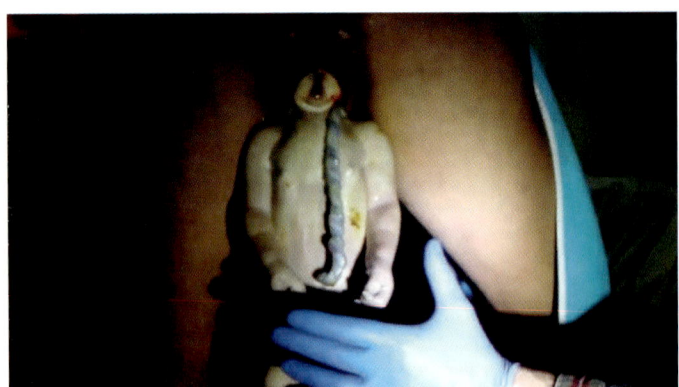
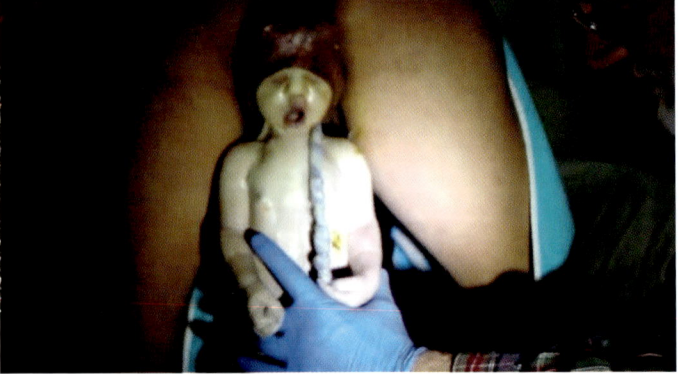

In Example 1 (primip frank breech), the head was assisted with a shoulder press and gluteal lift.

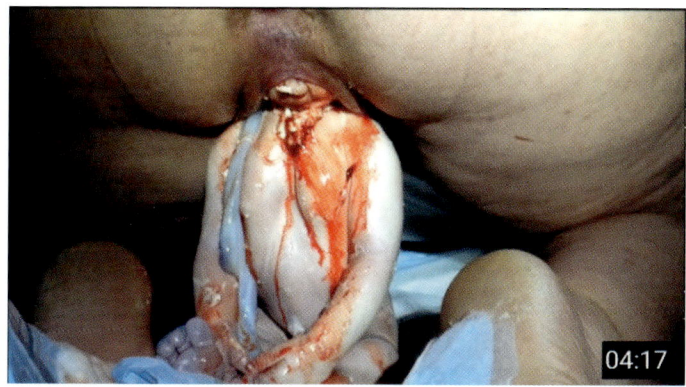 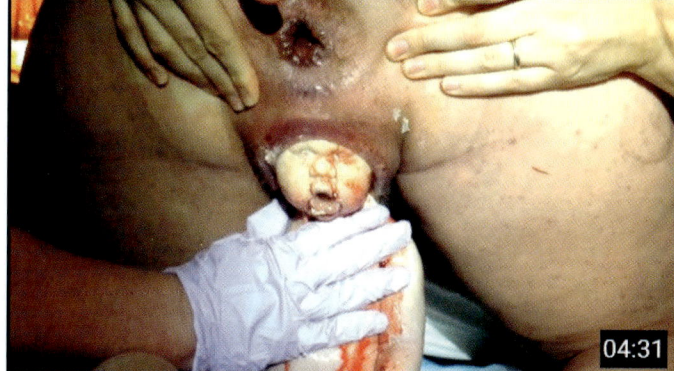

In Example 5 (incomplete breech), the head was assisted by a shoulder press.

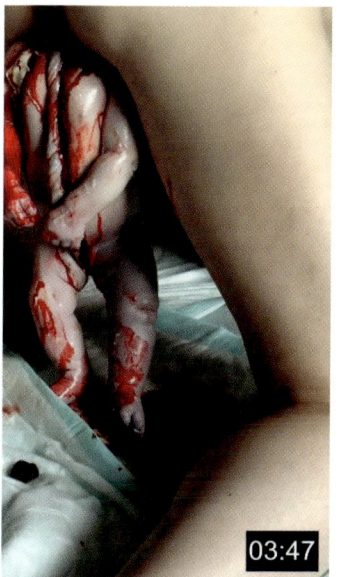 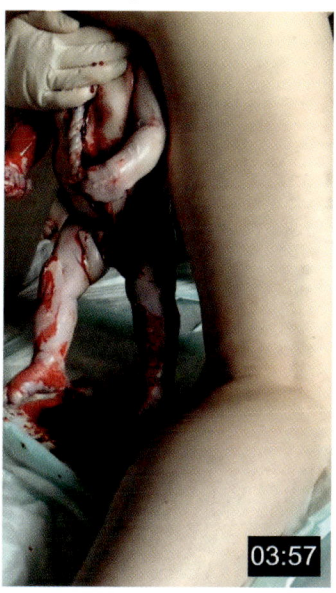 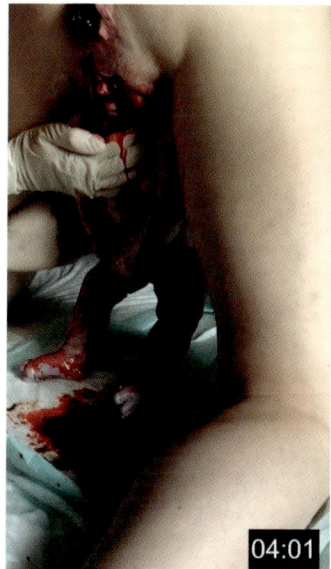 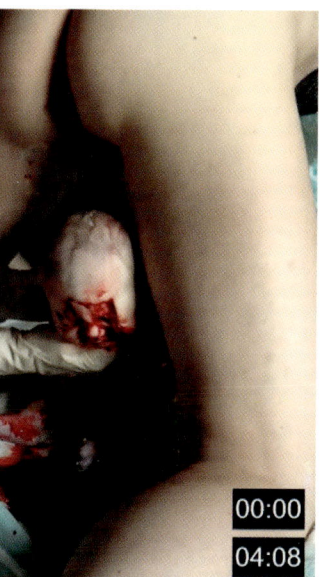

Conclusion

That concludes the lesson on normal breech birth. We've covered normal mechanisms from engagement to rumping to birth with both frank and complete breech presentations. Now hopefully you have a good clinical picture of what normal vaginal breech birth looks like.

In the next lesson, I'm going to switch gears and talk about selection and exclusion criteria for vaginal breech birth. Who are good candidates for vaginal breech birth? I think you'll find it interesting and enlightening.

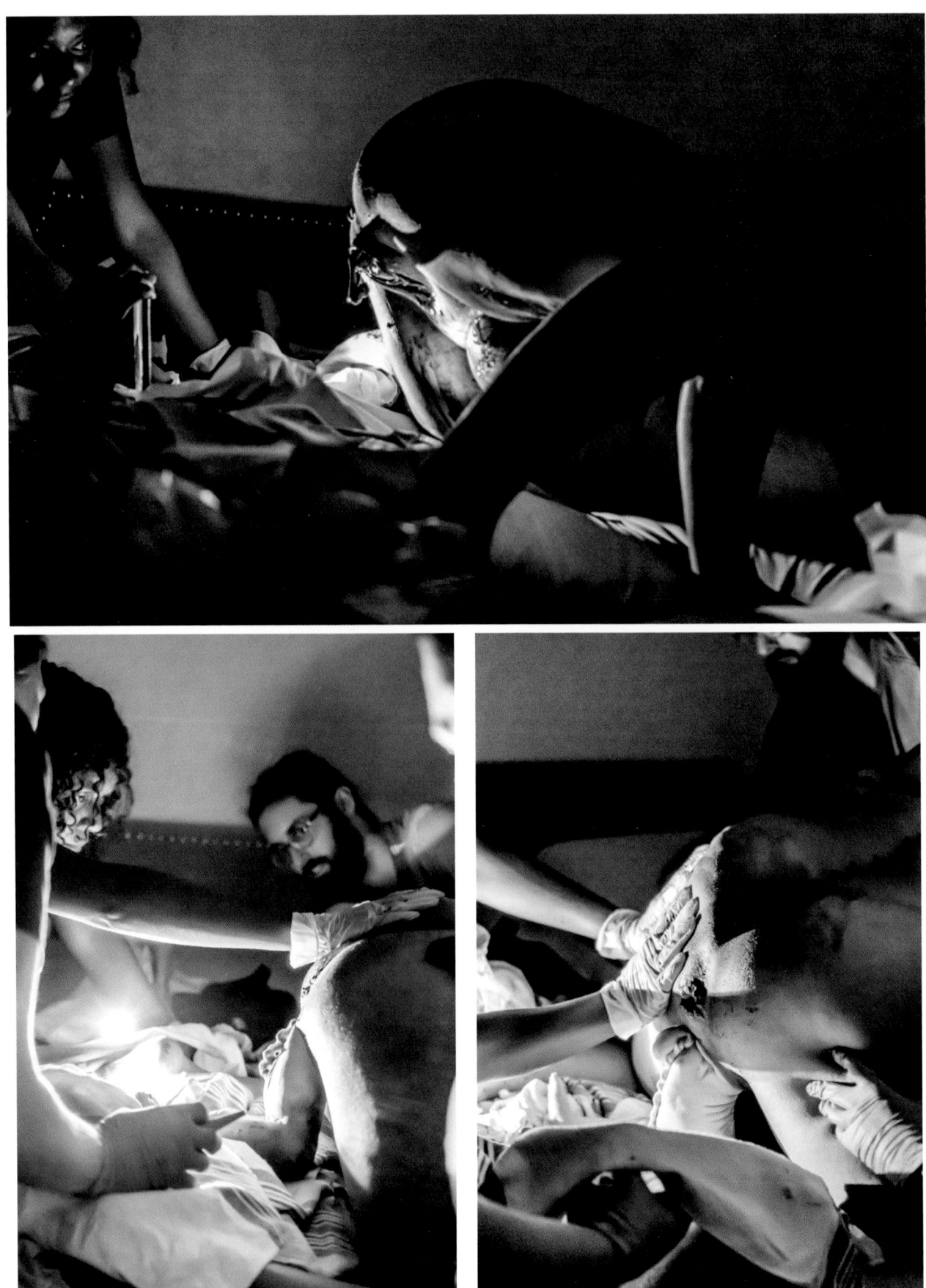

Shatamia Webb, Baby Catcher Birth Center. Undiagnosed frank breech assisted virtually by a BWB clinician

Lesson 9: A Review of Clinical Practice Guidelines
Clinical Aspects, Part 2
By David Hayes, MD

This lesson teaches you how to evaluate the mass of conflicting information on vaginal and surgical breech birth. I hope you can use this information to offer your clients risk-benefit data that accurately reflect the current state of breech birth research. We're going to take a close look at the information offered by various medical societies and groups, where that information comes from, and how research informs or fails to inform that information. If you love reading about research, you're going to enjoy this lesson. If you're not passionate about this topic, you can skim through the main points.

Candidates for vaginal breech birth

Clinical Practice Guidelines: The documents developed to recommend selection and exclusion criteria

Selection criteria: Characteristics recommended to be present to have a vaginal breech birth

Exclusion criteria: Characteristics recommended to be absent to have a vaginal breech birth

Candidates for breech birth are selected or excluded based on a set of criteria: selection criteria and exclusion criteria. Those criteria are developed by professional organizations like the ACOG (USA), the RCOG (UK), the SOCG (Canada), and the Fédération Internationale de Gynécologie et d'Obstetrique (FIGO), which is a European obstetrical group. We're going to spend a lot of time going through this information in some depth, and hopefully you will have something to take to your clients when we're done.

Clinical practice guidelines

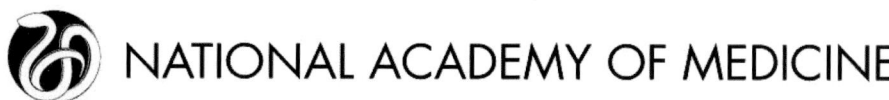 NATIONAL ACADEMY OF MEDICINE

1. Transparent process for CPG development and funding
2. Guidelines for managing conflicts of interest
3. Developed by experts, clinicians, and affected populations
4. Based on systematic reviews of the literature
5. Summary of the strength of the evidence
6. External reviews of all CPG
7. Schedule for updating CPG

1-2. The US National Academy of Medicine offers guidelines for how to construct clinical practice guidelines. The first two concern us less, but they are important nonetheless. As you might imagine, the way medicine is practiced in the United States is of great interest to private companies that develop medical devices or pharmaceuticals. Many of the doctors, experts, and clinicians who practice in the United States also consult for these companies, which makes sense. You want your company's product to be driven by what the medicine says and ideally not vice versa. But obviously, it raises concerns over how much influence people who stand to benefit financially have over the way that medicine is practiced. The first two guidelines are there to say, "Yes, we're going to hold you accountable, especially if you have financial reasons to recommend a certain treatment."

3. Clinical practice guidelines should be developed by **experts**, which makes sense. Obviously, the people who do most of the research and are considered the experts in the field should be people who contribute to any clinical practice guidelines. **Clinicians** are the doctors, midwives, and nurses who use guidelines to inform their work and to inform their clients and who are in the trenches doing the work. So, yes, they should definitely have some input into what those clinical practice guidelines say.

And then finally: **affected populations** should also have a say. In the case of breech birth, that means pregnant women. In an ideal world, there would indeed be pregnant women on guideline creation committees. There is little evidence that that takes place in the US. These are the ideals and unfortunately, we don't always live up to them.

4. Guidelines should be based on **systematic reviews of the literature**. A systematic review of the literature is actually a fairly specific and well-defined thing. It involves considering what your question is, defining the areas of medicine, the fields of research, the countries, the languages, the specific journals that you would intend to use to draw your information from. And then it involves evaluating all that information in a systematic manner. (It's what Rixa Freeze does for Breech Without Borders; she tells me that she has a "high tolerance for boredom" because it is very tedious work!)

5: Guidelines should include a **summary of the strength of the evidence**. That's the labor-intensive part of this process. You classify how good the evidence is on each study you read.

6. Guidelines should include **external reviews** of all clinical practice guidelines. Once you've developed your clinical practice guidelines with your in-house team, it then goes to other people who are familiar with aspects of medicine, such as research, epidemiology, biostatistics, statistical analysis, or research design (all highly technical specialties). You farm it out to these people, who are independent but knowledgeable, to review and give you back their take on what you've done and how good it is.

7. Finally, and very importantly, clinical practice guidelines should always include a **schedule for being updated**. Research doesn't wait. It moves on. Studies are published, and a good study will raise more questions than it answers. Then other people read that research and answer those questions. The current state of knowledge is always changing—hopefully for the better but sometimes for the worse. Obstetrics in particular is full of practices that, instead of advancing, seem to go around in circles.

Classification of evidence levels		Grades of Recommendation	
1 + +	High-quality meta-analyses, systematic reviews of randomised controlled trials or randomised controlled trials with a very low risk of bias	**A**	At least one meta-analysis, systematic reviews or RCT rated as 1 + +, and directly applicable to the target population; or a systematic review of RCTs or a body of evidence consisting principally of studies rated as 1 +, directly applicable to the target population and demonstrating overall consistency of results
1+	Well-conducted meta-analyses, systematic reviews of randomised controlled trials or randomised controlled trials with a low risk of bias		
1–	Meta-analyses, systematic reviews of randomised controlled trials or randomised controlled trials with a high risk of bias	**B**	A body of evidence including studies rated as 2++ directly applicable to the target population, and demonstrating overall consistency of results; orExtrapolated evidence from studies rated as 1++ or 1 +
2 + +	High-quality systematic reviews of case–control or cohort studies or high-qualitycase–control or cohort studies with a very low risk of confounding, bias or chance and ahigh probability that the relationship is causal	**C**	A body of evidence including studies rated as 2+ directly applicable to the target population, and demonstrating overall consistency of results; orExtrapolated evidence from studies rated as 2 + +
2+	Well-conducted case–control or cohort studies with a low risk of confounding, bias or chanceand a moderate probability that the relationship is causal	**D**	Evidence level 3 or 4; orExtrapolated evidence from studies rated as 2+
2–	Case–control or cohort studies with a high risk of confounding, bias or chance and asignificant risk that the relationship is not causal	**Good Practice Points**	
		✓	Recommended best practice based on the clinical experience of the guideline development group
3	Non-analytical studies, e.g. case reports, case series		
4	Expert opinion		

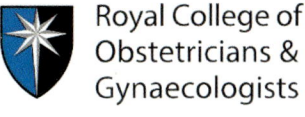

Royal College of
Obstetricians &
Gynaecologists

The RCOG (UK) puts the above chart in every clinical practice guideline they issue, called Green-top Guidelines. These two rating systems inform their clinical practice guidelines. On the left you see classification of evidence levels. All studies identified during the research process are then classified as to the quality of evidence.

The best evidence, according to this column, is "high-quality:" meta-analyses, systematic reviews of randomized controlled trials, or randomized controlled trials with very low risk of bias. As you go down the list and as the ratings go higher, this means that the quality of the evidence is lower.

Then on the right-hand column, we have grades of recommendations. The guideline authors look at the data and examine it closely. They draw their conclusions from it, and they make recommendations. That is done by grading each recommendation. If there is a recommendation that gets an A-grade, that means it drew upon high-quality evidence (a rating of 1 or higher on the left-hand list). We have B-grade recommendations, C-grade recommendations, D-grade recommendations, and then at the bottom, good practice points. Good practice points are basically committee opinions. They are recommended best practice based on the clinical experience of the guideline development group.

Green-top Guideline 20b

Why the RCOG guideline?

- Good example of a well-designed and executed guideline
- Takes into account emerging information and moves guidance toward best practices
- A reasonable starting point for clinicians looking for information

Now we will move ahead to the RCOG (UK) Green-top Guideline #20b. Why the Green-top Guideline? Breech Without Borders is a US-based organization, although we teach around the world. Why are we looking at the RCOG guidelines? It is a good example of a well-designed and well-executed guideline. They are very transparent about their process. The RCOG guideline takes into account emerging information and moves previous guidance toward best practices.

As we go through this guideline, I'm going to point out things that I may or may not agree with. There are going to be recommendations that run counter to some of the research that's currently out there, so I will point those things out. But this guideline, developed in 2017, took what was known at that time and tried to bring practice from where it had been previously up to that level.

Organizational change is hard. Getting doctors to change practices that they've been trained in and that they've been practicing all their life, is hard. I recognize that, and they recognize that. I have to give them credit for dragging the field in the right direction, even if we don't always get there.

And finally, these guidelines are a reasonable starting point for clinicians looking for information. Whether you are attending breech births, or you have breech clients and you want to give them the best information possible, you will likely find the following information very useful.

Let's go ahead and jump into the recommendations of the Green-top Guideline. The first one is as follows:

Women should be informed that planned caesarean section leads to a small reduction in perinatal mortality compared with planned vaginal breech delivery. Any decision to perform a caesarean section needs to be balanced against the potential adverse consequences that may result from this.

A 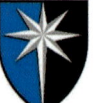 Royal College of Obstetricians & Gynaecologists

Adverse consequences may result from any surgery, actually, not just C-sections. They have good evidence to support that. That's considered an A-grade recommendation and you don't see very many of these A-grade recommendations. That's absolutely correct. Cesarean section does indeed have a lower perinatal mortality risk in a first pregnancy, especially compared to term vaginal breech delivery. There's no question about that.

> Women should be informed that the reduced risk is due to three factors: the avoidance of stillbirth after 39 weeks gestation, the avoidance of intrapartum risks, and the risks of vaginal breech birth and that only the last is unique to a breech baby. **[New 2017]**

B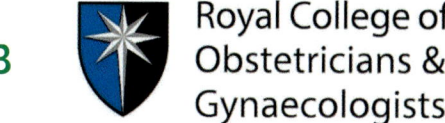

This recommendation was a new addition to the 2017 guidelines. I like this thought process a lot. Basically, they're saying there are three things that increase the risks associated with a vaginal breech birth, but only one of them is unique to breech birth. There are two other things that also increase the risk: a) being pregnant longer than 39 weeks and b) having a vaginal birth regardless of the position of the baby.

> Women should be informed that when planning delivery for a breech baby, the risk of perinatal mortality is approximately 0.5/1000 with a caesarean section after 39+0 weeks of gestation; and approximately 2.0/1000 with planned vaginal breech birth. This compares to approximately 1.0/1000 with planned cephalic birth.

C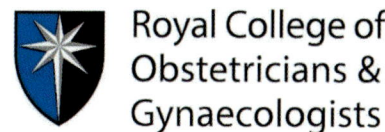

Above, we talked about the avoidance of intrapartum risks, the avoidance of stillbirth after 39 weeks, and the risks of a vaginal breech birth. The additional time being pregnant and the risk of having a vaginal birth of any kind account for the difference between 0.5/1000 and 1.0/1000, which Rixa discussed in an earlier lesson. That's double the risk for any vaginal birth. And then you double the risk again for a planned vaginal breech birth. Only 50% of that risk is due to the baby is breech.

> Selection of appropriate pregnancies and skilled intrapartum care may allow planned vaginal breech birth to be nearly as safe as planned vaginal cephalic birth. **[New 2017]**

C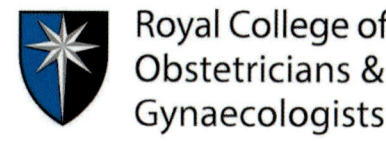

This was a new recommendation in 2017, one I was glad to see. It recognizes the fact that the maneuvers and the management of vaginal breech birth are evolving and undergoing a revolution. What that statement suggests, and what I think the literature suggests, is that once there are enough trained people to do vaginal breech birth and enough data collected on physiological breech birth, there will likely be no difference in mortality rates between vaginal cephalic birth and vaginal breech birth. I agree with this wholeheartedly.

> Women should be informed that planned vaginal breech birth increases the risk of low Apgar scores and serious short-term complications but has not been shown to increase the risk of long-term morbidity. **[New 2017]**

B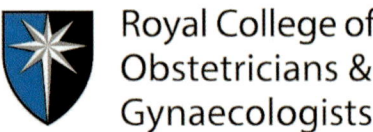

This is another new addition that has solid B-grade evidence supporting it. And yes, it does indeed seem to be the case that there is an increased risk of low Apgar scores. There is an even more increased risk of low Apgar scores of first-time moms, but there has not been shown to be an increased risk in long-term morbidity.

> Clinicians should counsel women in an unbiased way that ensures a proper understanding of the absolute as well as the relative risk of their different options. **[New 2017]**

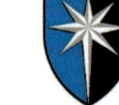 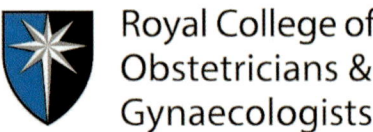

This is not an evidence-based statement. This is a committee opinion statement, as shown by the mortarboard hat on the side. Counseling for informed consent needs to be unbiased, and it needs to be presented honestly. If you counsel women that vaginal breech birth is 4 times more likely to result in the death of the baby compared to a planned C-section, that is an accurate statement—technically. But that reflects only the *relative* risk. It does not reflect the fact that any vaginal birth has at least twice as much relative risk compared to a planned C-section. And it does not reflect the *absolute* risk of any of the three scenarios, which in all three cases is actually very small.

> Women should be informed that planned caesarean section for breech presentation at term carries a small increase in immediate complications for the mother compared with planned vaginal breech birth.

A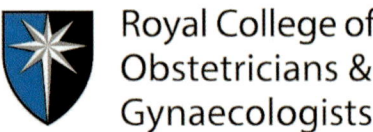

There is a risk of complications for any surgery: post-operative wound infections, hemorrhage, and damaging bowels or bladders. It is simply the nature of surgery or any intervention, for that matter, that it comes with some risk. That risk needs to be communicated to anyone who is making this decision, obviously.

> Women should be informed that maternal complications are least with successful vaginal birth; planned caesarean section carries a higher risk [of maternal complications], but the risk is highest with emergency caesarean section which is needed in approximately 40% of women planning a vaginal breech birth. **[New 2017]**

B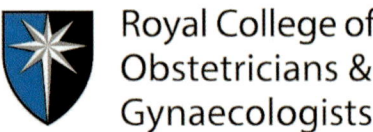

They're saying that 40% of women planning a vaginal breech birth require an emergency cesarean section. There are a number of studies that do not agree with those numbers. Most significantly would be the PREMODA study, which had a successful vaginal birth rate of 71% and an in-labor C-section rate of 29%. In my own experience, 100% of my breech labors so far have ended in vaginal births; these have taken place in hospitals, homes, and in low-resource settings. Several of my highly experienced colleagues have vaginal breech birth rates around 98%. This is not likely for a less experienced provider, but vaginal breech birth rates can be quite high with enough skill and experience.

> Women should be informed that caesarean section increases the risk of complications in future pregnancy, including the risks of opting for vaginal birth after caesarean section, the increased risk of complications of a repeat caesarean section and the risk of an abnormally invasive placenta.

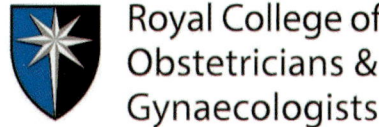

An "abnormally invasive placenta" means placenta accreta, percreta, or increta. This is also a new addition in 2017. I only wish that there had been more information presented about the increased risk for maternal mortality that comes with repeated C-sections, because it is dramatic. I don't believe they have included that fact. But still, what they have included is accurate and useful.

> Women should be given an individualized assessment of the long-term risks of caesarean section based on their individual risk profile and reproductive intentions, and counseled accordingly. **[New 2017]**

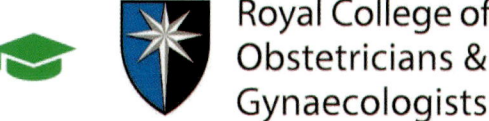

I am so happy to see that statement in any obstetric guidance. I have never seen that sort of information presented in that manner, and I'm very, very pleased to see it. "Individual risk profile" means: what is the particular person's risk for surgery in general? If you're going to have a cesarean section, do you have a clotting disorder? Do you have a pulmonary disorder? Do you have a cardiac disorder? Have you had previous abdominal surgeries? Previous uterine surgeries? There are so many individual characteristics that influence how much risk there is in a surgery.

Up until this point, that seems to have been totally ignored. The phrase "reproductive intentions" assumes that everyone's plans pan out the way that they intended for them to. And we all know life doesn't quite work that way. I think "reproductive lifetime" would be a better target for counseling: *These are the possibilities. You are now X years old; you could have this number of pregnancies and this number of babies. What would be the impact on future pregnancies and babies if you decided to have a vaginal birth or a C-section in this pregnancy?* It has not ever been approached like that, but definitely should be. So that's a wonderful addition.

> Women should be informed that caesarean section has been associated with a small increase in the risk of stillbirth for subsequent babies, although this may not be causal. **[New 2017]**

C 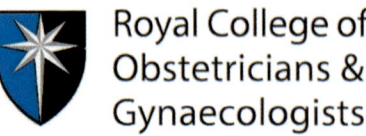 Royal College of Obstetricians & Gynaecologists

This is an accurate statement, but I don't think it goes far enough. At the 2016 Amsterdam Breech Conference, Rixa listened to a researcher, Thomas van den Akker, who calculated the long-term risks for breech birth using Dutch data. He estimated that a breech C-section in the first pregnancy would prevent 24 perinatal deaths from occurring out of 10,000 births. But in the second pregnancy, there would be an excess of 27 perinatal deaths out of 10,000 subsequent births due to the uterine scar (IUFD, uterine rupture, etc.). Everything saved by doing the C-section was lost in the second pregnancy, plus there would be four maternal deaths and many additional cases of SAMM (severe acute maternal morbidity) among those 10,000 women with uterine scars. The downstream consequences of decisions made during a current pregnancy should always be taken into consideration.

Now we're getting to the actual exclusion criteria that the RCOG uses. This is a C-grade recommendation, which acknowledges that the risk factors are not terribly clear and that there's definitely some controversy and disagreement in the field.

> Women should be informed that a higher risk planned vaginal breech birth is expected where there are independent indications for caesarean section and in the following circumstances:
> - Hyperextended neck on ultrasound, High estimated fetal weight, (more than 3.8 kg)
> - Low estimated fetal weight (less than the tenth centile)
> - Footling presentation
> - Evidence of antenatal fetal compromise
>
> **[New 2017]**

C 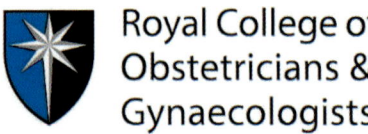 Royal College of Obstetricians & Gynaecologists

"Independent indications for caesarean section" would mean things like a previous uterine surgery or other factors not associated with the breech presentation. Those are the RCOG exclusion criteria. In a moment, I'm going to go into each of those a little bit deeper, in conjunction with looking at some other organizations' exclusion criteria.

> The role of pelvimetry is unclear.

C Royal College of Obstetricians & Gynaecologists

I'm glad to see that statement. Pelvimetry is a method of measuring the size of the pelvis to determine if the pelvis is adequate. The number of things wrong with pelvimetry are really too vast to count. But let's start with the fact that a pelvis is not a static structure. It is flexible. It moves with the mother's movement. It moves with the baby's movement. A measurement of the size of that pelvis at one point in time and in one position does not necessarily give you much information about the size of that pelvis during labor when the mom is mobile. So that's one piece of it.

The other piece is that physicians have been trying to perfect pelvimetry forever. Clinical pelvimetry—where you take your hands and put them inside of the vagina and use your fingers to guess the distance from the sacral promontory to the inferior aspect of the symphysis pubis—is not repeatable. Very few people can do it within any reasonable degree of accuracy.

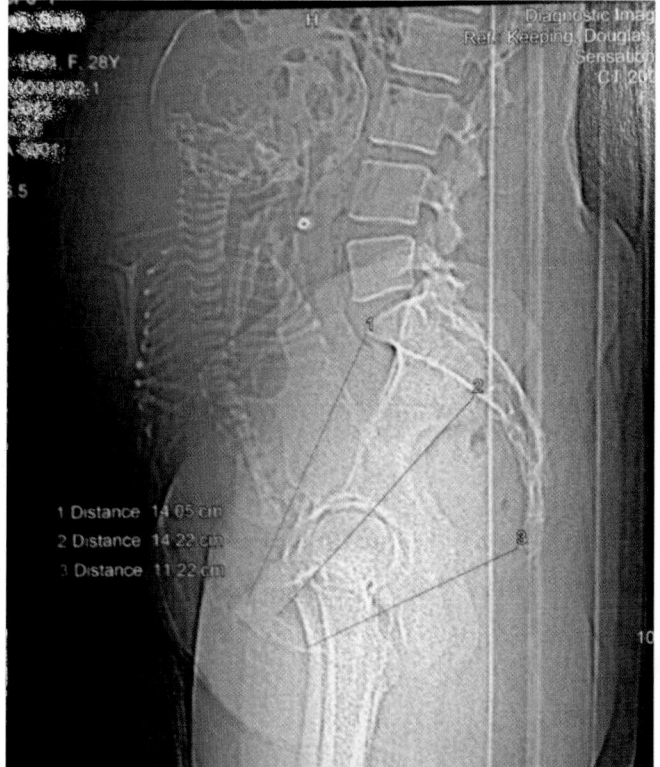 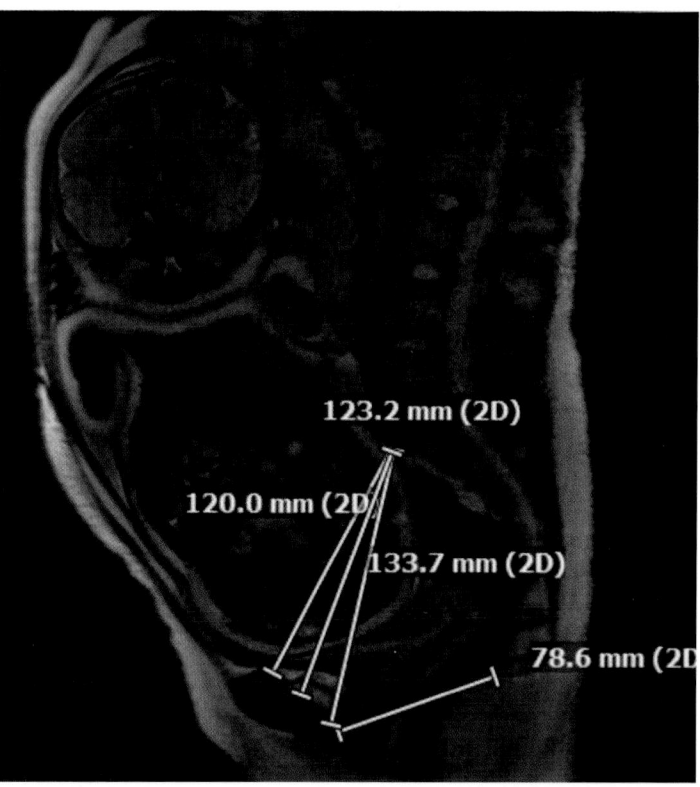

X-ray pelvimetry

MRI pelvimetry, courtesy of Annette Fineberg.
Note the triple nuchal cord on the left

Recognizing the problems with clinical pelvimetry, the medical field has attempted to define pelvimetry by radiologic means since the 1950s or earlier. The first tries at it were with x-rays. Besides the dangers of x-rays, they were unable to determine any benefit from using a certain size pelvis as an exclusion criterion. It did not improve perinatal outcomes to exclude women with certain smaller pelvic measurements and require them all to have C-sections.

When pelvimetry didn't work with x-rays, it was repeated with ultrasound, which has fewer radiologic concerns. But there is no evidence that ultrasound pelvimetry improves outcomes. The same thing has been done with CTs and is currently being attempted with MRIs. In all cases, there is yet to be any significant evidence that radiologic pelvimetry improves perinatal outcomes.

Exclusion criteria

I'm going to focus on the exclusion criteria now from three obstetrical societies: the RCOG (UK), SOGC (Canada), and RANZCOG, which is the Australia and New Zealand obstetrical society. I've collected the exclusion criteria in each of their documents.

Exclusion Criteria	RCOG	SOGC	RANZCOG
Hyperextended head on ultrasound	X		X
EFW > 3800 g		X	X
EFW < 10th percentile	X	X	X
Fetal anomaly (likely to interfere with vaginal birth)		X	X
Any non-frank or non-complete presentation	X		X
Footling presentation	X	X	X
Evidence of antenatal fetal compromise	X		
Lack of recent ultrasound		X	
Cord presentation		X	X
Clinically inadequate pelvis (CT not required; poor labor progress)		X	X

Hyperextended head on ultrasound: I both disagree and agree. If you have a fetus in utero that has a *persistently* hyperextended head, that strongly suggests that the baby is neurologically compromised. Why? Babies don't usually have persistently hyperextended heads; they like to remain flexed in a fetal position. However, a hyperextended head on a single ultrasound is a static image of something dynamic happening in the mother's womb. I think it's a little extreme to use a single ultrasound finding as a contraindication to vaginal birth. Hyperextension should be consistently verified through multiple ultrasounds before being used to exclude VBB.

EFW > 3800 g: All three organizations agree that 3800+ g babies should be excluded. The current literature does not support that recommendation; we will talk about that later in this lesson.

Fetal anomaly (likely to interfere with vaginal birth): That's from SOGC and RANZCOG. I don't want to be overly picky, but that is a vaginal birth exclusion criterion, not unique to vaginal breech birth. A fetal anomaly likely to interfere with birth is likely to interfere with any birth *whether it's breech or cephalic.*

Any non-frank or non-complete breech presentation: This is casting a wide net for RANZCOG. "Any non-frank or non-complete breech" is likely to leave out breeches that would be considered for a vaginal birth in other non-RANZCOG countries—such as France, Belgium, and Norway. I'm going to go past that issue and come back to it briefly in a moment. Rixa also addresses it in her nomenclature lesson.

Footling presentation: All three of them eliminated footling presentation. Almost any textbook or most research that you read on footling presentation says that footling presentations have a higher rate of cord prolapse. So, of course, nobody needs to even look further. *We have a higher rate of cord prolapse; therefore, we must do C-sections to prevent poor outcomes.*

However, the evidence suggests that nonfrank breeches with cord prolapse don't tend to have compromised cords. It's one thing to say that there's an increased risk of cord prolapse, ergo, we must do a cesarean section. If you say there's an increase in cord prolapse, which results in an increase in neonatal morbidity and mortality, then you've got a case I can listen to. But there's no evidence that nonfrank cord prolapse leads to worse outcomes. Just because we're used to thinking of cord prolapse as a dangerous thing doesn't imply that it always is.

With a footling breech, the torso has a narrower anterior-posterior dimension. And you have a less uniform dilating cone, so that there's much less of an opportunity for the cord to get compressed between the baby and the pelvis. It appears that nonfrank breeches, with their increased rate of cord prolapse, do not have an associated increased rate of perinatal mortality or morbidity. We need to reexamine some of our assumptions on that. On the other hand, cord prolapses with frank breeches are definitely associated with an increase in morbidity and mortality.

Evidence of antenatal fetal compromise: Absolutely, 100%, no question, no argument. I will say that hyperextended head on ultrasound is apparently intended to be that evidence of antenatal fetal compromise. Whether that's accurate or not was my question. That was my issue with that first recommendation.

Lack of a recent ultrasound: Lack of a recent ultrasound should not be sufficient to exclude someone from a vaginal breech birth. The impetus for requiring an ultrasound is to verify that the fetal head is not extended. In an otherwise normal pregnancy, assessment of fetal condition (fetal heart rate and pattern, fetal activity counts) should be sufficient to infer that the fetus maintains a normal pattern of flexion, which may include intermittent, but not persistent, extension. There is no evidence that excluding women from attempting a vaginal birth on the basis of a single ultrasound depicting head extension in an otherwise normal fetus improves outcomes in any way.

Cord presentation: I find it fascinating that RCOG doesn't have that in there. Typically, prolapsed cords are considered an emergency situation. In certain types of breech, prolapsed cords are more common. But there's interesting literature that suggests that cord prolapses are not always going to result in a compromised cord, and therefore don't always necessarily require emergency management. Rixa also addressed this in her nomenclature lesson.

Clinically inadequate pelvis (CT not required; poor labor progress): I've already given my opinion on the idea of a clinically inadequate pelvis, so I won't belabor the point here. **CT not required:** When saying that a CT is not required, I think they're giving cover to people who believe there's a clinically adequate pelvis but don't have access to a CT. But what about **poor labor progress**?

We commonly allow labor to go on in cephalic births for a very long time: 12 hours, 24 hours, 36 hours. The suggestion here is that long labors; or labors with pauses, plateaus, or stalls; are not appropriate for breech-presenting babies. One advocate for this position was Mary Cronk, a UK midwife with extensive breech experience.

Please note that there is vigorous debate among physiological breech providers about whether breech labors should progress differently than cephalic. I have not seen sufficient evidence, either in the literature or in my clinical experience, that extended labors in breech presentations have any worse outcomes than extended labors in cephalic presentations. I don't think it's justified to hold breech to a higher standard than you're holding cephalic birth, and I'll leave it at that.

Next, we're going to go through some literature that directly contradicts some of the information that is in these guidelines. But before we move on, I want to point out something that you all may have been wondering, and that is: where is ACOG? Why did I not include ACOG's breech practice guideline in our review?

Where's ACOG?

Org	# References	Year
RCOG	**76**	2017
SOGC	**82**	2019
ACOG	**16**	2006 (2018: ECV)

There is no ACOG practice guideline for breech birth, vaginal or otherwise. What we have is the ACOG Committee Opinion #745. Committee opinions, as we've already talked about, are a group of experts sitting around and creating guidelines where there is not the literature available to pull good information from. That's clearly not the case with breech birth, and so it raises the question: why is there no ACOG practice guideline for breech birth?

I want to point out that the Green-top Guideline (RCOG) did a systematic review, which included 76 references when it was done. It was published in 2017 and is usually updated every 3 years. In its most recent guideline update, SOGC included 6 more studies published between 2017 and 2019, for a total of 82. In contrast, ACOG has cited 16 references *total*.

ACOG Committee Opinion #745:
July 2006/July 2018
16 references

Committee Opinion #745 was issued in 2006 and updated in 2018. Of the 16 total references, 6 were added in 2018, of which 4 address ECV only. Three references do not address breech birth outcomes; 4 references are about the Term Breech Trial data; and 4 references address non-TBT studies.

Four papers added in 2018 address ECV only:

1. **ACOG Practice Bulletin No. 161** (2016). External cephalic version.
2. **Hofmeyr, 2015:** Cochrane review on ECV for breech presentation at term
3. **Goetzinger, 2011.** Article about regional anesthesia and ECV.
4. **Magro-Malosso, 2016:** Article about regional anesthesia and ECV.

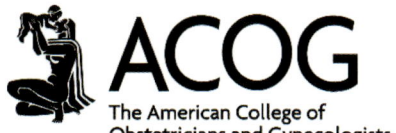

One paper added in 2018 looks at the Cochrane Database findings on term breech

1. **Hofmeyr, 2015.** Planned CS for term breech delivery.

Three papers provide no data on breech birth outcomes:

1. **Martin, 2003.** US Vital Statistics Report for 2022
2. **Lavin, 2004.** Survey of faculty attitudes toward VBB
3. **Kotaska, 2004.** Methodologic critique of the TBT

There were three papers that provided no data on breech outcomes. **Martin 2003** is just the US Vital Statistics Report. That was their source for statistical information on the rate of C-sections. **Lavin 2004** did a survey of faculty attitudes toward vaginal breech birth.

> Even in academic medical centers where faculty support for teaching vaginal breech delivery to residents remains high, there may be insufficient volume of vaginal breech deliveries to adequately teach this procedure. (citing Lavin 2004)

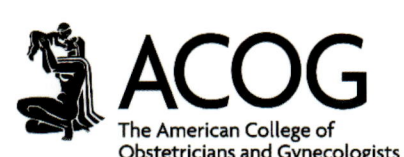

Let me comment about the above statement from C.O. #745. Having been a resident during the time in which the Term Breech Trial was released and during which Lavin published those results, I strongly question if there is an insufficient volume of vaginal breech deliveries to adequately teach this procedure.

And then the last one of the three, **Kotaska 2004**, is a methodological critique of the Term Breech Trial. It's very well written. It's worth a read if you're interested in this topic. Kotaska points out that the rate of breech presentation is about **4%** in the US at term. In contrast, the rate of cesarean-hysterectomy in the USA is **0.12%.** A cesarean-hysterectomy is a considerably more difficult surgery than a hysterectomy or a cesarean section alone.

There are roughly **33 times more breeches than cesarean-hysterectomies** to deal with. Yet every obstetrician in the country is expected to know how to do a cesarean-hysterectomy. You would not be considered adequately enough trained to get hospital privileges if you don't know how to do a cesarean-hysterectomy. It's disingenuous to then try and claim that residents are unable to get enough experience to learn how to do breeches.

Four papers from TBT data:

1. **Hannah, 2000:** The Term Breech Trial
2. **Whyte, 2004:** Outcomes of children at 2 years. "Planned cesarean delivery is not associated with a reduction in risk of death or neurodevelopmental delay in children at 2 years of age."
3. **Hannah, 2004:** Outcomes of mothers at two years. "Maternal outcomes at 2 years postpartum are similar after cesarean section and planned vaginal birth for the singleton breech fetus at term."
4. **Su, 2004.** "The increased risk of a composite measure of perinatal and neonatal morbidity and mortality between planned C/S and planned BB was greatest during labor (RR 0.14 p<0.001) and much less during birth (RR 0.37, P=0.03)."

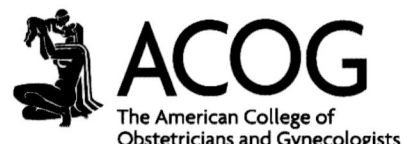

The next 4 papers in C.O. #745 are all from the Term Breech Trial.

Hannah 2000: that is the Term Breech Trial, which randomized 2,000 women to either VBB or CS.

Whyte 2004: they looked at the outcomes of Term Breech Trial children at 2 years of age, so it's data from the same study 2 years after the birth. Their conclusion was that by 2 years of age, any differences in mortality or morbidity were erased. The big outcome of the Term Breech Trial (significantly better outcomes after CS than after VBB) disappeared when the data was reexamined at 2 years of age.

Then there's **Hannah 2004**. This was the outcome of mothers at 2 years after the Term Breech Trial. They're saying there was not a significant difference in vaginal pain and urinary incontinence and abdominal pain from surgical adhesions, those kinds of things.

I find that questionable, just intuitively. Based on a lot of other research we have about long-term outcomes from cesarean surgeries and just abdominal surgeries in general, I question those conclusions. It is also worth noting that they looked at maternal outcomes, but they did not look at maternal morbidity and mortality with the next pregnancies. Granted, the mothers were only 2 years postpartum, but people do get pregnant less than 2 years postpartum. I think what they *didn't* include in their data is as telling as what they did.

And finally, **Su 2004**. They are saying that avoiding birth has far less impact than avoiding labor. That is counter intuitive. If breech *birth* were dangerous, you would not expect to see that finding. That does not support the position that breech birth is inherently dangerous. They're saying that the danger is from letting people with breeches *labor*.

But let's assume for a moment that this is a legitimate finding. If you go back to the first recommendation of the Green-top Guideline, when they were talking about the three contributors to neonatal morbidity and mortality, they referred to avoiding post-39 week morbidity and mortality, avoiding intrapartum events not specifically related to breech, and then avoiding intrapartum events relating to breech.

This finding suggests that the actual process of labor somehow contributes more to the perinatal mortality and morbidity than the actual birth itself, which is incredibly counterintuitive. I'll leave that there for now.

Four non-TBT studies:

1. **Reitberg, 2005.** Dutch national registry retrospective study.
   - pVBB vs pCS before and after TBT
   - CS rate increased from 50% to 80%
   - Perinatal mortality decreased from 0.35% to 0.18%

2. **Alarab, 2004.** Irish single center retrospective study
   - Outcomes from strict selection criteria at Dublin Maternity Hospital
   - < 3800 g, < 41 weeks, no induction/augmentation, low threshold for CS
   - Of 641 breeches, 54% pre-labor CS, 23% in-labor CS, 23% VBB

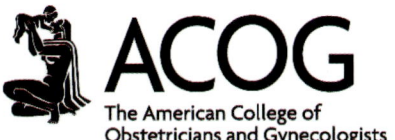

3. **Guiliani, 2002.** Australian single center retrospective study.
   - pVBB vs pCS prior to TBT (1993-1999).
   - No perinatal or neonatal deaths, no cerebral palsy, no difference in developmental delay
4. **Berhan & Haileamlak, 2016:** Meta-analysis of pCS vs pVBB. **(added 2018)**

At this point we have looked at 12 of the 16 references. Of the 16, there are only 4 non-TBT related studies about term breech outcomes considered in C.O. #745.

One was **Reitberg 2005**, a Dutch retrospective study from a national birth registry. It studied planned vaginal breech birth versus planned cesarean section both before and after the Term Breech Trial. They found that breech C-sections increased from 50% to 80%. During this same time, the dependent variable was perinatal mortality, which decreased from 0.35% to 0.18%, likely because of the increase in C-sections. That's one study supportive to the TBT findings.

Second study: **Alarab 2004** is an Irish single center retrospective study from the Dublin Maternity Hospital. They went back through their data and found something different from Reitberg's conclusions. They argued that you can still do breech births with strict guidelines. Their selection criteria were as follows: estimated fetal weight < 3800 g, maximum 41 weeks of gestation, and no induction or augmentation. If you went past 41 weeks with your breech, then you didn't have the option. They specifically noted that they had a "low threshold for a C-section." Of 641 breeches, there were 54% who had pre-labor C-sections, so they did not meet the strict selection criteria. 23% had in-labor C-sections, which left them with a 23% vaginal breech birth rate. Having 23% of your population successfully have a vaginal breech birth is not a strong recommendation for their approach.

And the third one, **Giuliani 2002**, is an Australian single center retrospective study. They looked at planned vaginal breech birth versus planned C-section, all prior to the Term Breech Trial. To give you the timeline here, in 2002, which was 2 years after the Term Breech Trial came out, these people had gone back through their 1993-1999 data. A lot of people in Europe and other countries were scratching their heads about the Term Breech Trial because it offered results that they weren't seeing in their centers. Sure enough, they looked back at their pre-Term Breech Trial data, and they found no perinatal neonatal deaths, no cerebral palsy, and no difference in developmental delays.

Finally, there was one new study added in 2018 about vaginal breech birth by **Berhan & Haileamlak 2015**, a meta-analysis that calculated an estimated risk of perinatal mortality of 3/1000 for pVBB and 0.5/1000 for pCS. This is close to the RCOG estimates of 2/1000 and 0.5/1000, respectively. This meta-analysis is referenced in lessons 3 and 4.

So those are the studies that the ACOG Committee on Obstetric Practice chose to make their case for failing to promote training and for supporting the cessation of breech birth and the deskilling of breech birth providers.

This comes from the ACOG Committee Opinion recommendations:

> The decision regarding the mode of delivery should consider patient wishes and the experience of the health care provider.

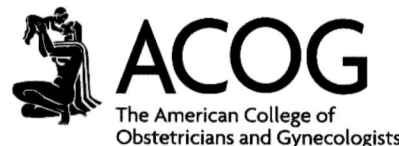

Okay, fair enough.

> Obstetrician-gynecologists and other obstetric care providers should offer external cephalic version as an alternative to planned cesarean for a woman who has a term single term breech fetus, desires a planned vaginal delivery of a vertex-presenting fetus and has no contraindications.

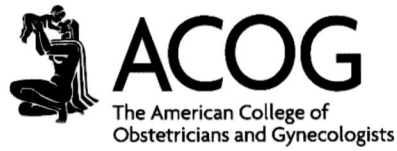

They of course don't offer any contraindications, which is probably a probably good thing. They just throw that statement out there and say, "External cephalic version should be attempted only in settings in which cesarean delivery services are readily available." I have always done ECVs in my office (outside of the hospital) under direct ultrasound. I have never had a complication or hospital transfer after ECV, so I think that that is an unnecessary restriction.

That recommendation probably has something to do with the fact that external cephalic version has changed fairly dramatically. They now give tocolytic pharmaceuticals (uterine relaxants). They now strongly recommend epidural anesthesia, which makes it more comfortable for the mom, but it also lowers the mom's blood pressure and may not give the baby as much oxygen reserves as it might need.

> Planned vaginal delivery of a term singleton breech fetus may be reasonable under hospital-specific protocol guidelines for eligibility and labor management.

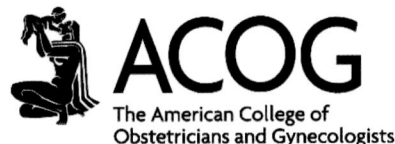

Where do they anticipate that hospitals will draw these protocol guidelines from, if not from ACOG? To me, it is the height of absurdity to assume that a group of obstetricians and a local hospital is better equipped to do a systematic review of the literature and create a policy that reflects that literature, when ACOG themselves have failed to do so.

> If a vaginal breech delivery is planned, a detailed informed consent should be documented—including the risk that perinatal or neonatal mortality or short-term serious neonatal morbidity may be higher than if a cesarean delivery is planned.

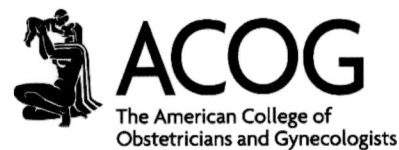

Is that adequate informed consent? They specify mentioning morbidity and mortality differences between a vaginal breech birth and a cesarean breech birth. Does the counseling for vaginal cephalic birth require this language in it? I would submit to you that it does not.

I've never seen a consent form that said: "If you come into our hospital to have a vaginal delivery, you have to understand that the risk of your baby dying is twice as high than if you had a C-section." We as a society have chosen to accept a perinatal mortality rate of 1/1000 for vaginal cephalic births over a C-section perinatal mortality rate of 0.5/1000. It seems very disingenuous to include that relative risk information for vaginal breech birth versus breech cesarean delivery and not for vaginal cephalic birth versus cephalic cesarean delivery.

In sum, ACOG is missing true clinical practice guidelines for breech. We would be in a much better place if ACOG were to follow the process recommended by the National Academy of Medicine, creating well-researched and consistently updated guidelines as other countries have done.

The literature

Macharey 2017: Finnish national registry retrospective case-controlled study

- Subjects were all planned VBBs between 2005-2014
- Compared births with any adverse outcomes against those with normal outcomes
- Adverse perinatal outcomes were associated with fetal growth restriction, oligohydramnios, previous CS delivery, gestational diabetes, nulliparity, and epidural anesthesia.

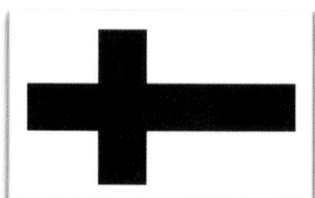

We're going to move on and consider a couple of studies that have come out since the 2017 RCOG guidelines. One of them, **Macharey 2017**, is a nationwide Finnish retrospective case control study. They went back and looked at all of their vaginal breech birth outcomes between 2005 and 2014. Now, this is a population study, and that's important because it means this is not a small sample from which we are inferring things about the general population. This is the *whole population of Finland*—to the extent we can assume that Finnish pregnant women respond and have outcomes that are similar to pregnant women in the rest of the world. There may be some question about that. This should be more widely applicable than many studies, based on that criterion alone.

The subjects were all planned vaginal breech births between 2005 and 2014. They compared those that had any adverse outcomes with those that had normal outcomes. Then they went through their charts and extracted all of the comorbidities: the complicating factors in their pregnancies and labors and births. This is what they found to be associated with adverse outcomes in vaginal breech birth:

1. **Fetal growth restriction**. Fetal growth restriction implies that a baby may or may not be neurologically intact. That's one issue. In addition, asymmetric growth restriction (very small trunk and very large head) is a phenomenon where, due to poor placentation, typically for the duration of the pregnancy, the baby's developing body invests all of its available resources in making the brain work (see the photos below). You tend to have a normal-sized brain and normal-sized upper torso, and the growth restriction is limited to the trunk and lower extremities. In that case, obviously, there would be concern about whether the aftercoming fetal head was the biggest part to come out. There's some suggestion in the literature that there's an increase in perinatal morbidity and mortality from asymmetrically growth restricted babies. Asymmetrical IUGR comprises 70-80% of all IUGR diagnoses.

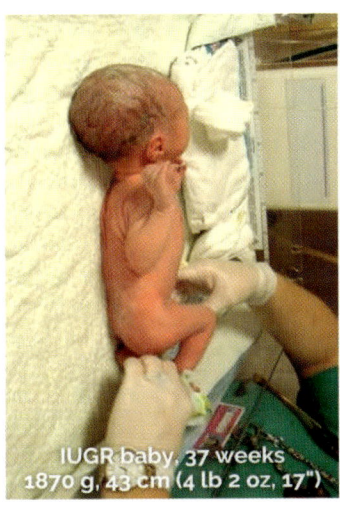
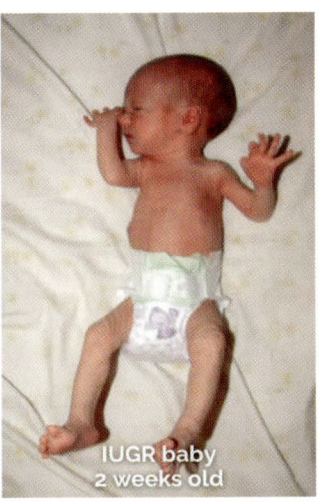
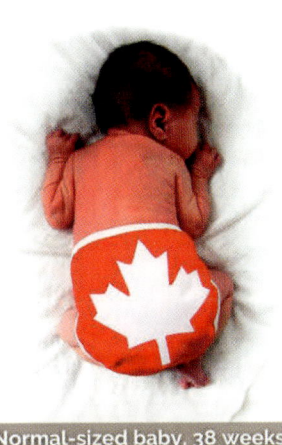
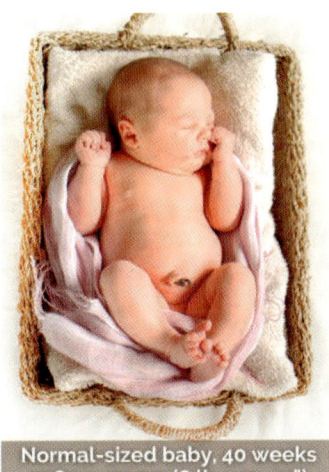

IUGR baby, 37 weeks
1870 g, 43 cm (4 lb 2 oz, 17")

IUGR baby
2 weeks old

Normal-sized baby, 38 weeks
3150 g, 49.5 cm (7 lb, 19.5")

Normal-sized baby, 40 weeks
3760 g, 53 cm (8 lb 4 oz, 21")

2. **Oligohydramnios**: with oligohydramnios, there's a concern that something may be neurologically not intact. Certainly, that doesn't apply to everyone with oligohydramnios. Some of them are just dehydrated, but they found oligohydramnios to be correlated with adverse outcomes.

3. Also, **previous cesarean deliveries**, we've already talked about and is no big shock at all. The more C-sections you have, the worse the outcomes for future pregnancies are going to be for mother and baby.

4. **Gestational diabetes:** again, not a surprise. Babies of mothers who have gestational diabetes, particularly if it's not well-controlled, tend to have worse outcomes than babies that don't. It's not particularly surprising that they would have worse outcomes in a breech presentation as well.

5. **Nulliparity**: I don't know other recent data that suggests nullips have worse outcomes, although it certainly may be out there. They certainly have a higher C-section rate, and I think that's a failure of the system as much as anything. But to the extent that there's an increase in adverse outcomes associated with the first-time moms, it also applies as much to vaginal *cephalic* birth as it does to vaginal breech birth.

5. Finally, which I'm really happy to see, **epidural anesthesia**. There are many studies, generally done by anesthesiologists, which suggest that epidural anesthesia does not result in worse outcomes. As a practitioner, I have seen way too many women get an epidural, drop their blood pressure and crash the baby, and we end up going for a C-section. You're never going to convince me that epidural anesthesia does not increase the length of labor, does not increase perinatal morbidity and mortality, and does not increase C-section rates. Particularly in physiological breech birth, labor and birth are a collaboration between the mom and the baby. The baby makes its difficulties known by getting stuck in places that cause exceptional amounts of pain, and the pain is specific and localized. Moms that can feel that and are mobile enough to respond to it can relieve that pain, which also relieves the obstruction that caused it. It's a very collaborative process that is severely disrupted by epidural anesthesia.

Jennewein 2018: German single center retrospective cohort study

- Subjects were all planned VBBs in Goethe University Hospital between 2004-2016
- Compared outcomes of babies < 3.8 kg at birth with those ≥ 3.8 kg.
- Morbidity was not significant between the groups (< 3.8 kg 1.8%, ≥ 3.8 kg 2.6%)
- Babies weighing ≥ 3.8 kg were significantly more likely to be delivered by CS (OR 1.57, P=0.0001)
- There was no difference in maternal birth injury among women who delivered vaginally

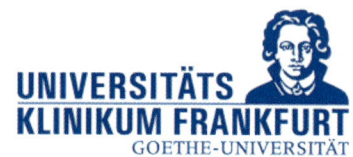

Next we will look at **Jennewein 2018**, a German single center retrospective cohort study. This is, in fact, Frank Louwen's clinic and lab at Frankfurt, where they do large numbers of upright breech births. The subjects of this study were all planned vaginal breech births at Goethe University Hospital between 2004-2016. You'll note that this study is from 2018. It followed the publication of the 2017 RCOG guidelines, and it was designed specifically to test the veracity of the 3.8 kg upper weight limit in the RCOG guidelines, which Dr. Louwen and many others of us disagree with.

They compared the outcomes of babies that weighed < 3.8 kg with babies that weighed ≥ 3.8 kg. They found that the morbidity between the two groups was not significantly different. Babies ≥ 3.8 kg had a perinatal morbidity of 1.8%, whereas babies < 3.8 kg had a perinatal morbidity of 2.6%, so even higher. This doesn't surprise me because that's where you're going to capture your more growth-restricted babies that aren't thriving as much as they might.

It is true that babies weighing > 3.8 kg were significantly more likely to be delivered by C-section. It is also true that this was not a double-blind study and that the people calling the C-sections knew how much the baby's estimated fetal weight was, and that probably had some impact on the decision to go to C-section.

Be that as it may, interestingly, there was no difference in maternal birth injury between those who delivered a baby ≥ 3.8 kg and those who delivered a baby < 3.8 kg.

We have gone through what some of the major generators of clinical practice guidelines have to offer. We have looked at ACOG's failure to contribute anything meaningful to clinical practice of breech birth. We have taken a look at some of the literature since the Term Breech Trial to the 2017 RCOG Green-top Guideline and 2018 ACOG Committee Opinion. We have pointed out where the research now seems to be veering away from the existing clinical practice guidelines.

You can also see the RANZCOG guidelines (from Australia and New Zealand).

RANZCOG recommendations (excerpts):

For women with suspected breech presentation in late third trimester, an ultrasound should be performed to confirm the examination findings.

Women with a breech presentation at or near term should be informed about external cephalic version (ECV) and offered it if clinically appropriate.

ECV should only be performed by suitably trained health professionals where there is facility for emergency caesarean section.

[Lists absolute and relative contraindications for ECV]

1

Where there is maternal preference for vaginal birth, the woman should be counselled about the risks and benefits of planned vaginal breech delivery in the intended location and clinical situation.

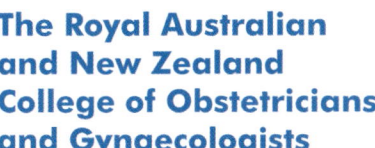

The Royal Australian and New Zealand College of Obstetricians and Gynaecologists
Excellence in Women's Health

[Lists contraindications to vaginal breech birth]

Planned vaginal breech delivery must take place in a facility where appropriate experience and infrastructure are available [including CFM, immediately available CS, and an experienced OB]

When breech presentation is first recognized in labour, the obstetrician should discuss the options of emergency caesarean section or proceeding with attempted vaginal breech birth.

There are also non-governmental organizations that have created clinical practice guidelines from their own independent reviews of the literature. FIGO—the equivalent of ACOG or RCOG, but Europe-wide—has breech guidelines, as does Doctors Without Borders. Another one of these organizations is ALARM International.

Vision: To improve the health and status of women and their newborns globally by advancing awareness and respect of sexual and reproductive rights of women among health care providers, policy and program decision makers.

GLOWM: The Global Library of Women's Medicine
glowm.com

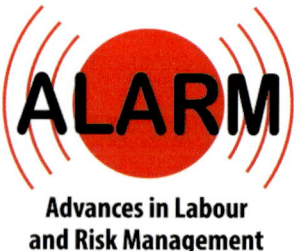

ALARM stands for Advances in Labour And Risk Management. Their information is available at the Global Library of Women's Medicine (GLOWM), glowm.com. It's also a very good reference for many things in women's medicine outside of just pregnancy and birth.

ALARM Selection Criteria

- Insufficient data to recommend for or against frank or complete breech birth when EFW > 4000 g
- Frank or complete breech > 36 weeks and/or EFW 2500-4000 g
- Frank or complete breech 31-35 weeks and/or EFW 1500-2500 g
- **Ultrasound:** AFT, cord presentation, anomalies, placenta location "useful" but not required
- **Criteria examined and excluded as unimportant:** parity, maternal age, pelvimetry, medical and/or obstetrical complications
- **Implied exclusion criteria:**
  - EFW < 1500 g or gestational age < 31 weeks
  - Non-frank or non-complete presentation

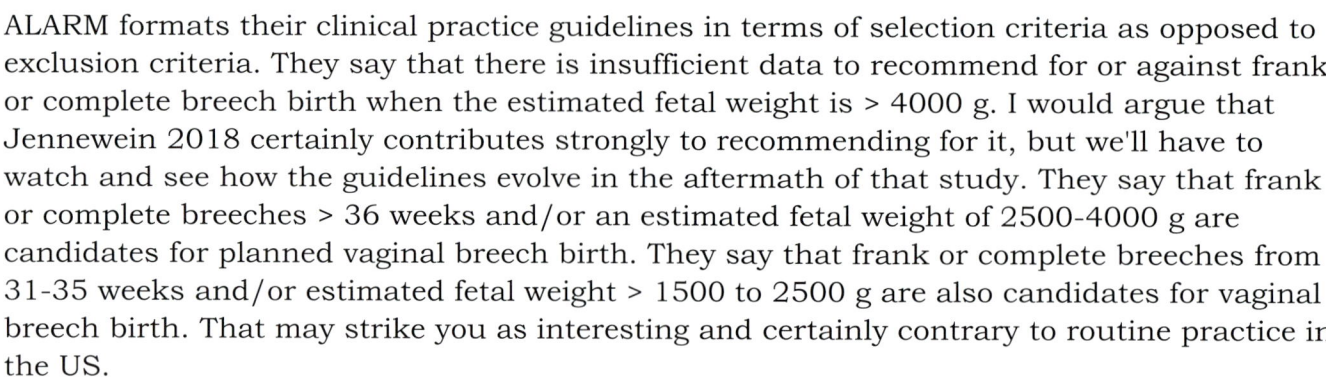

ALARM formats their clinical practice guidelines in terms of selection criteria as opposed to exclusion criteria. They say that there is insufficient data to recommend for or against frank or complete breech birth when the estimated fetal weight is > 4000 g. I would argue that Jennewein 2018 certainly contributes strongly to recommending for it, but we'll have to watch and see how the guidelines evolve in the aftermath of that study. They say that frank or complete breeches > 36 weeks and/or an estimated fetal weight of 2500-4000 g are candidates for planned vaginal breech birth. They say that frank or complete breeches from 31-35 weeks and/or estimated fetal weight > 1500 to 2500 g are also candidates for vaginal breech birth. That may strike you as interesting and certainly contrary to routine practice in the US.

But indeed, 31-35 week babies don't seem to have any higher morbidity and mortality delivered vaginally as when delivered by cesarean section, so that makes them appropriate candidates. (Of course, these babies would not be born at home!)

They examined the role of **ultrasound**. Their position was that it was useful for determining amniotic fluid index, determining cord position, discovering fetal anomalies, and locating the placenta. But there was no evidence that those things improved outcomes, so their conclusion was that ultrasound was not required.

I agree that ultrasound is not required for most routine vaginal breech birth or vaginal births of any kind. I don't personally require an ultrasound.

You have to consider ALARM's criteria in the context of their audience, which is intended to be the entire world. They're trying to standardize selection criteria across the globe. They examined certain criteria—**parity, maternal age, pelvimetry, medical and/or obstetric complication**s—and excluded them as unimportant, with the understanding that "unimportant" means unimportant to the mode of delivery, not unimportant to the outcome of the pregnancy or the birth. While those things individually can have an impact on the pregnancy, they apparently don't have a selective impact on vaginal breech birth. On that basis, they were excluded as unimportant. That leaves ALARM's exclusion criteria as estimated fetal weight < 1500 grams, gestational age < 31 weeks, and a presentation that is not frank or complete.

Dolichocephaly

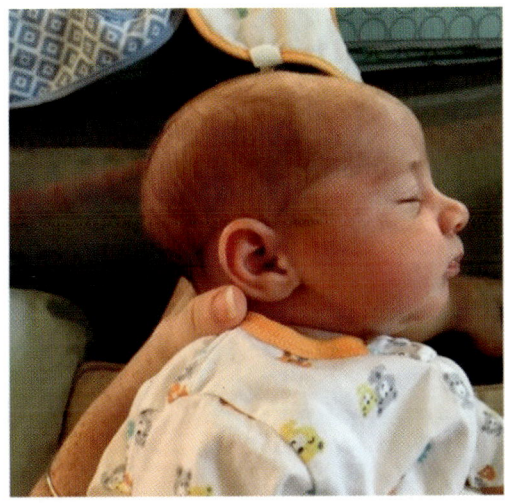

Before I try to tie all this together, there's one other piece of information that I want to slip in about dolichocephaly. Dolichocephaly refers to the flattening of the baby's head side to side and the lengthening of it front to back. This was one of my breech babies. This was a more dramatic dolichocephaly than it appears on this picture. But you get the idea at least.

Dolichocephaly is not specifically in anyone's exclusion criteria. However, there are exclusion criteria that address congenital malformations, and this unfortunately is often included in that class.

Dolichocephaly is a phenomenon that occurs primarily in breeches that have been persistently breech for a long time and that have a posterior fundal placenta. In that situation, of course, the baby's head will be using the placenta for a pillow. There's less space there and the head has a tendency to grow to fit that space.

Anecdotally, many people have used dolichocephaly as an exclusion criterion based on the fact that it was a congenital anomaly. There is no evidence to support that. And as long as the baby's head is properly flexed, it does not have a larger presenting diameter than a non-dolichocephalic baby.

My takeaway: Greatest risk factors for vaginal breech birth

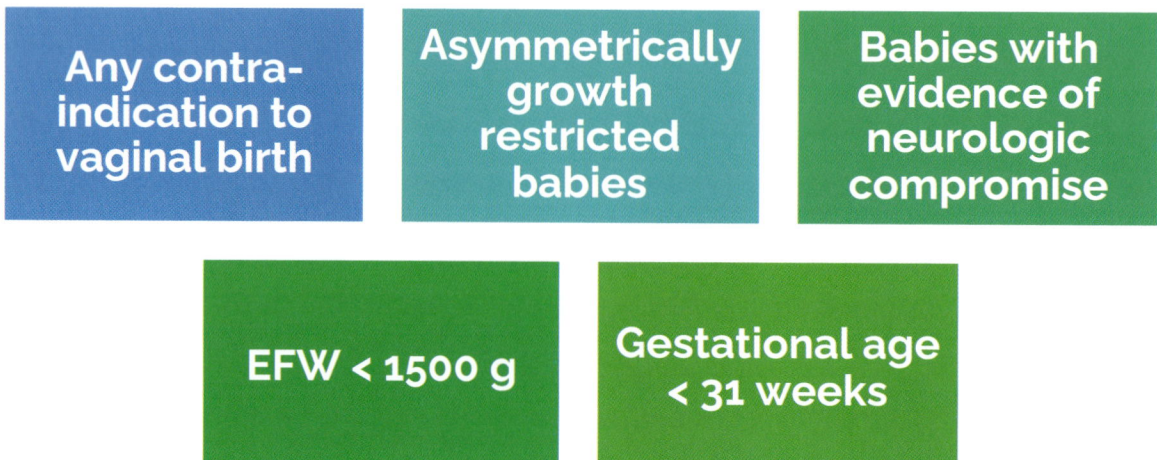

This is my summary of things that I would consider greater risk factors for a vaginal breech birth. I don't exclude people per se. I inform them and try to support them. But this is what stands in for exclusion criteria, in my practice.

- **Any contraindication to vaginal birth:** Obviously.
- **Asymmetrically growth-restricted babies:** For obvious reasons, which we have already talked about.
- **Babies with evidence of neurologic compromise:** If they can't participate in their birth, if they can't maintain head flexion, at the very least you're in for a very difficult breech birth and probably an increase in morbidity and mortality.
- **Estimated fetal weight < 1500 g**. There are certainly viable babies that are < 1500 grams, and I have issues with the type of cesarean sections that are done on those mothers. That becomes a very difficult set of risks and benefits to balance.
- Same thing with the next one: **gestational age < 31 weeks.** Those are excluded based on the best literature available, but with the caveat that the cesarean that is typically done in very premature babies carries much greater risk going forward for the mother and for future pregnancies, so it warrants a discussion. Most of the risk of a preterm breech birth still comes from the prematurity, not the presentation or mode of birth.

ECV vs. vaginal breech birth

ECV is the current approach that ACOG is taking, as opposed to promoting the reskilling and retraining of breech skills. ECV is a procedure by which you externally turn the baby head-down. I offer it to all my clients because it is an option with proper informed consent.

Having to change providers at term in order to achieve a vaginal birth is obviously very disruptive to someone's plans. It may be less disruptive to some people than to others, but it certainly can be disruptive to be in a different town, in a different hospital, or in a different home setting after nine months of planning. I do offer ECVs, which I consider part of informed consent and supporting my clients. I have an 80% success rate with my ECVs, unless the placenta is anterior. Among women with anterior placentas, my success rate drops to about 25%, so there's a dramatic difference depending on where the placenta is located.

Kew et al, 2007: Australian single center retrospective data	rate
447 attempted ECVS, with 165 successful	37%
Of the 400 for which data was available (47 lost to follow-up)	
202 planned CS	50.5%
43 in-labor CS for medical indications	10.8%
30 in-labor CS for breech presentation	7.5%
3 "emergency" CS for fetal bradycardia during ECV	0.8%
112 vaginal births out of 400 breech presentations	**28.0%**
112 cephalic births of 165 cephalic presentations	67.9%
PREMODA 2006: 1796 VBBs of 2526 attempts	**71.1%**

What is the impact of ECV in a population of women who have breech-presenting babies? **Kew et al.** is a 2017 Australian single center retrospective study. They looked at all of their attempted ECVs and then mapped out what the ultimate outcomes were.

They found 447 attempted ECVs. Of those, 165 were successful, or 37%. This is not a very impressive ECV rate. Of the 400 for which data was available (47 were lost to follow up), 202 had planned C-sections, just over 50%. Forty-three (10.8%) had an in-labor C-section for a medical indication, presumably non-reassuring fetal heart tones or nervous obstetrician. Take your pick.

Thirty or 7.5% had in-labor C-sections for breech presentation alone. That would include people who did not have a successful ECV, planned a C-section, but went into labor prior to their planned C-section. That would also include people who had a successful ECV whose cephalic baby decided it wanted to be breech and flipped back, so they were discovered in labor to be breech again.

And then there were 3 "emergency" C-sections (I have that in quotations: maybe they were emergencies, maybe not) for fetal bradycardia during the ECV. That does suggest that the ECV might carry some risk of its own of 0.75% or 3/400.

In total, there were 112 vaginal births in 400 breech presentations. That's a 28% vaginal birth rate. Of the 165 successful ECVs, 112/165 equals a 67.9% vaginal birth rate.

By way of comparison, the PREMODA study from France and Belgium had 2,526 attempted vaginal breech births, of which 1,796 were successful. So that gives the PREMODA study a successful vaginal birth rate of 71.1%. That does not provide very encouraging data for the use of ECV as an alternative to offering vaginal breech birth.

Leung et al., 1999: BJOG
Undiagnosed breech

- Compared outcomes of undiagnosed vs. known breeches
- **46%** of undiagnosed breeches delivered vaginally
- **11%** of breeches diagnosed during prenatal care delivered vaginally
- Including women who had a successful ECV, **26%** of breeches diagnosed prenatally delivered vaginally

One more study by **Leung et al. in 1999**. This was prior to the Term Breech Trial when, in theory, hospitals were still doing vaginal breech births. They were interested in the question of undiagnosed breeches. They compared the outcomes of breeches diagnosed in labor with breeches diagnosed during prenatal visits. In this study, **46%** of the undiagnosed breeches delivered vaginally. That's considerably higher than the 28% overall vaginal birth rate in the Kew study we looked at previously.

But only **11%** of the breeches diagnosed during prenatal care delivered vaginally. That tells you something about their environment towards vaginal breech birth. If you also include women who had successful ECVs, still only **26%** of all breeches that were diagnosed prenatally delivered vaginally.

There may be a very small benefit to ECV in situations where vaginal breech birth is not an option, but there's no evidence that ECV increases the rate of vaginal birth or improves outcomes, if there are experienced breech providers available.

Furthermore, the rate of vaginal birth among those who attempted ECV is exceptionally low. The rate of vaginal births among those who've had successful ECVs (**67.9%**) remains far below the rate of successful vaginal birth among those with access to trained breech providers (71.1% in the PREMODA study, around 98-100% among me and several of my very experienced colleagues). This means offering ECV is not an acceptable alternative to offering vaginal breech birth.

On that note, we will conclude Part 2: Clinical Practice Guidelines. In the next lesson, we will focus on the maneuvers used to assist during vaginal breech birth.

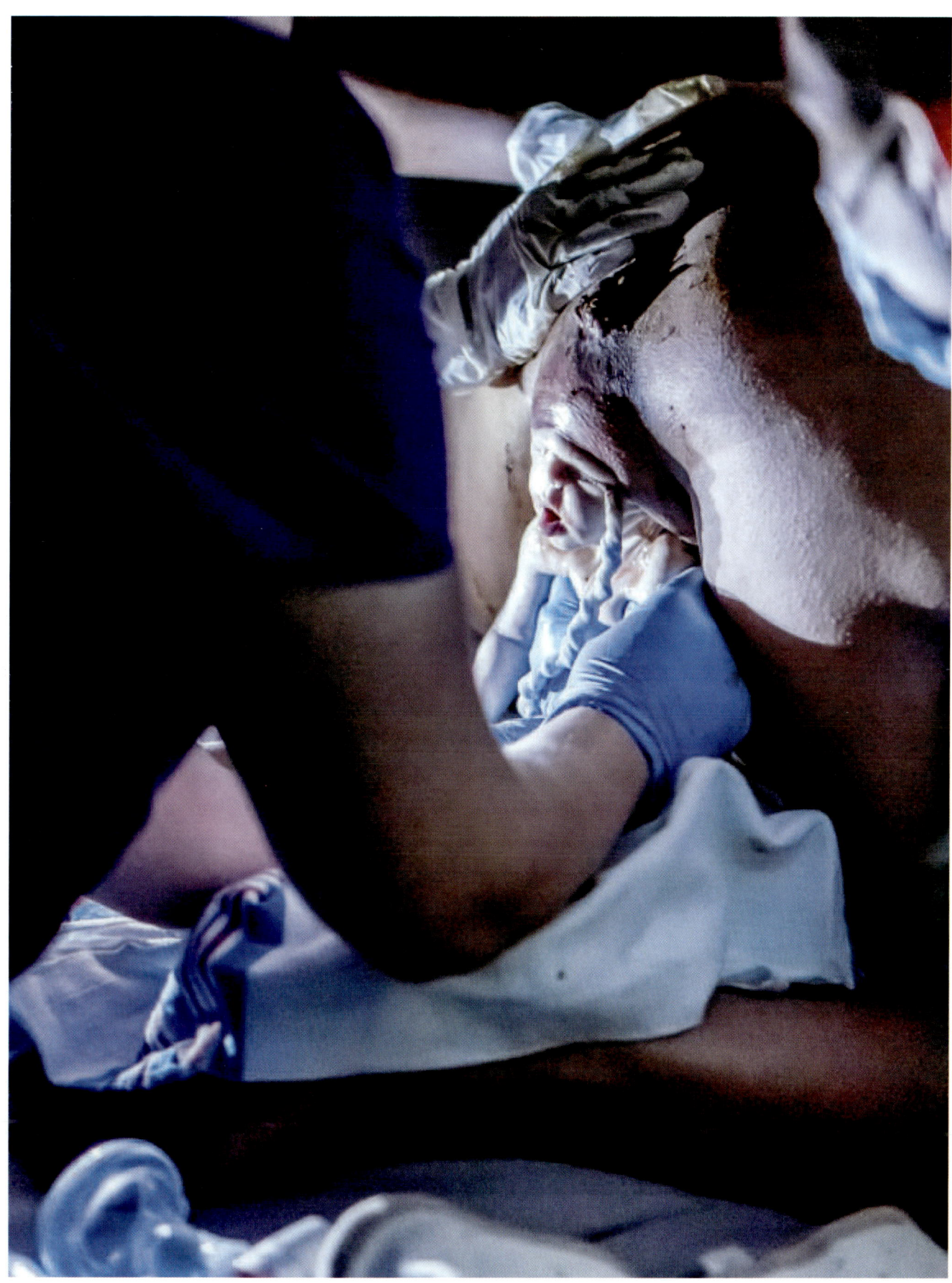

Shatamia Webb, Baby Catcher Birth Center. Undiagnosed frank breech assisted virtually by a BWB clinician

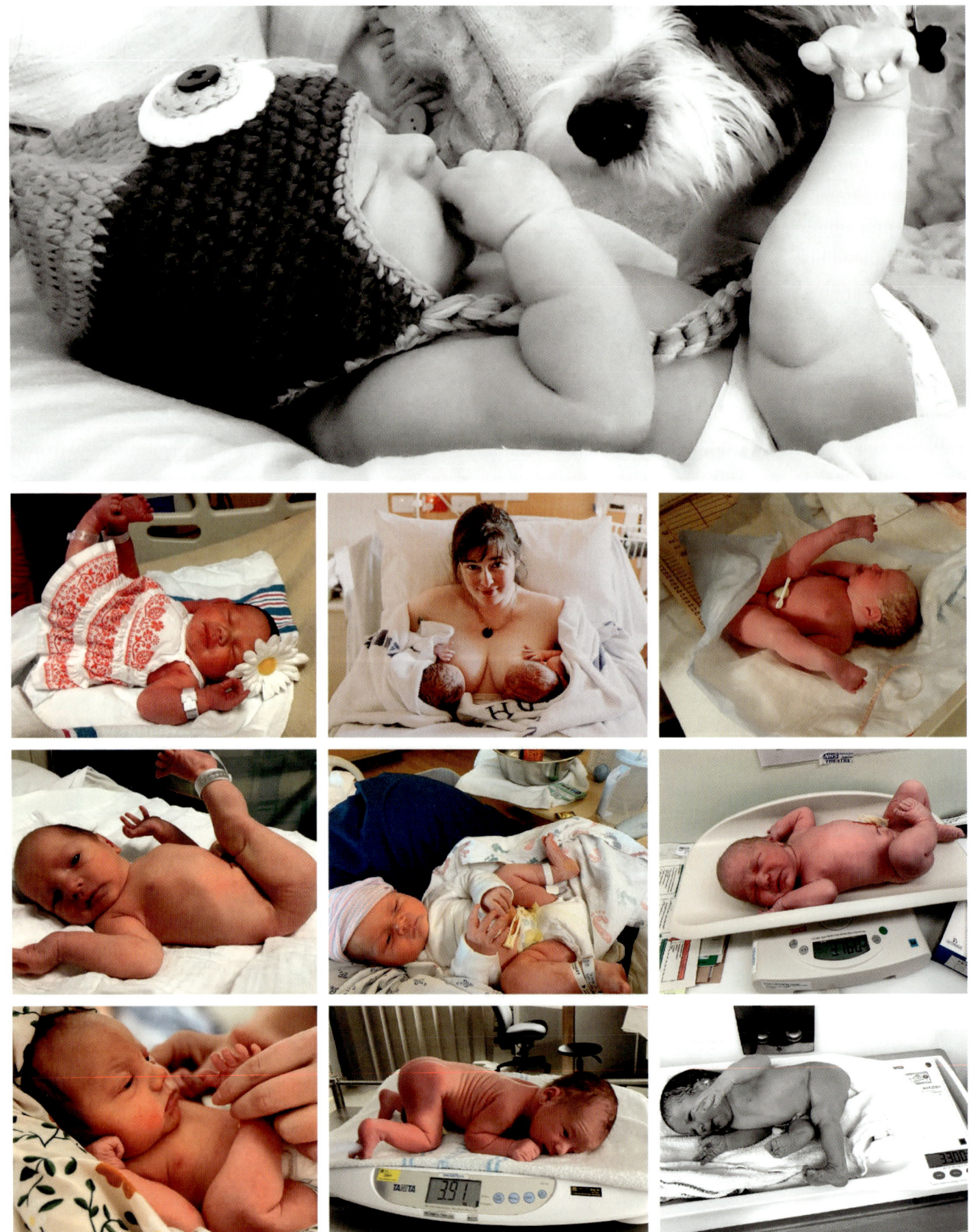

Lesson 10: Vaginal breech management & maneuvers Clinical Aspects, part 3

By David Hayes, MD

Welcome to Part 3 of Clinical Aspects: Vaginal Breech Management and Maneuvers. In this session, we're going to pick up where we left off in Part 1, going through normal vaginal breech birth with the recognition that vaginal breech birth, like all birth, isn't always normal. We'll briefly touch on the basic principles of managing breech labor and birth and then spend most of the session emphasizing a subset of six essential maneuvers to employ when breech birth doesn't go smoothly.

Characteristics of vaginal breech birth

Labor length is variable, just like cephalic birth. There is no evidence to support holding it to a different standard than cephalic birth.*

An undisrupted active second stage, from "rumping" (appearance of the bitrochanteric diameter) to birth is quick, normally requiring less than seven minutes.

Physiologic birth requires active cooperation between the person giving birth and the baby being born; therefore, a vigorous, neurologically intact baby is essential.

Management of VBB: General principles

- Labor should not be a selection criterion*
- The time elapsed since rumping for 2nd stage should be regarded as one piece of information contributing to your assessment of the baby, **not a hard time** limit to "get the baby out."
- Consider the appearance of the mechanism, the condition of the baby, the progression of the birth, the contraction pattern, and the total elapsed time in deciding whether to intervene.
- The baby can be seen and directly assessed during second stage
- The mechanism can be inferred from direct visualization.
- The baby is directly accessible to perform necessary maneuvers

Management of vaginal breech birth

Manage first stage like any vaginal labor:

- Encourage movement
- Provide support, hydration, and nourishment
- Assess fetal well-being

From the birth of the bitrochanteric diameter:

- Encourage "all fours" or upright positions
- Watch descent, rotation, and elapsed time carefully
- Observe fetal activity, tone, and heart rate
- Avoid unnecessary intervention: The baby should be pushed out, not pulled out, if at all possible

Why do we prefer upright positions?

Being in an upright forward-leaning position (standing, hands & knees, kneeling, etc.) is something women have been doing for as long as humans have existed. Look at this beautiful artwork from around the world, spanning thousands of years.

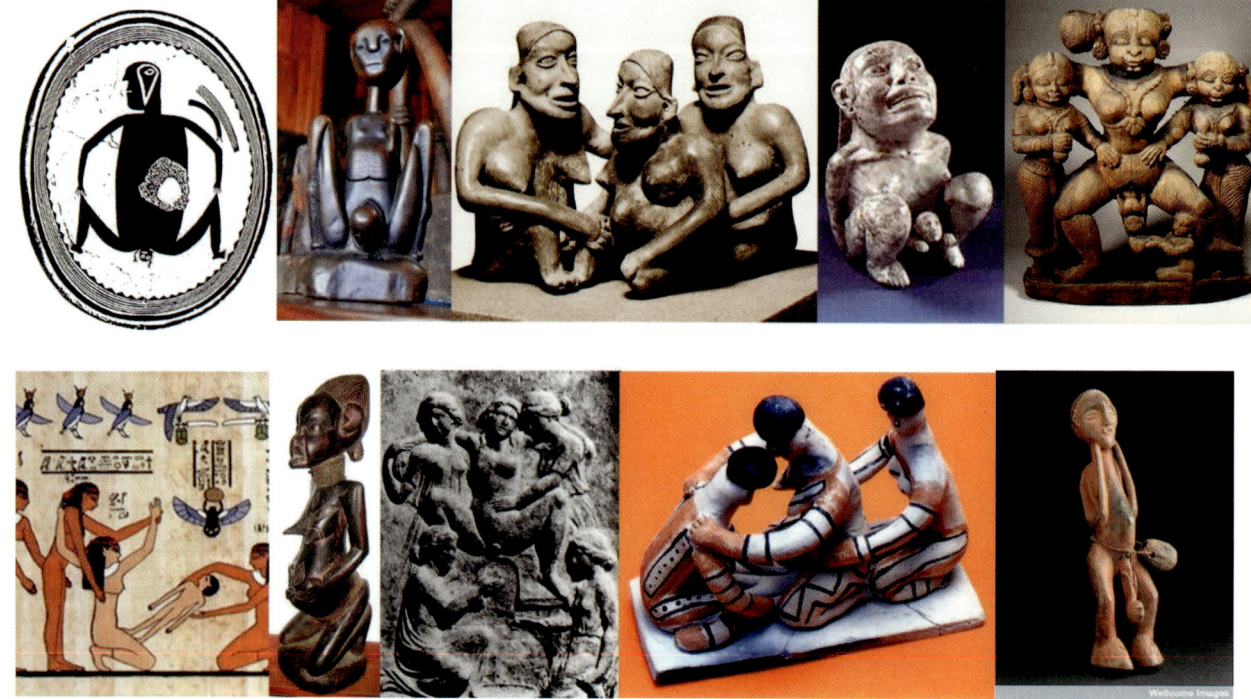

We also have several recent studies on upright breech birth that prove what women have always known intuitively: upright or physiological birth works better. One large study from a breech center in Frankfurt, Germany found that being upright, compared to lying down, leads to a shorter pushing stage, fewer neonatal injuries, fewer maternal injuries, fewer maneuvers required, and fewer in-labor C-sections (Louwen 2017).

Thanks to MRI studies of the pelvis in both pregnant and non-pregnant women, we also know, that the mid-pelvis and pelvic outlet are significantly larger when women are in upright positions, compared to lying down (Reitter 2014). Of course, midwives have "known" this long before MRIs existed, but it helps to have scientific evidence to convince the skeptics.

Intervene at your own risk.

Countless generations of midwives preserved and passed on the knowledge and practice that form the backbone of physiological breech birth as it is emerging in 2020. There is strong evidence that improper intervention causes more problems than it fixes. The key factor to understand is that breech birth has lower morbidity when the baby is pushed out, rather than when it is pulled out.

Most of the interventions and maneuvers that have been used by obstetricians, prior to the advent of physiological breech birth, have involved some variation of trying to pull the baby out. Pulling the baby out extends the baby's head. A neurologically intact baby is capable of flexing its head if it gets extended. But getting a head extended is the most common way to get it stuck. So yes, there is lower morbidity when the baby is pushed out, than when it is pulled out. Ideally that should be by the person giving birth, rather than the person supporting the birth.

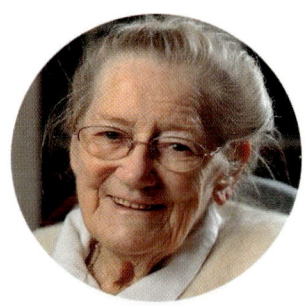

We have mentioned Mary Cronk previously. She is the Grande Dame of British midwifery. She was famous for her saying, "Hands off the breech. Sit on them if you must."

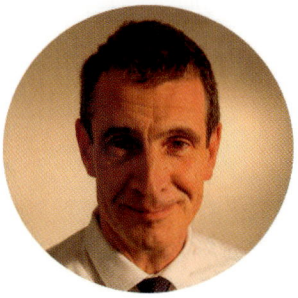

Lawrence Impey is a maternal fetal medicine specialist and the lead author of the 2017 Green-top Guideline on breech birth (from the Royal College of Obstetricians and Gynecologists in the UK). The question was put to Dr. Impey, "Well, what do you do if you're on duty and there is no one who is breech experienced on the service, and someone comes in with a breech presentation?" His answer was, "Put them in all fours and have a cup of tea." Lawrence Impey recognizes, as much as anyone, the need to have trained, experienced breech providers available. But he emphasizes that doing the wrong thing is often worse than doing nothing.

Plentl & Stone, 1953

> "The more manipulation is performed and the earlier this manipulation is instituted, the greater the fetal mortality and morbidity..."
>
> Plentl AA, Stone RE. The Bracht Maneuver. *Obstetrical & Gynecological Survey*. 1953; 8:313-25.

Plentl & Stone, obstetricians from Columbia University in the 1950s, recognized that manipulating a breech birth led to greater morbidity and mortality. Clearly it has been recognized that intervention in breech birth is a bad thing unless absolutely necessary. We're going to build on that by showing you how to do it more safely when it is necessary.

John William Burns, 1934

This is John William Burns, the obstetrician who developed the Burns-Marshall Maneuver. In 1934, he wrote this passage on the right. Now we could extend that to the past 90 years! We are going to try to offer you some new ideas here.

> That new principles of treatment have not been expressed and that each writer has simply perpetuated the teachings of his predecessor is clearly evident from the perusal of the textbooks published during the past twenty or thirty years. On no important point does the treatment ever appear to be questioned, and the paucity of new ideas is everywhere remarkable."
>
> Breech: A Method of Dealing With the Aftercoming Head. *BJOG*. Vol 41:6 December 1934.

Anatomy & orientations

Be comfortable with your orientations. Sacrum is on the same side of the baby as the occiput. Obviously, we are used to talking about *occiput posterior, occiput anterior*. It's easy to get confused when we're talking about breech.

- **Sacrum** = occiput = back side of the baby
- **Posterior** = back side of the mama
- **Anterior** = front side of the mama
- **Transverse** = maternal left-right diameter

You may be in a position that may be unfamiliar to you, if you're used to dorsal lithotomy position births. Sacrum occiput equals the back side of the baby. The posterior is the backside of the mom, which would be facing you. The anterior is the front side of the mom, which would be facing away from you. The mom is on all fours or in a supported upright leaning forward position, occasionally a supported squat. Her right is your right. Her left is your left. The baby is opposite the mom, making a mirror image, what Shawn Walker refers to as "tum to bum."

Assessing fetal well-being

If you're not seeing tummy crunches, you can touch the baby's foot and elicit a reflex. If it has muscle reflexes, that's a good sign. But you also have the cord accessible to you. I can't emphasize enough how valuable a tool this is. You can palpate the cord to feel a pulse. Contrary to what you may have been taught, it will not spasm. There is no mechanism for it to spasm. You can also look at the cord. If the cord is tumescent and full, if the Wharton's jelly structure is intact, if the coiling is still tight, and if there's no laxness in the cord, you can be almost 100% assured that the baby is still oxygenated.

Fetal heart rate is a very sensitive indicator of acid-base balance in the blood and of acidosis due to hypoxia. It's extremely sensitive. If you have a baby that is becoming acidotic, that will absolutely be reflected in the fetal heart rate pattern. There will be decreased variability and, if it's severe enough, bradycardia. The problem with fetal heart rate—and more specifically with continuous fetal monitoring—is that it is a notoriously *nonspecific* test.

Continuous fetal monitoring is sensitive and nonspecific. It has a false positive rate of 99% for hypoxia. And even when it works, it is a *lagging* indicator of fetal oxygenation. You can cut off the fetal oxygen supply, and it won't be reflected as hypoxia or as acidosis for a couple of minutes.

The information that you have by observing breech babies directly gives you a 2 or 3 minute head start on what a continuous fetal monitoring strip would tell you. You will know ahead of time that the baby is losing its oxygenation and that you have a couple of minutes to get this baby out still kicking and healthy. Learning to look at the cord and understanding when it's actually full is crucial. Cords start going flaccid just like the rest of the baby starts going flaccid. You have to you learn to recognize it early on. You can intervene at a point that will give you a perfectly healthy baby.

When to intervene or not

There is some difference of opinion in the physiological breech world about indications for doing interventions. There is a group that is heavily promoting a time-based algorithm for intervening. We and many other breech professionals are concerned about that approach. It's functionally recreating the Friedman curve, which was never a good thing and took us 60 years to get rid of. We're hesitant to say that a baby should be born in a certain time frame— whether 2 minutes or 5 or 7. Each case is individual. You can have a baby that crashes 2 minutes past rumping. You can have a baby that is vigorous and kicking at 10 minutes past rumping.

Time alone is not a very good predictor of fetal outcome. Instead, we focus on assessing the baby and being ready to intervene when you see any sign that it's starting to lose oxygenation. That being said, the risk of compromise goes from extremely low when the baby first enters the pelvis to significantly high once the shoulders and head are in the pelvis. Not many babies are going to survive being low in the pelvis for 20 minutes.

You have to look at your presentation and project how many more contractions and how much more time will likely elapse, given the rate at which the birth has been occurring. If the answer is more than another few minutes, you probably want to do something to speed that birth up. There are other situations in which you might shorten the time to birth: deep variable decels or repetitive early decels, for example. Even though both of those things are almost always false positives, there is still some indication of fetal risk in them. You might consider an intervention—fundal pressure—that could shorten the time to birth and make the baby available for manipulation if you needed to do a maneuver.

If you have a bigger baby, and the baby is moving and trying to free itself, it often will. By being patient, you can avoid unnecessary interventions. But it is also true that each successive contraction with no progress makes the following contraction exponentially less likely to result in progress.

Often, when you have a stuck anterior arm, the posterior shoulder will pivot and continue to descend, while the trapped anterior shoulder will stay in place. Sometimes what looks like progress is actually dystocia because the anterior shoulder is still locked into place.

Tight pelvic floor musculature

Let's say you have a primip who is an Olympic gymnast, ballerina, tennis player, or CrossFit athlete. The voluntary muscles of her pelvic floor musculature have a resting tone tighter than I can ever make mine, no matter how hard I try. If you're lucky enough to get this person into your practice at ten weeks, be a wise obstetrician or midwife and refer her to a pelvic floor physical therapist. They will identify the muscles and teach her how to relax them individually. In just two or three sessions, you will see a dramatic difference.

Among these athletes who have done physical therapy, their births tend not to be as primipy. If these highly athletic women have not had pelvic floor physical therapy, you might encounter significant soft tissue dystocia. If descent is significantly delayed during the expulsive phase and the heart tones aren't as good as you would like, you might consider using fundal pressure.

Dropped foot breeches

Let's discuss the stage in a dropped foot or footling labor where the legs are out but the rump is still not on the perineum and is higher in the pelvis. At that point, there's a low risk of cord compromise. It's perfectly acceptable to sit and wait for the legs to descend. 15 minutes, 30 minutes, or an hour is not unusual. You just keep watching the baby and listening to heart tones. The risk of compromise increases as the shoulders and head enter the pelvis.

When the legs are out, remember that the intrathoracic pressure is higher than the atmospheric pressure. As a result, when a baby is exposed to these pressure differentials for a significant amount of time, blood will pool in the baby's extremities. The legs will start to turn interesting shades of purple. It's perfectly normal and will resolve in a few days.

Frank vs nonfrank mechanisms

Let's briefly review the mechanisms. In a frank breech birth, the baby will to rotate from ST to SA on the first contraction after rumping. The rotation is driven by the shoulders entering the pelvic inlet and encountering the sacral promontory. The posterior shoulder slides away from the promontory, causing the rotation to SA.

In a nonfrank breech—complete breech in particular—the legs and feet tend to get caught inside the pelvis. The pelvis is widest in the transverse diameter. But as you go down toward the outlet, it gets narrower. When these long bones of the legs go down through the pelvis alongside the buttocks, the feet and knees will start to impinge on the walls of the pelvis. The baby keeps descending because it has flexible joints. However, it's not unusual for the legs to be stuck for a while until there's enough tension to release a foot.

During this whole process of descent, the shoulders are entering the pelvis. The posterior shoulder still wants to slide off the sacral promontory, but rotation may be restricted because of the legs splinted below. As contractions continue, the shoulders are going to compress and enter the pelvis squished into whatever position the torso is locked into—usually somewhere between oblique and transverse. After the shoulders enter the pelvis, there's nothing left to drive rotation. Sometimes the legs will descend without getting too wedged, and that baby will rotate to SA just like a frank. If a nonfrank baby remains completely transverse, I would suspect arm impingement. That will become evident once the baby is born to the armpits and you can visualize the presence or absence of a chest crease. Complete arrest of descent at this point, despite a good contraction, would suggest a trapped nuchal arm.

Six essential maneuvers to master

My goal in this lesson, and in our in-person trainings, is to make a bridge between the information in previous lessons and actual practice. I think that you are best served by mastering a smaller subset of tools—a toolbox, if you will—that you can immediately call on when you need them. With that in mind, here are the 6 tools that will allow you to manage nearly any breech situation you might encounter:

1. Side to Side maneuver
2. Shoulder press
3. The Crowning Touch
4. Ritgen
5. Fundal pressure
6. A set of maneuvers for resolving a hyperextended head in the pelvic inlet: a maneuver we call "Flex, flop, & drop" plus a Løvset maneuver

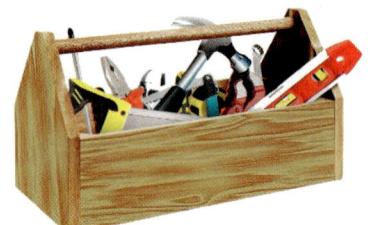

There are two rotational maneuvers for resolving trapped arms—the Side to Side and the Front to Back. They use different hand grips and rotate in different directions. After seeing participants confusing the two maneuvers and mixing up the hand grips, I decided to teach just one. You're better served to learn one and learn it well.

Why have I selected the Side to Side maneuver rather than the Front to Back? The flat hands grip associated with the Front To Back maneuver is tricky to maintain, especially when the baby is slippery and space is tight inside the vagina. During both simulations and video peer reviews, we have seen participants having difficulty maintaining the proper hand grip. They inadvertently move their hands around on the baby, trying to get a better purchase, grabbing in places that are not protected by bony structures and taking up valuable time in order to get a good grip (see the two pictures below). We also know that the Side to Side maneuver has been studied in a large cohort (Louwen 2017) and comes out very well compared to other methods of breech birth.

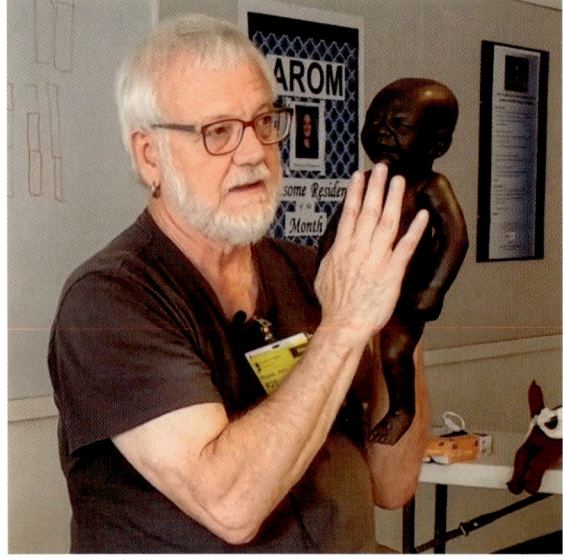
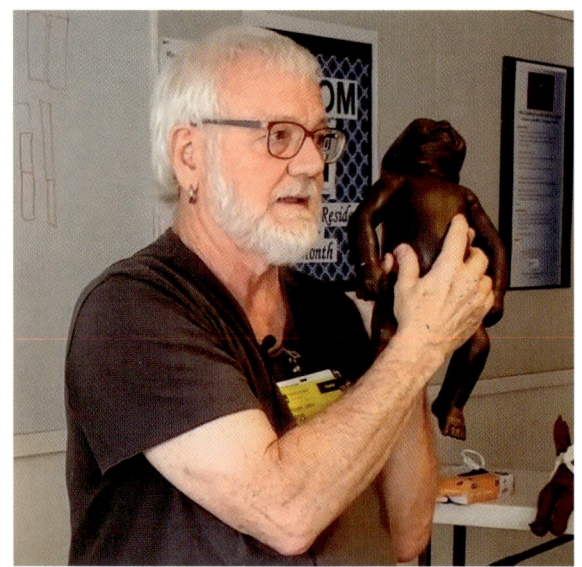

One of the potential drawbacks of the Side to Side maneuver is that you're taking the bulk of your hands and adding them to the lateral aspects of the baby. With that in mind, I have altered it for my use by using a scissor grip. This gives you a narrower profile as well as a good purchase on the baby to do your disimpaction. Some prefer the shoulder grip, others the scissor grip, depending on the size of their hands and the strength of their fingers.

When doing maneuvers—whether shoulder press, Side to Side, or Løvset—you always place your thumbs anteriorly if the mother is upright and you are behind her. If you are in front of the mother (birth stool or supine), your thumbs will be on the baby's back. Proper hand placement will ensure that you can only rotate in the proper direction because otherwise you'd have to stand on your head to do the rotation!

Upright = thumbs on front   **Supine/birth stool = thumbs on back**

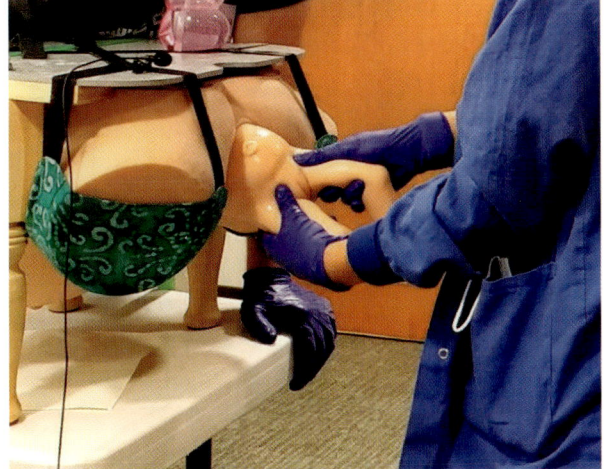 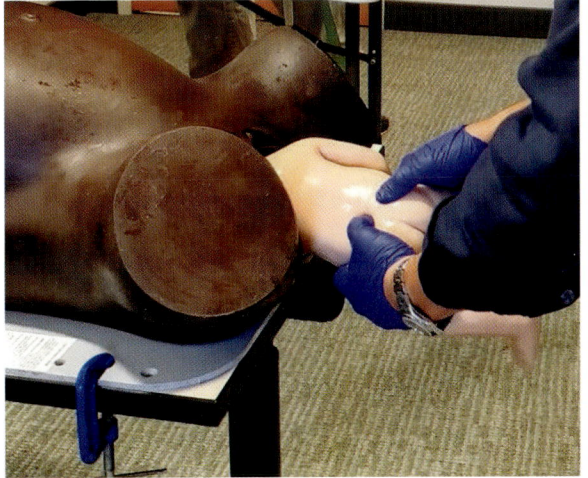

I also want you to master three head flexion maneuvers: shoulder press, the Crowning Touch, and Ritgen. Next, your toolbox should include fundal pressure, a maneuver that allows you to diagnose an obstruction, to shorten the time to delivery if you have baby that is compromised, to give contractions additional power, or to bring the baby down far enough so that you can access to it to do the other maneuvers.

The final tool that I'm going to give you is a set of maneuvers for extracting the baby. Physiologic breech maneuvers work very well as long as you have a baby that is neurologically intact and has good muscle tone. Once the baby has lost tone, it becomes significantly more difficult to get the baby out and the maneuvers tend to be less effective. I will present a two-person technique for disimpacting a hyperextended head in the pelvic inlet, then bringing the baby down and doing a Løvset maneuver to extract the baby quickly.

In her earlier lesson, Rixa introduced these six maneuvers. I will briefly review the main points in this lesson and supply more details where appropriate.

1. Side to Side

Indication: Arrested rotation and descent

- Shoulder grip: fingers on the posterior shoulders, thumbs on the anterior shoulders
- Scissor grip: make a V with your index and middle fingers. The armpit will fit into the "V"
- Disimpact and rotate 180° to the opposite side, then 90° back to SA
- Arms are **NOT** swept as part of this maneuver, but may be swept after successful completion, if indicated.

The indication for a Side to Side maneuver is arrested rotation and descent. Grab the baby by its shoulder girdle, thumbs in front and fingers in back. Alternatively, insert scissor fingers underneath each armpit. Next, disimpact significantly, then rotate 180° from the side you're on all the way to the other side, and then 90° back to sacrum anterior. That is done typically in one smooth motion: disimpact, rotate, rotate. It should only take a few seconds to complete. This illustration of the Louwen maneuver comes from the Louwen 2017 article describing upright breech birth in Frankfurt, Germany.

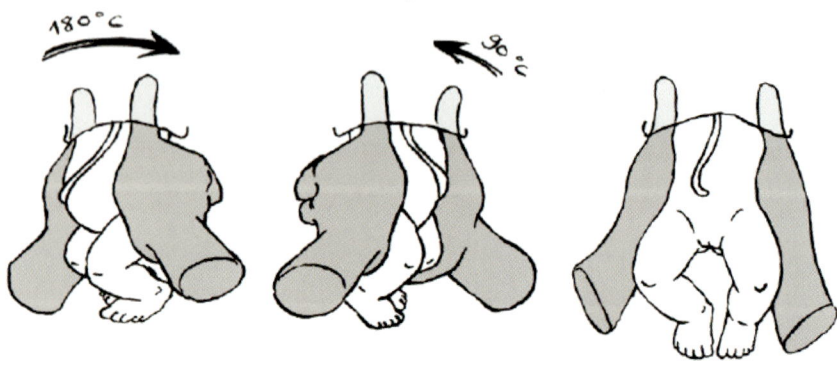

The arms will usually deliver themselves during that maneuver; if not, you can sweep them, but sweeping them is not considered to be part of the maneuver the way it's taught. If you've decided that you need to intervene, the best option is to try one maneuver, then go to the next maneuver in quick succession.

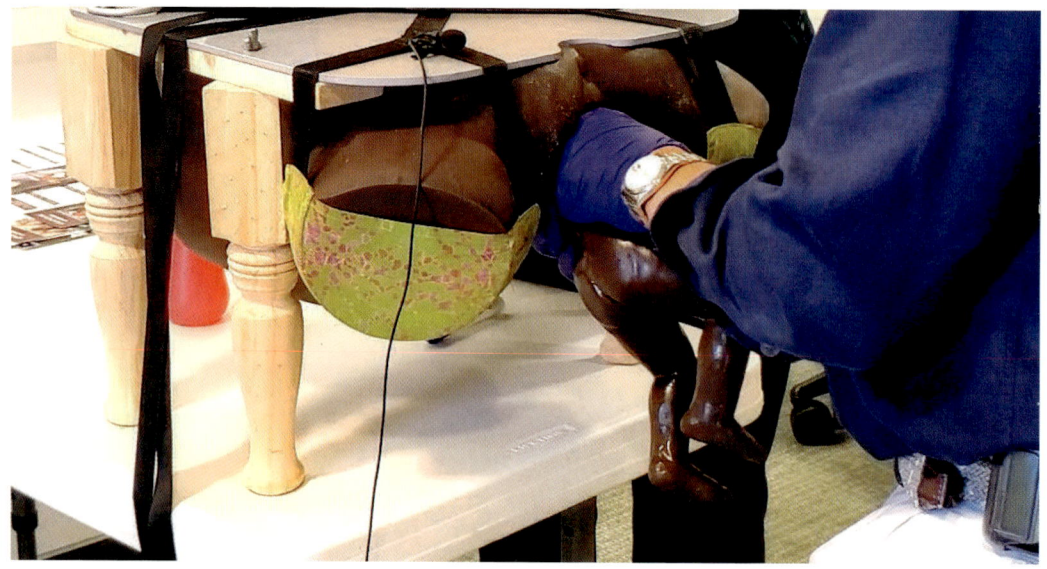

2. Shoulder press

Indications:

1. Extended head on the perineum
2. Shorten time to delivery

Pressing the occiput against pubic rami flexes the fetal head and facilitates birth.

Two techniques:

1. Place flat hand on the chest and press directly anterior
2. Grasp the shoulder girdles and press directly anterior

May be combined with a gluteal lift

The shoulder press seems very minor, and it is not a particularly invasive maneuver. But it is actually quite elegant and powerful. If you have an extended head on the perineum or if you need to shorten the time to delivery with the head already on the perineum, this is your go-to maneuver.

In dorsal lithotomy breech births, MSV is used to flex the baby's head. The shoulder press maneuver is infinitely more elegant, easier to do, less invasive, and more effective. It is, however, designed for upright births when you have access from behind the mother.

The shoulder press works by pressing the back of the baby's head against the pubic symphysis. Here is your situation: you've got a baby whose head that may be extended. If the head is caught on anything, it's caught on the perineum. The back of the baby's head is right on the symphysis pubis (pubic bone). That forms a barrier to the baby and causes its head to flex when you push the baby backwards towards the pubic bone. If you are doing a flat hand shoulder press, it's easy to add the Crowning Touch or the Ritgen and do both at the same time.

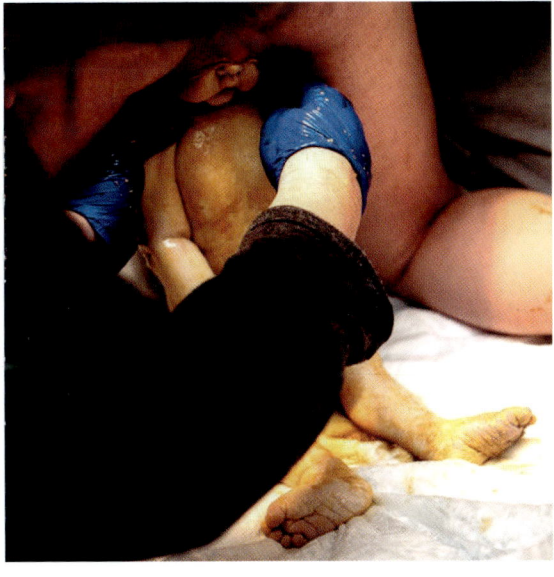 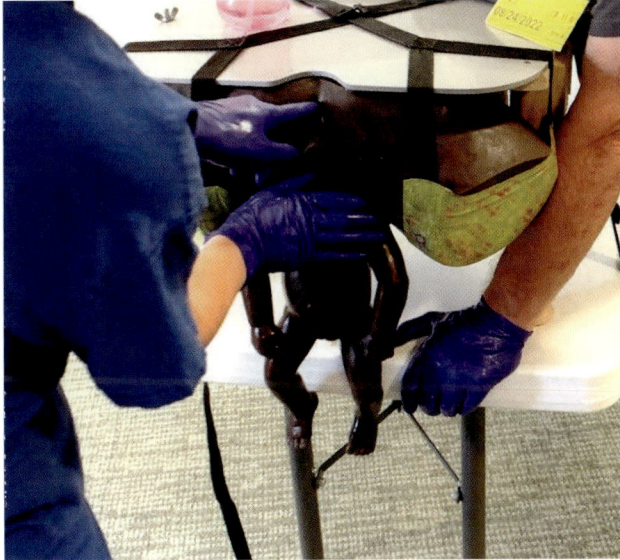

3. Crowning Touch

This maneuver is becoming my flexion maneuver of choice. Most of our trainees remark on how elegant, simple, and intuitive it is. Put two fingers beside the baby's check, then go back until the tips of your fingers feel the ear. Then cock your fingers downward and go down so your middle finger is at the nape of the neck and your first finger is on the occiput. Your 3rd and 4th fingers act as a fulcrum. They push against the baby's chest as you flex your wrist forward.

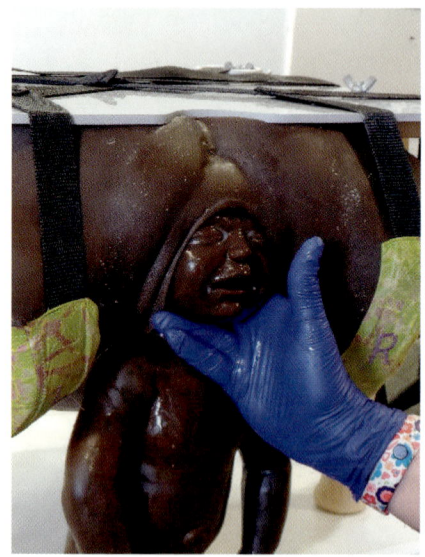
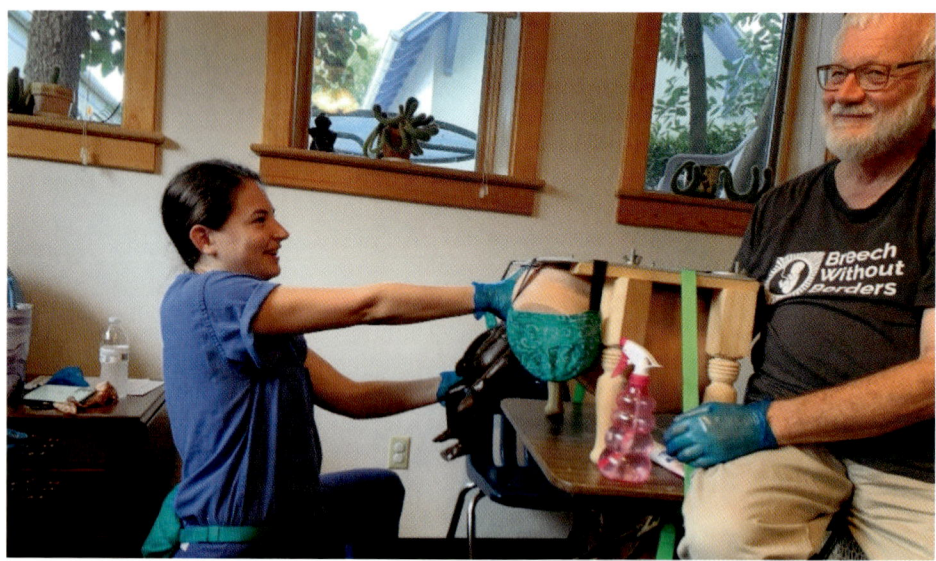

4. Ritgen

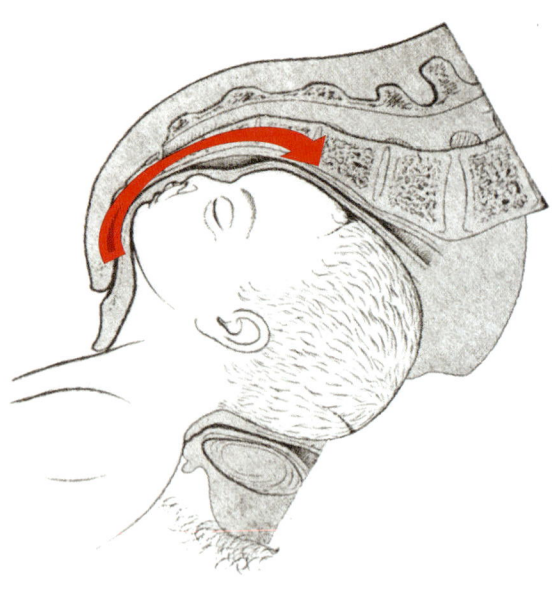

The classic Ritgen maneuver is used most often for occiput posterior cephalic babies. I came up with a variation for assisting an aftercoming breech head. It involves putting one or two fingers in the rectum. As you can see in this illustration, if you put your fingers in the rectum, you can easily reach the top of the baby's head without adding any bulk into the vagina. A Ritgen will give you good access and the ability to exert much more force to flex the baby's head. Ritgen can be done upright or supine. I vastly prefer Ritgen to MSV for supine births and hope to never again use MSV in my career.

5. Fundal pressure

Now we're going to switch gears and talk about fundal pressure. Fundal pressure, as the name sounds, is putting pressure on the fundus of a pregnant woman in labor to help move her baby down.

There's not a lot of information in the literature about it, but this whole section arose out co-teaching with Betty-Anne Daviss, a breech expert midwife in Canada. Betty-Anne studied with Frank Louwen in Frankfurt and learned his techniques and his information. While she was there, she noticed people doing fundal pressure—not just a little, but a lot. She told me: "Fundal pressure was so common it wasn't considered an intervention. No one documented it. My own observational data on 53 planned vaginal breeches that I attended in Frankfurt is that it was used about 35-40% of the time."

It wasn't just my interactions with Betty-Anne. It was also Dr. Louwen's paper on physiological upright breech in 2017, Appendix S 1 that said:

> "We never pull, only push the breech...We rely on the mother's contractions, but sometimes proceed to the use of oxytocin, and fundal pressure (the Kristeller maneuver)...
>
> The Kristeller maneuver (fundal pressure) is sometimes used in the unit, but has not been well captured."
>
> Louwen et al, 2017, Appendix S1, Footnote Table 5d

Bogner, who authored an Austrian study on breech birth in 2015, reported: "Delivering on the back nearly 100% need fundal pressure." Obviously, fundal pressure is something that is being done very commonly in some European countries during breech births, even if it's not considered a maneuver or being captured.

Indications for fundal pressure

1. Non-reassuring fetal heart tracing
2. Maternal exhaustion/poor expulsive effort
3. Diagnosing an obstruction

> "If fundal pressure is being used once the baby has emerged to past the umbilicus in order to assist with the shoulders, and the baby does not turn to face the practitioner but instead remains at sacral transverse, it is a sign that one of the shoulders is caught. This is the signal to the practitioner to stop using fundal pressure and to do a rotational maneuver instead."
>
> Betty-Anne Daviss, *Rethinking the Physiology of Vaginal Breech Birth*, 13th ed p. 13

> "If the baby is direct posterior, fundal pressure can be used to see which way the baby appears to be turning to guide the practitioner as to which way they might help the rotation."
>
> Betty-Anne Daviss, 2019. Personal correspondence

Indications for fundal pressure are non-reassuring fetal heart tracing, maternal exhaustion or poor expulsive effort, or diagnosing an obstruction. Now, by diagnosing an obstruction, I mean if you put pressure on the baby and it doesn't go down, then that gives you a strong suggestion that there's an obstruction. Getting that information by doing fundal pressure makes a lot of sense. It tells you whether the baby is stuck and/or if the baby wants to rotate a certain way. Again, I'd like to see data on it, but that certainly is very intuitive.

This next section comes from a video I obtained from Betty-Anne where she is describing fundal pressure and how and why they do it. These are her words:

"I want to give you the indications that we use for fundal pressure. The first indication is if there's a fetal heart tone that's going awry in second stage. We never do this in first stage. We wait, and we never do it until we actually see the baby's rump. Certainly, we do it when the baby is turned out at three o'clock (RST) or nine o'clock (LST). You have to have the mother fully dilated and the baby should be quite low already, almost on the perineum.

"What do we do it for? It's not just if the fetal heart tone is low. It's also if the mother has really been pushing and she's just really exhausted. I've done it a couple times when the physicians come in the room and say, 'Okay, we'll need to section. She can't do this.' And the mother is getting exhausted. And I just push and get the baby out in two minutes.

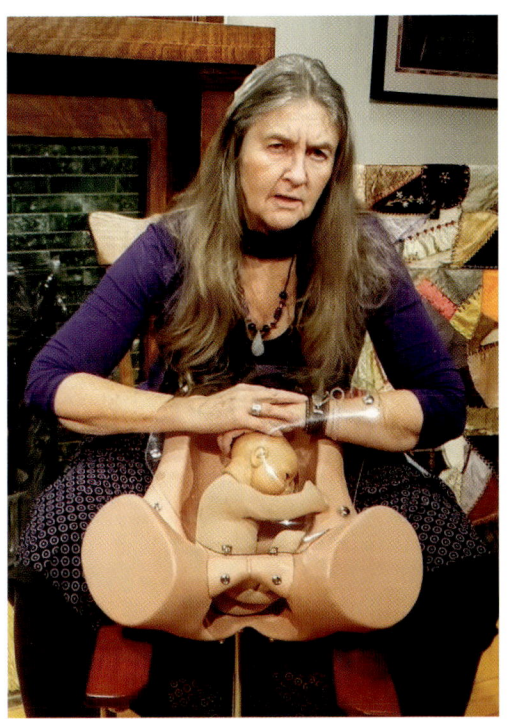

"It's similar to the Heimlich maneuver, but smoother and in reverse. The Heimlich maneuver is jerky, right? You do it to get something lodged in your esophagus out. Fundal pressure uses a very similar technique. You put one hand on top of the baby's head and the other hand on top of that, and then you press downward. It is incredible how easily this works. Just as you start to do press on the top of the fundus, the baby starts to come out and starts to do the maneuvers it needs. It just speeds up the process.

"On the other end, you're going to be seeing this baby come right down, and usually it comes right down to the arms.

"The third indication, besides low fetal heart tone or maternal exhaustion, is sometimes if you don't know what's going on, you can use it as a diagnostic tool. Because if fundal pressure doesn't work, then you might have some real dystocia that you need to do a section for. Or, conversely, if you have an incomplete breech, where the baby has come out with one leg and not the other, sometimes because of that position, it's harder to get the baby out and fundal pressure can help."

Controversies with fundal pressure (Kristeller)

- Use of the Kristeller maneuver in cephalic presentations has been associated with an increased incidence of Anal Sphincter rupture (uncertain incidence) and Levator Ani Muscle avulsion of 17-38%. It is also claimed in a high percentage of successful malpractice actions and has been banned in multiple countries.

- There is no data to suggest that fundal pressure increases maternal morbidity in breech presentations; however, there is very little data available.

- The Wolfgang Goethe University Hospital in Frankfurt began collecting data on their use of Kristeller in 2016.

The use of fundal pressure to assist second stage has been controversial for a number of decades, actually. In cephalic presentations, it has been associated with an increased incidence of anal sphincter rupture. There's a recent paper that shows an incidence of levator ani muscle rupture, of avulsion (tearing it off), of 17-38%. That's a very high morbidity for a maneuver. It is also claimed in a high percentage of successful malpractice actions and is actually banned in many countries. The US doesn't actually ban things as a country, but I think that in most jurisdictions in the US, you would get into a lot of trouble doing Kristeller in a cephalic birth.

Having said that, there is not data to suggest that fundal pressure increases maternal morbidity in breech presentations, but there isn't very much data. So that's why Wolfgang Goethe University (that's Frank Louwen's group) began collecting data on their use of Kristeller at Betty-Anne's suggestion in 2016. I hope to see some data come out to support this, because otherwise I think it's going to be very difficult to get it in wide use—even if, in fact, the data supports using it, which I suspect that it will.

How to do fundal pressure

We've talked about the indications for doing fundal pressure and some of the concerns associated with it, but we haven't really talked at all about how to do it. It's fairly straightforward, yet it needs to be done with a certain amount of caution. First of all, you need to understand that you only do fundal pressure if the woman is in second stage; that means that she is contracting, pushing, preferably with the rump visible on the perineum. That's the situation that you're looking for. If you've got a baby that's higher in the abdomen, I would not recommend doing fundal pressure.

Under this circumstance alone, you can use fundal pressure as a diagnostic tool to determine whether the baby is hung up on something or has the freedom to move. You can use it to shorten the time to delivery if you've got a non-reassuring fetal heart rate. What you want to make sure of, first and foremost, is that the baby is presenting in a proper position in the pelvis. In order to do that, you generally need to have a sacrum that's available to see.

It can be done in any kind of breech presentation: frank, incomplete, complete, etc. All of those are possible. But you need to have enough awareness of exactly where the baby is, so that you understand what position the baby is in. That's important for several reasons. If it's not in an appropriate position, then that increases the risk of the maneuver itself. Also, if you understand where the sacrum is, then you understand where the head is and which direction the head is pointed. When you're putting pressure on the fundus and on the fetal head, you want to do so in such a way that you're increasing flexion on the head rather than creating extension on the head.

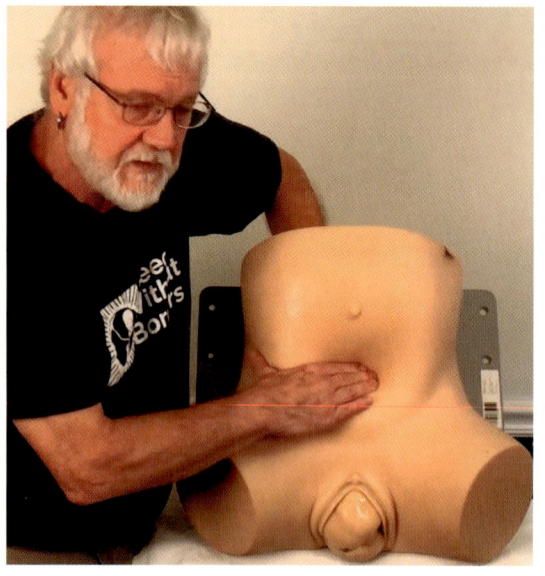

In this situation, we have a baby in RST. You can see the mom has pushed it down almost to the point of rumping. That's your clinical situation. Maybe it's taking a little longer than you're comfortable with. Maybe fetal heart tones are not reassuring. Maybe mom is just getting exhausted and there's a reason to want to shorten the time to birth. You palpate abdominally and you find the fundus of the uterus and the head. When you find that, you put your hand on it. (Some people prefer using two hands, as Betty-Anne Daviss has demonstrated.)

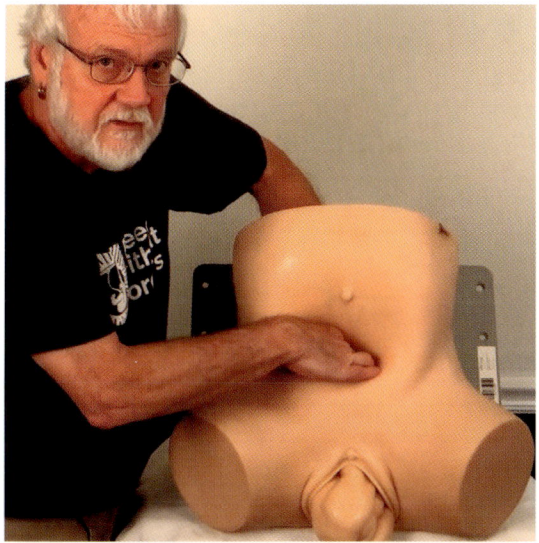

Press gently downward, and it should come fairly easily. It takes some pressure to do, of course. If you see something like this happening and preferably also a rotation going along with it, then you've improved your situation.

If you get resistance to your descent and if you get no rotation of your baby, then it's time to stop doing fundal pressure and do a rotational maneuver instead.

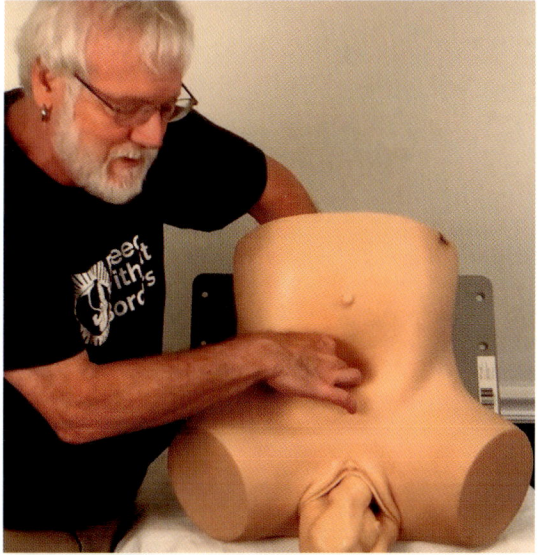

This baby has descended significantly with fundal pressure. The legs are out past the knees.

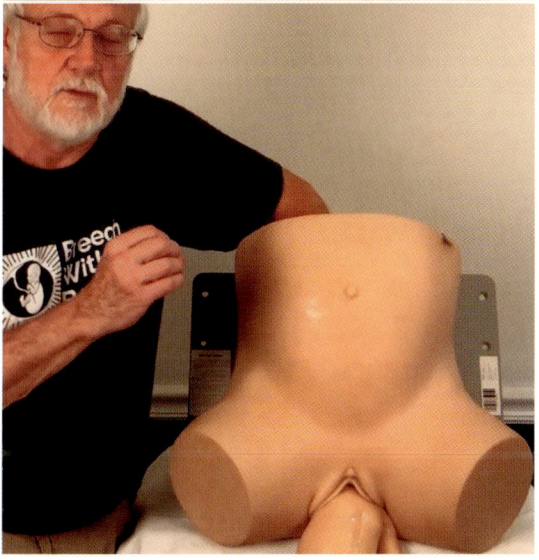

With a bit more fundal pressure, the baby's legs and one of the arms released. The baby also rotated normally during the fundal pressure.

6. Pelvic inlet arrest: Flex, flop, & drop + Løvset

Next, we're going to be looking at a maneuver that involves pressure on the fetal head, but it is with the intention of turning or flexing the fetal head, not with the intention of pushing the baby out. This situation is an extended head at the pelvic inlet. This is rare, and I hope you will never run across it.

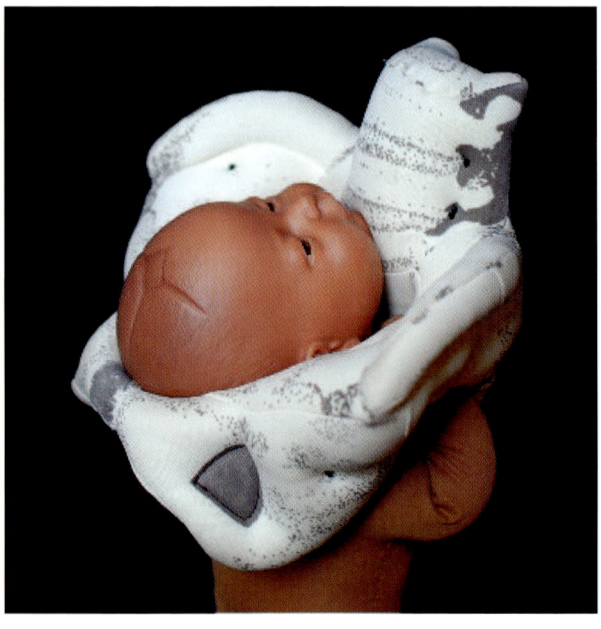

There are three salient interconnected points with a pelvic inlet entrapment. First, the baby descends direct sacrum anterior. This is unusual and is significant because it means the head is in the anterior-posterior orientation. Second, the baby is profoundly compromised. It has no muscle tone at all until, and the heart rate will likely be low. Third, the baby is caught very high up. The umbilical cord may not even be out. When you see that constellation of things—and indeed, it can *only* occur when you have that constellation of things—you should immediately think *hyperextended head in the pelvic inlet.*

How does this happen? When the baby descends sacrum anterior with an extended head and the mentum catches on the sacral promontory, the head hyperextends and the occiput then runs into the pubic symphysis. This impedes any further descent. You cannot push this baby out. You cannot pull this baby out.

The maneuver is fairly intuitive: you grasp the baby by the femurs and elevate. At the same time, your assistant cups the top of the fetal head and applies gentle counterpressure. As the head elevates, it encounters that counterpressure and flexes against that barrier, then flops to one side of the sacral promontory. You let go of the baby, and the assistant follows the head down until it drops into the oblique of the pelvis. While this maneuver is unnamed, we are calling it "**flex, flop, & drop**." You may have heard us refer to it previously as "elevate, flex, & rotate" but we feel the new name more accurately reflects what the maneuver does.

How to correct a hyperextended head in the pelvic inlet (Flex, flop, & drop)

1. Confirm your diagnosis: Palpate above the pubic bone and then feel directly superior to it. You will feel the entire head above the pubic bone (this might be difficult if the mother has a lot of adipose tissue on her abdomen).
2. Call for backup assistance (peds/NICU if you are in a hospital, EMS or equivalent if you are at home)
3. Call an assistant to help you. Tell the assistant that you have a hyperextended head in the pelvic inlet. Ask your assistant to cup two hands and apply counterpressure to the *top* of the baby's head (not the back of the head). The assistant should confirm that their hands are in position.
4. Grasp the femurs and disimpact the baby significantly. This will cause the baby's head to

push up against the counterpressure and flex. Your assistant will feel the head **flex and flop** to one side of the sacral promontory. Ask your assistant to confirm when they feel a change.
5. Let go of the baby completely. Instruct the assistant to continue providing downward pressure on the baby's head, following it downward as far as it will go. The head will **drop** into the oblique of the pelvis and you should see significant descent (to mid-chest or lower).
6. Be prepared to do a Løvset maneuver to extract the baby as it will likely be compromised.
7. To deliver the head, do a Crowning Touch or Ritgen if the mother is upright. If the mother is supine, do a Burns-Marshall or Bracht to elevate the fetal body, then use Ritgen to deliver the head.

This can be done upright or supine as illustrated in the photos below.

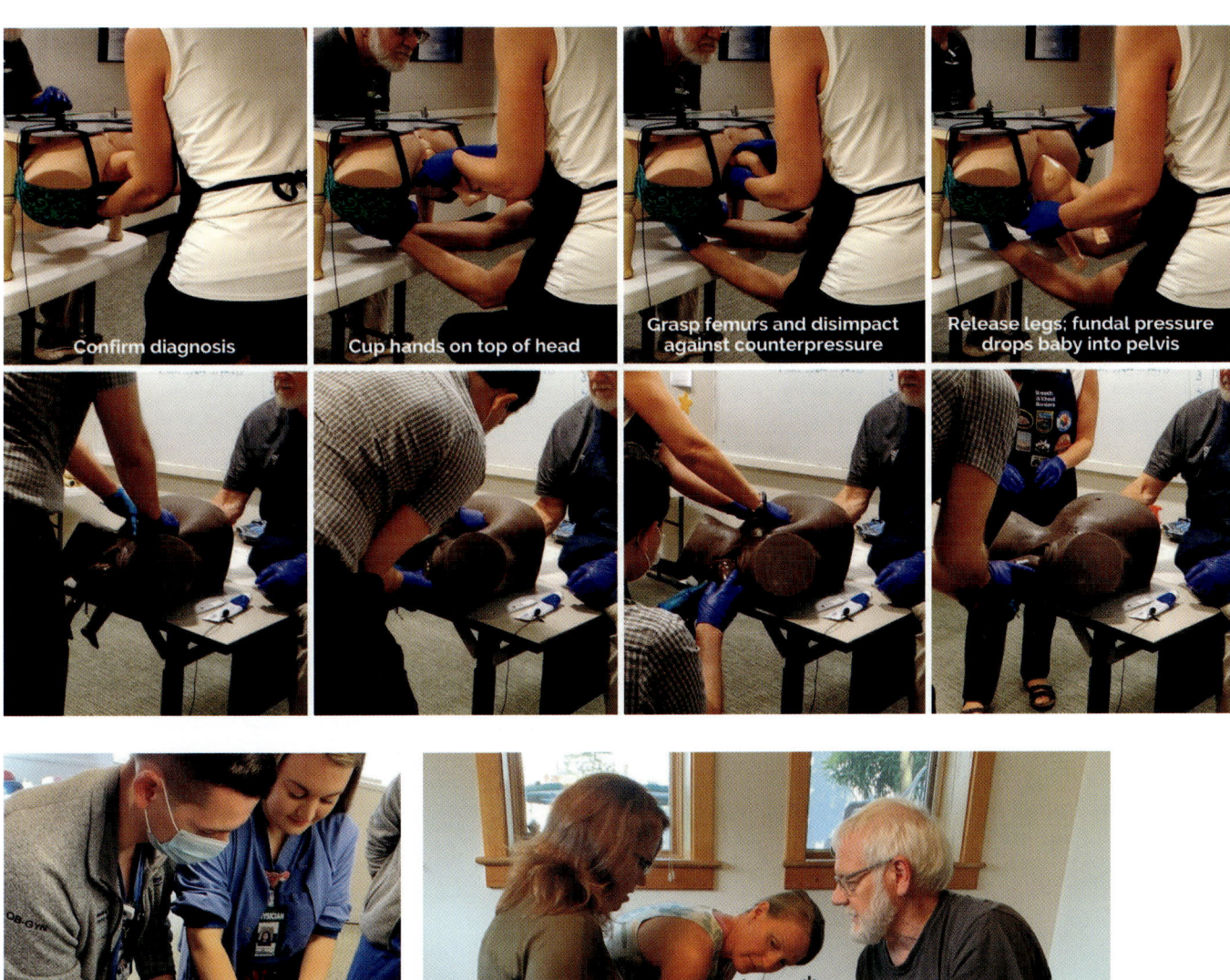

Walker & Reitter describe a similar technique done internally rather than externally. In their words: "Head at the pelvic inlet: Elevate and rotate: (1) The birth attendant runs a finger up to identify that the chin is high; the head is extended and trapped at the inlet to the pelvis. (2) Using 'flat hands' (also called 'prayer hands'), the birth attendant shifts one hand onto the chest of the newborn. Another hand, on the back of the newborn, shifts up to elevate and lift the occiput off the maternal pubic bone. If necessary, the occiput would be rotated at this point into oblique or transverse to assist engagement. (3) Once engaged in the pelvis, the neonatal head is flexed and realigned in the pelvis. The head is then delivered by a shoulder press or variation of Mauriceau" (Reitter, Halliday, & Walker 2019).

Løvset

After finishing steps 1-5, the baby will be low enough to perform a Løvset maneuver, which is an extraction maneuver: Løvset's maneuver has been around for a long time. It is still in common use in areas that routinely do vaginal breech birth. The procedure automatically corrects any upward displacement of the arms.

These illustrations below are from Løvset's original article, published in 1937.

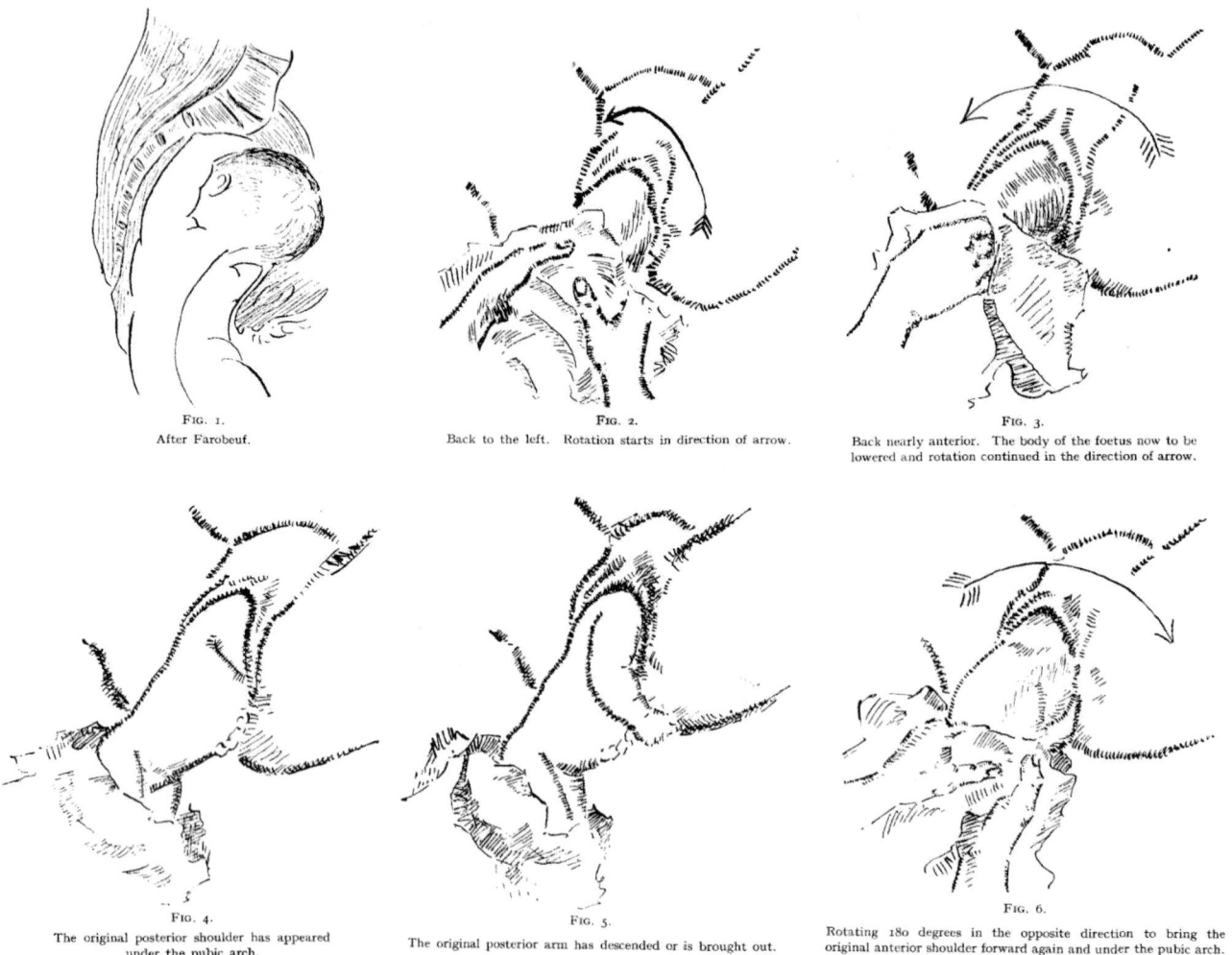

FIG. 1.
After Farobeuf.

FIG. 2.
Back to the left. Rotation starts in direction of arrow.

FIG. 3.
Back nearly anterior. The body of the foetus now to be lowered and rotation continued in the direction of arrow.

FIG. 4.
The original posterior shoulder has appeared under the pubic arch.

FIG. 5.
The original posterior arm has descended or is brought out.

FIG. 6.
Rotating 180 degrees in the opposite direction to bring the original anterior shoulder forward again and under the pubic arch.

The idea of the maneuver flies in the face of everything that we've taught you so far. You are going to pull the baby down and corkscrew it out.

To review, first you laterally flex the baby towards the mother's pubic bone. That pulls the posterior shoulder down into the sacrum. When you have that accomplished, you rotate the baby 180°. That helps the original posterior shoulder rotate and come completely out of the perineum, and it also disimpacts the anterior shoulder. You've now delivered the posterior shoulder underneath the symphysis. Your stuck anterior shoulder is now posterior. Then you do the same thing again: you laterally flex the baby to pull that posterior shoulder down, then you rotate 180° back where you came from. You have now delivered both shoulders. This maneuver is not intended to correct the mechanisms. It is absolutely intended to extract the baby from the woman.

When you do the Løvset maneuver, you are pulling down on the baby and you deflex or even hyperextend the head. Then you are left in a position where you have to flex the baby's head and deliver it. Now that we know other maneuvers for flexing the head, we may never need to resort to the MSV. The Crowning Touch or Ritgen would be recommended in this situation, because the shoulder press is less likely to work on a compromised baby. Ritgen is particularly useful as it can be used in both upright and supine positions, while the shoulder press and the Crowning Touch can only be done from behind when the mother is in some variation of upright.

Conclusion

That wraps up Part 3 of Clinical Aspects of Physiological Breech Birth. We focused on 6 maneuvers that will comprise the bulk of your breech practice. If you master these, you will be prepared for almost any situation that may arise.

In the next lesson, we'll focus on diagnosing abnormal breech birth and develop a framework for determining if, when, and how to intervene.

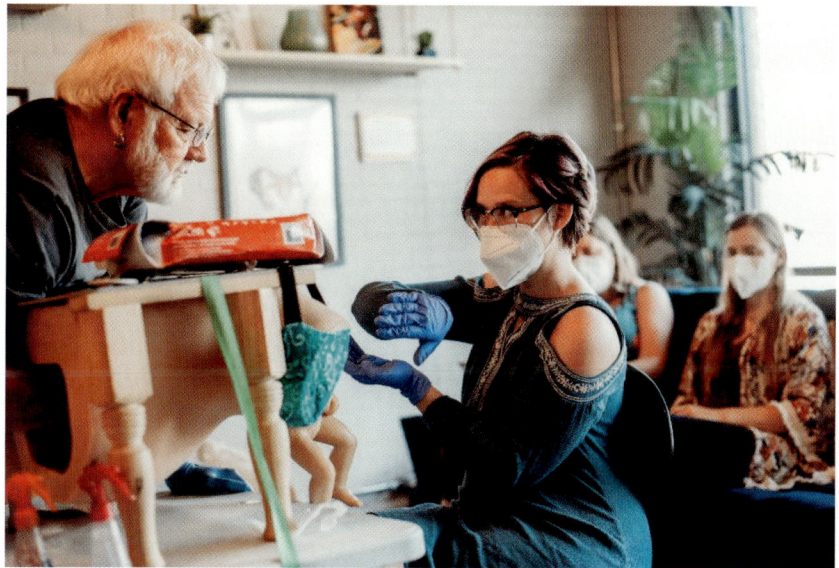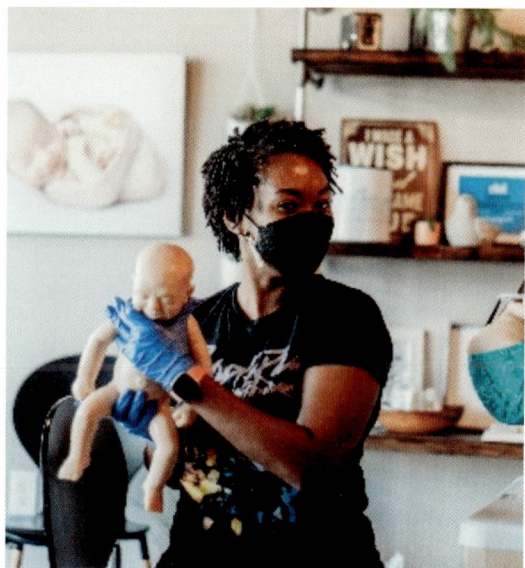

Hands-on training with Dr. Hayes

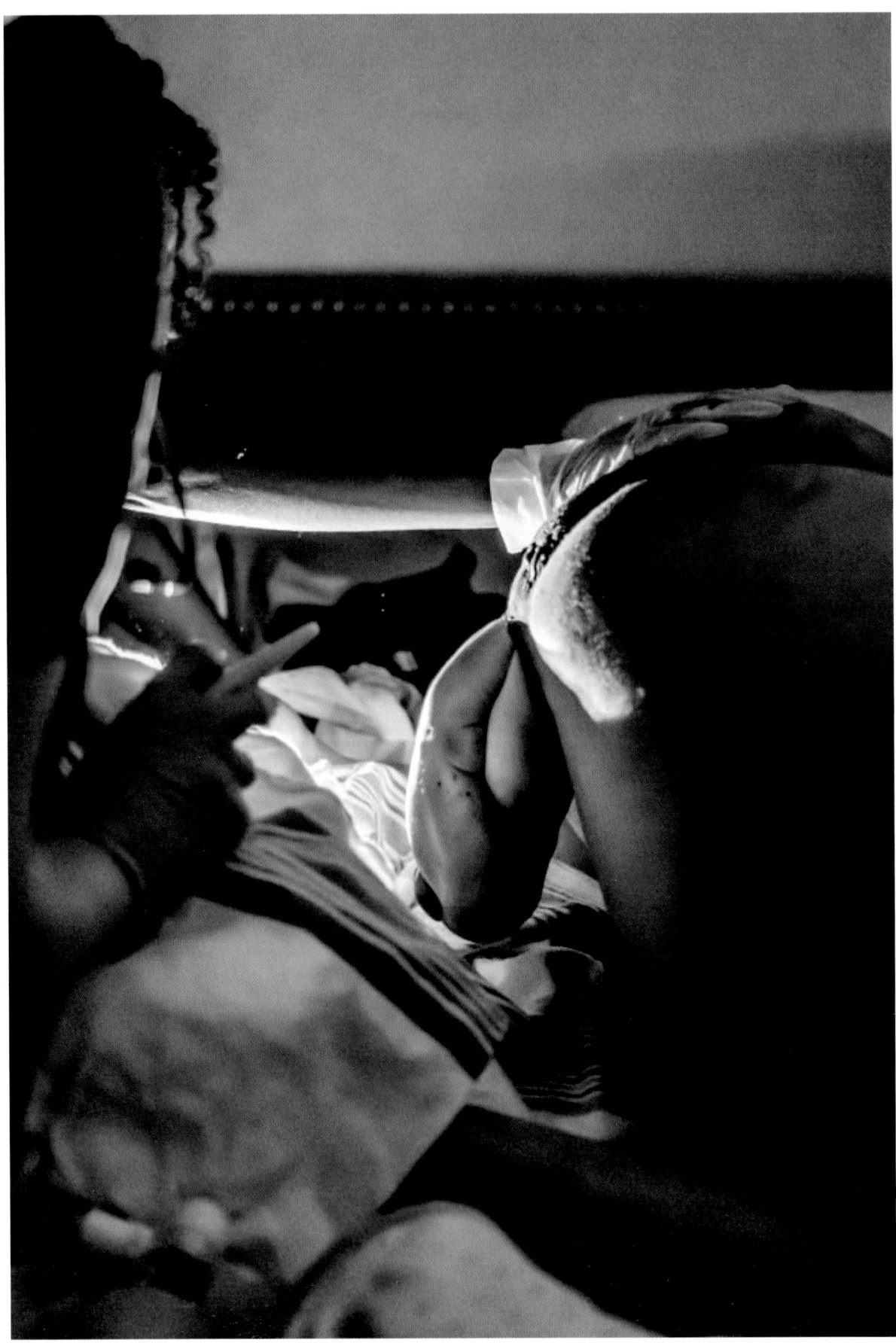

Shatamia Webb, Baby Catcher Birth Center. Undiagnosed frank breech assisted virtually by a BWB clinician

Lesson 11: Abnormal Breech Birth
Clinical Aspects, Part 4

By David Hayes, MD

Welcome to the final lesson of Clinical Aspects: Session 4 on Abnormal Breech Births. This is where we examine births, identify what's happening, and what, if anything, to do about it. Hopefully by the end you'll feel as though you can identify most problems as they arise and know how you would manage them. Then, in the hands-on portion, you will have a chance to put your newfound knowledge and skills to the test. So let us move on.

An approach: Questions to ask

Identify the deviation – What looks abnormal?

Identify the mechanism – What is causing the deviation?

Assess the impact – Is the deviation interfering with birth?

Is the baby tolerating labor well?

How much time has elapsed since rumping?

(rumping = birth of bitrochanteric diameter)

What condition is the baby in?

Is intervention necessary?

If so, determine the goal of your intervention: restore the mechanism or extract the baby?

I'm suggesting that you adopt something like the following approach. Ask yourselves these questions:

1. Identify the deviation: what looks abnormal?

2. Once you see that and you figure out what doesn't look right, identify the mechanism: what's causing that deviation? It won't always be possible, but usually you'll have a really good idea.

3. The next step is to assess the impact: is that deviation interfering with the birth? Is the baby tolerating labor well? How much time has elapsed since rumping (since the birth of the bitrochanteric diameter)?

4. If you decide the deviation is interfering with the birth, is intervention necessary? If so, then you need to think about what the goal of your intervention is going to be. Is it to correct the deviation and the mechanism? This would be the physiological approach. Or is it to extract the baby? This may be necessary in certain cases.

Signs of mechanism disruption

- Incomplete/abnormal rotation
- Asymmetric leg delivery
- Absence of cleavage
- Slow or no descent of the thorax
- Shoulders birth with no head behind the perineum

One sign of mechanism disruption is **incomplete or abnormal rotation**. We talked about rotation a great deal in earlier lessons. We know that things can happen that interfere with that rotation, so that would be an abnormal sign or a sign of mechanism disruption, especially in a frank breech birth, less so or not at all in a complete or incomplete presentation.

Asymmetric leg delivery: The baby, particularly in a frank presentation, comes down out of the pelvis. If the legs are the same length and it's coming straight down, you expect that the delivery of the legs would occur at approximately the same time. That's symmetric delivery. If something is holding the baby up and the baby is presenting asymmetrically, or the baby is coming down and one leg comes out in the other leg doesn't, in many situations, that's a sign that something is hung up, usually on the side in which the baby has not come down.

Slow or no descent: Descent is always what we're looking for ultimately, rotation or no rotation. If there's a slow descent or no descent, that is definitely a sign that the mechanism may be disrupted.

Finally, **shoulders born with a hollow perineum or no indication that the baby's flexed head is behind the perineum**. Those are the signs that you're looking for.

Things That Get Stuck

Arms/Shoulders
  Most common
  Nuchal or raised
Heads
  Rare in mid-pelvis
  Common in pelvic outlet
  Extended
Legs
  Rare among frank breech presentations
  Common in nonfrank breech presentations

Arms and shoulders:

Arms are certainly the most common things that get stuck, usually nuchal or raised of some variety. Nuchal arms can certainly disrupt some rotation. They can also disrupt descent. Arms may be raised or even behind the head, sometimes both arms. Usually, when there's one arm involved, it's going to be the anterior arm or shoulder that is caught on the symphysis pubis. The symphysis pubis, internally, presents a bony shelf that things can get caught on. In the posterior part of the pelvis, there is the sacral promontory, but there are also large muscle masses coming down into the pelvis that create a fairly smooth plane for descent. There is not as much back there for baby parts to get stuck on. The vast majority of cases are going to be an anterior arm or shoulder causing the problem.

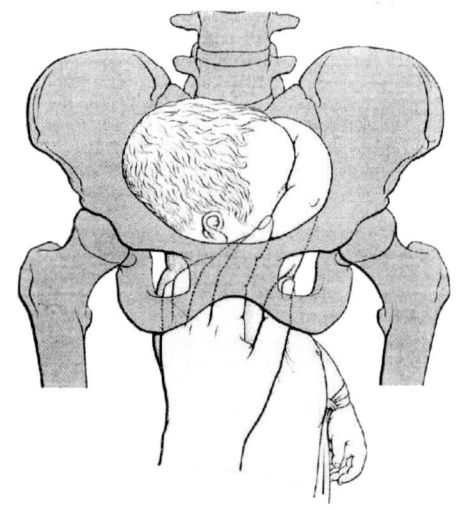

Heads:

Stuck heads are a rare complication in the mid-pelvis or pelvic inlet. But it's common on the perineum or at the pelvic outlet. With an extended head on the perineum, you know the maneuver to take care of that: a shoulder press. That is probably the most common maneuver that you will end up using because it is simple, because it is low-morbidity, and because it expedites the birth. The most patient of us sometimes feels like the baby needs to be out rather than in.

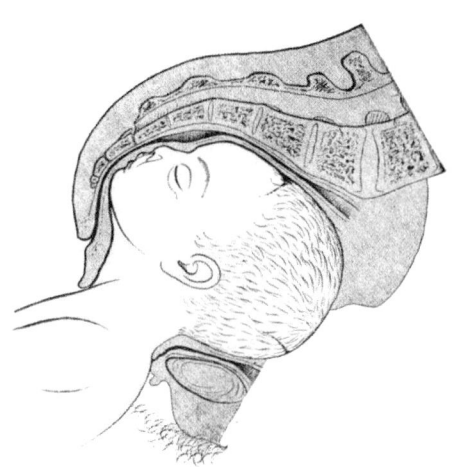

Legs:

Legs are very rarely a problem in frank breech presentations. However, legs commonly disrupt rotation in complete or incomplete breeches. Be aware of that when you see a complete breech, arrest of rotation may happen, but you should keep seeing descent.

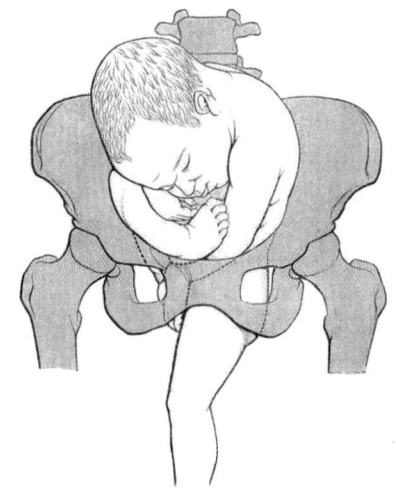

Places they get stuck

Pelvic inlet
  Pubic ramus to sacral prominence
Pelvic outlet
  Pubic ramus to coccyx
Perineum
  Soft tissue

Pubic ramus to the sacral prominence (pelvic inlet):

This is the smallest diameter in most pelvises. It's called the obstetric conjugate.

Pelvic outlet:

The pelvic outlet is the inferior aspect of the pubic ramus to the coccyx. There's a little more flexibility here and a little more length to start with. If you've made it past the pelvic inlet, there are very few reasons for a baby not to be able to come through the outlet.

Perineum:

Then finally, there is the perineum, which can create a soft tissue dystocia. The perineum may be very tight, or the baby's head may be deflexed and not presenting in a position that can easily come through the perineum.

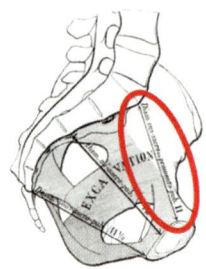

This is a summary of what I discussed earlier. When you're at a breech birth and you're watching like a hawk, ask yourselves these questions.

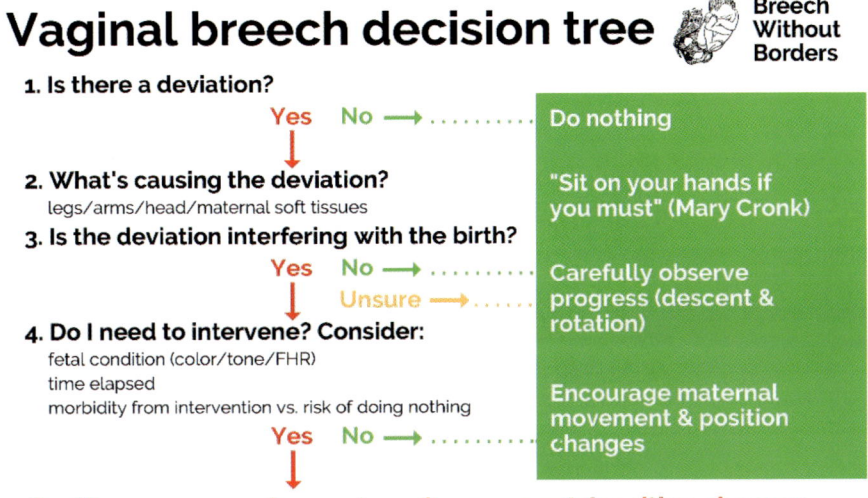

Vaginal breech decision tree — Breech Without Borders

1. Is there a deviation?
Yes   No ⟶ .... Do nothing

2. What's causing the deviation?
legs/arms/head/maternal soft tissues
"Sit on your hands if you must" (Mary Cronk)

3. Is the deviation interfering with the birth?
Yes   No ⟶ ....
Unsure ⟶ ......
Carefully observe progress (descent & rotation)

4. Do I need to intervene? Consider:
fetal condition (color/tone/FHR)
time elapsed
morbidity from intervention vs. risk of doing nothing
Yes   No ⟶ ....
Encourage maternal movement & position changes

Continue encouraging maternal movement/position changes

Is there a deviation?

If you see something that you think is a deviation, go down the list in your head.

What's causing this deviation?

We know it's most probably always going to be an anterior arm, but not always. What kinds of symptoms do we have that suggest that?

Is the deviation interfering with the birth?

There can be a deviation and the mechanism can be disrupted. But you have to ask yourself whether or not it's actually *interfering* with the birth. If you have an arrest of rotation and you think you have a stuck arm somewhere, but the baby is still descending, then depending on the other factors (time elapsed since rumping, baby's current status, strength & frequency of contractions), you may or may not decide that this deviation is interfering with the birth.

Do you need to intervene?

Again, you assess your baby, you factor in how much time has passed, and then you make a call as to whether the risks of intervention are worth the benefits.

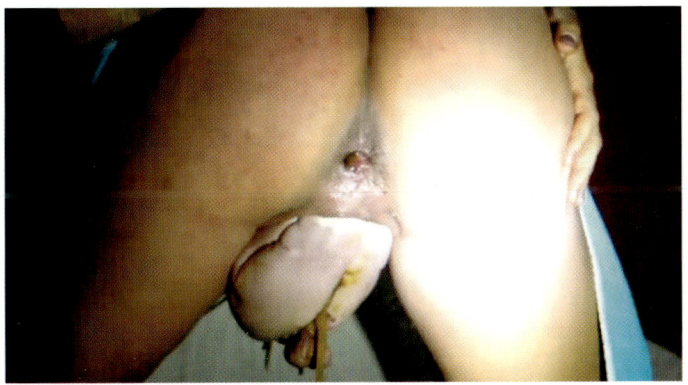

This is the woman from Example 2 earlier in the book from the lesson on normal breech birth. You're seeing the baby descending very nicely.

But what else are you seeing? Is there a deviation here?

Well, it's not entirely rotated to sacrum anterior. It doesn't always happen in one push, but most of the time it does, so I would be suspicious. But there's another clue as to whether or not this is abnormal. And that is the baby. Look at the baby's position: that is asymmetry personified. The baby is coming down, but it's being pushed dramatically to the mama's left side, and the baby's back is pressed into her thigh. So clearly there is a deviation.

What caused the deviation?
The anterior arm is almost always going to be your problem. Not always, but usually. Does this look like the anterior arm is your problem? It does not. That baby came down and got caught on something on its right side, which is indeed the posterior arm.

Would you intervene?
This is kind of an easy one, because you've already seen the birth in the normal section. But the other clue that you don't need to intervene, certainly not yet at least, is because with the last contraction, that baby was descending, and descending beautifully. Let's go on.

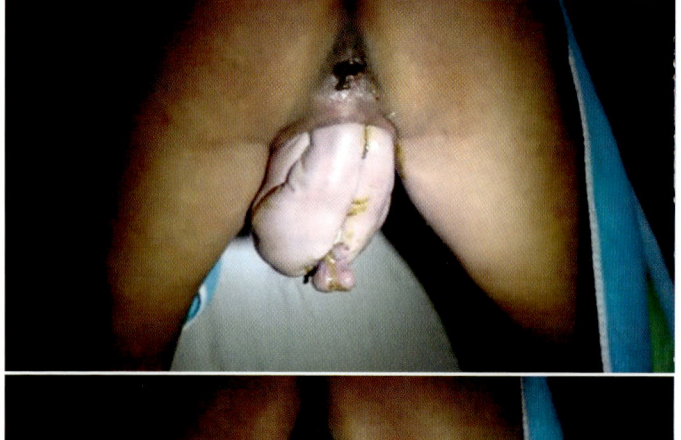
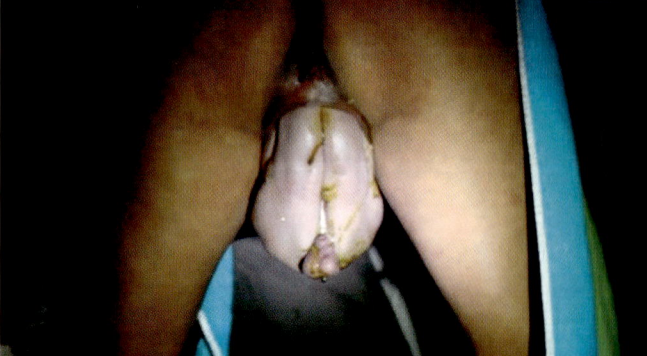

If you watch it, it feels like there's a little bit of rotation taking place, but it's also not being jammed so hard into the thigh. She's just pushing on her own because she feels probably something hanging up on that left side, and she's trying her best to respond to it. She is making all sorts of squatting movements; those are all her and not because I suggested them.

You see now that the baby is now completely away from her thigh; the baby is hanging much straighter. And you see a little crinkle on that side of the baby's chest. But look at that rotation. The mom is standing just a little bit sideways. This is a very clear demonstration of why the mom needs to be able to feel what's going on.

The baby has now rotated. With the next contraction and push, we will have a baby.

Here are the questions again. This will be a little bit more difficult than the last one. See what you think about it.

Questions

Is there a deviation?

What is causing the deviation?

Is the deviation interfering with the birth?

Do you need to intervene?

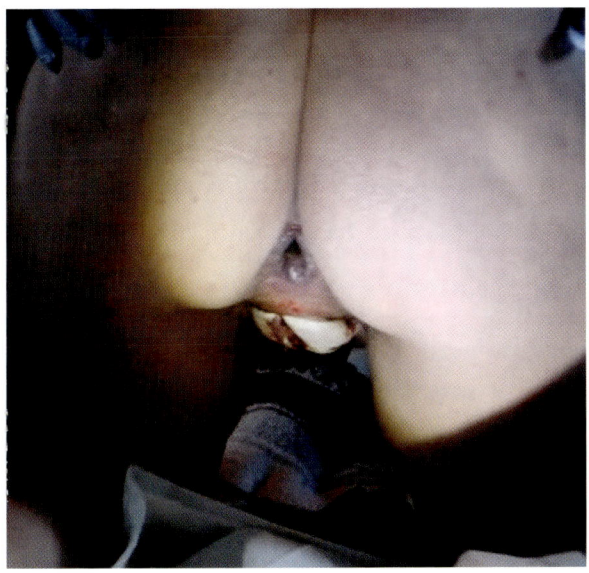

This woman is a primip. Do you see anything unusual about this image?

I'll give you a hint that there is something unusual.

Is there a deviation? Indeed, there is a deviation. The baby rumped sacrum anterior. It appears to have come a little bit from the right, because it's a little bit skewed to that side, but not much. That implies that something caused the baby to rotate *before* hitting the pelvic floor. That should definitely make you think.

What's causing that? Most likely not legs, because this appears to be a frank breech, almost certainly is a frank breech at this point. That leaves you with arms and heads. Heads don't generally interfere with rotation because heads have their own ability to rotate on an axis. If it gets stuck, the body can rotate separately. It's almost certain that the arms are causing the problem. It's difficult to say which arm, and in a situation like this that often means it is both arms.

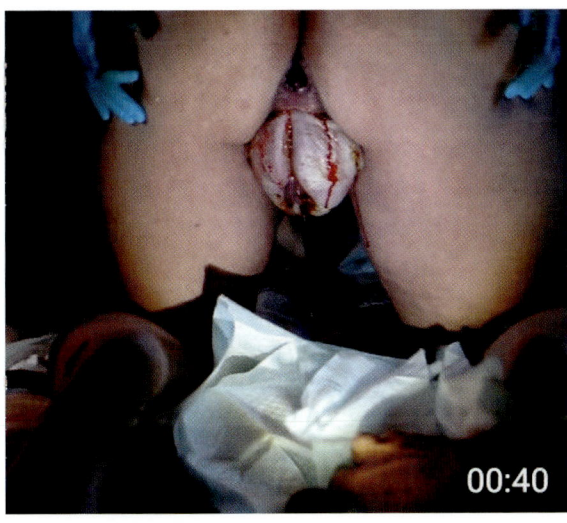

00:40

We don't know what the deviation is, and is it interfering with the birth? Keep in mind, this is a primip. She has never done this before.

And with her first push, she has the baby almost to the umbilicus, even though it presented originally in a sacrum anterior position, an abnormal position for rumping.

You can ask yourself if you would intervene at this point. My answer is going to be no. I can also tell you we're less than 40 seconds into the pushing phase here.

In the next picture, she is pushing. I see some progress.

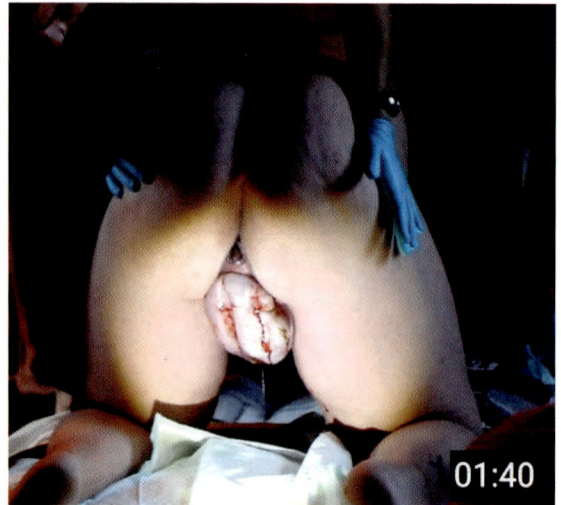

This is where she ended up after the last contraction. Compare that to where she started at 0:40 in the last picture, before this last contraction began. Clearly the sacrum anterior baby is now trying to rotate **back** to right sacrum transverse. Is that a deviation?

It absolutely is a deviation. What do you think is causing that deviation?

Well, as the baby is trying to come down, it's getting pulled back to the right. I'm going to guess that the baby's right arm, the one we usually think about, is hung up on the symphysis pubis. And as the baby goes down, the arm is pulling the baby in that direction because the arm isn't coming behind it. There may still also be something going on with the left arm. We will keep figuring this out as we go.

Would you intervene at this point? It seems to be interfering with the birth. However, this baby seems to have good muscle tone. And we're not even 2 minutes into this birth. The baby is currently still not in jeopardy. We're going to move on and see. I obviously elected not to intervene.

Let's look at this next image. The gluteal squeeze is probably not helping anything. Hip squeezes should be done on the femur heads and not by squeezing the buttocks together. You can also see another assistant wiping the mother's bottom (she did this multiple times during the birth). I imagine it's a distracting to have someone wiping your butt when you're trying to give birth. I made my feelings known to my assistants about that after this birth was over.

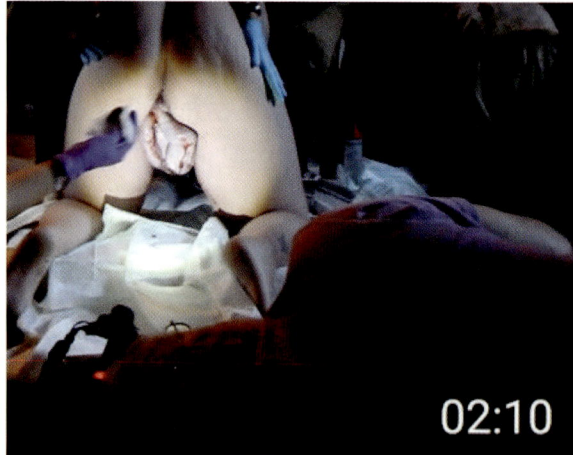

Look at the baby's left leg. You see that it seems to be doing something.

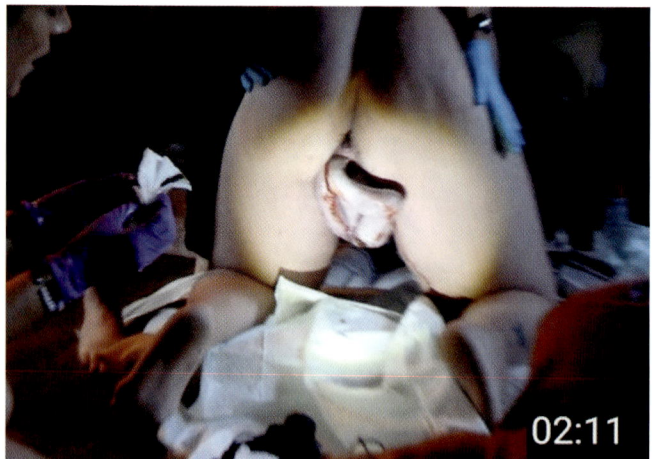

The rest of the baby isn't moving, but the left leg is. That's curious.

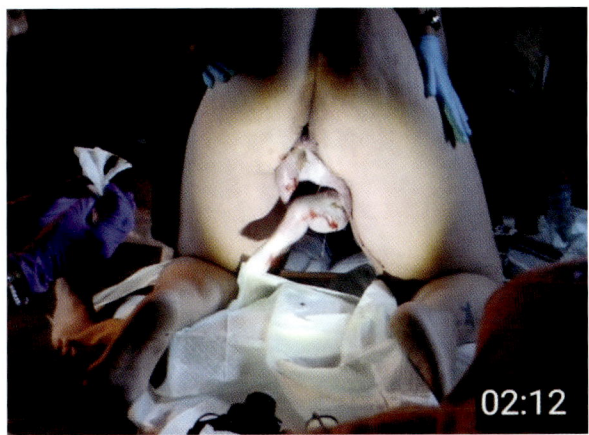

The leg came out. Is there a deviation? Yes, there is clearly still a deviation. The baby is still rotated off to the right a little bit and now seems to be pulled into mom's thigh on the left a little bit. There's asymmetry there. Is that the asymmetry of the leg delivery? I would argue no, that was not a passive delivery of one leg. **The baby pulled its own leg out.** That tells me tons about how vigorous that baby is.

Do you feel the need to intervene? I will let you think about your decision, and you will see what I decided to do.

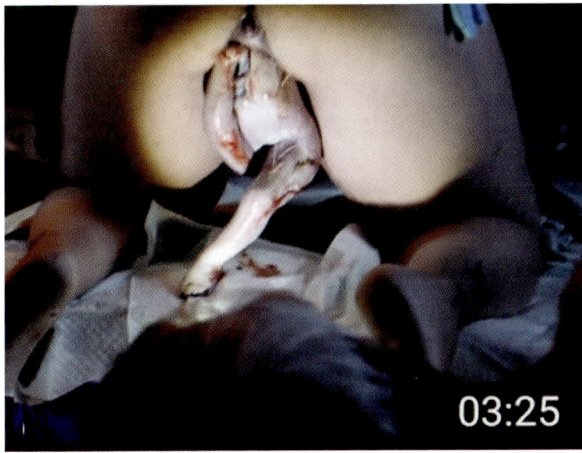

Obviously, I haven't elected to intervene yet. Let's look at what happens next.

To summarize, we're having a contraction. The mom is pushing, the baby descends.

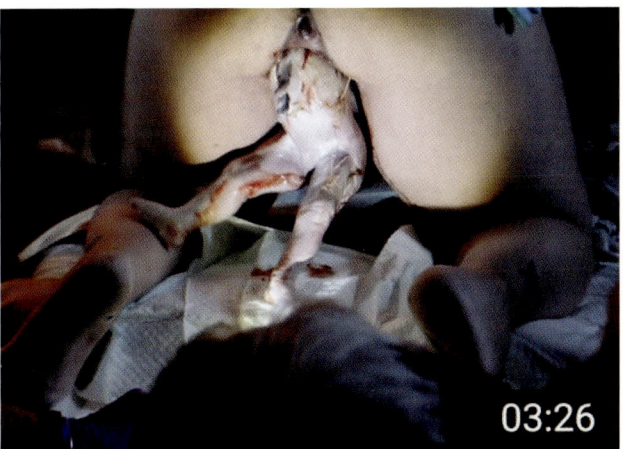

The right leg delivers spontaneously. You will note that the asymmetry in body posture that we were seeing in the last segment is now mostly gone, which suggests to me that the posterior arm has come away from whatever was holding it up.

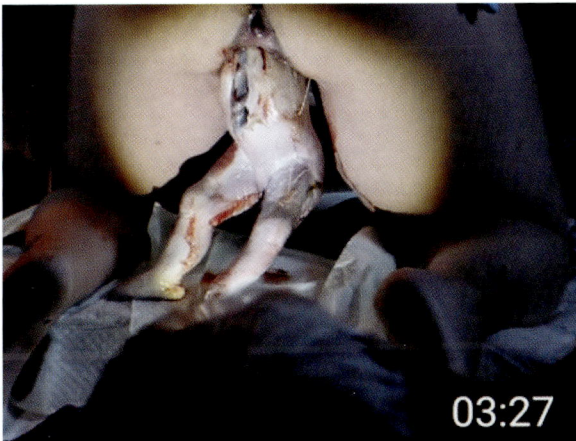

It's a bit hard to tell, but in this picture the baby has descended a bit more.

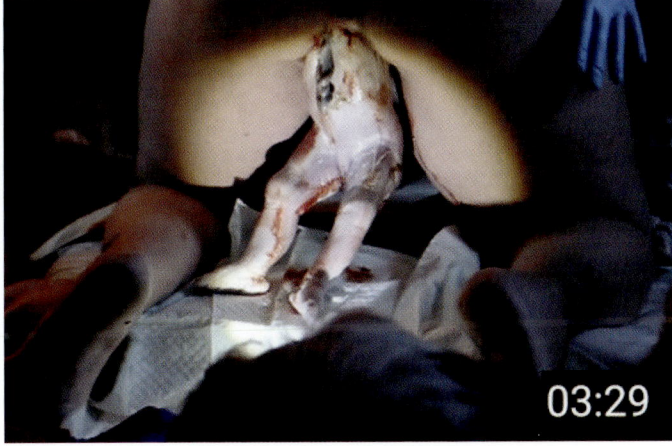

Baby has gone **upwards**! It's hard to see in the picture, but the baby has gone back up about an inch (2.5 cm).

Clearly there's still a deviation. What do you think about the baby ascending back into the pelvis? Maybe it just decided it liked it better in than out! But there is not a uterine mechanism for that baby going back up at that point in birth.

What could possibly have caused the baby to ascend like that, at the end of the contraction, too? Think about it for a second. I usually show these births in a classroom format. People get to throw out their guesses, and we have a raucous discussion about it.

My take on what we just saw is that the baby's arm was still caught. But with the relaxation after that last contraction, the baby was able to pull its own arm down, which had the effect of lifting it up into the pelvis. We will never know that for sure, but I can't think of another mechanism that would accomplish that and fit what we're seeing. If that's true, then we would expect the birth to follow shortly after because there are no longer any impediments to the birth.

Would you intervene at this point? I imagine, with everything I just said and seeing that the baby has good tone, everybody is going to say no. And indeed, I did not.

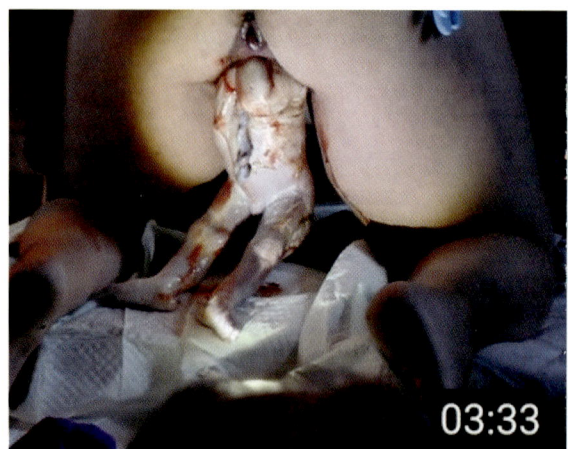
Baby pulls its left arm out.

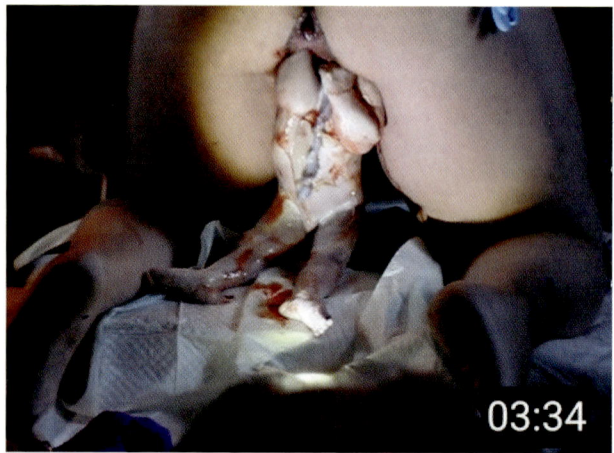
Baby pulls its right arm out.

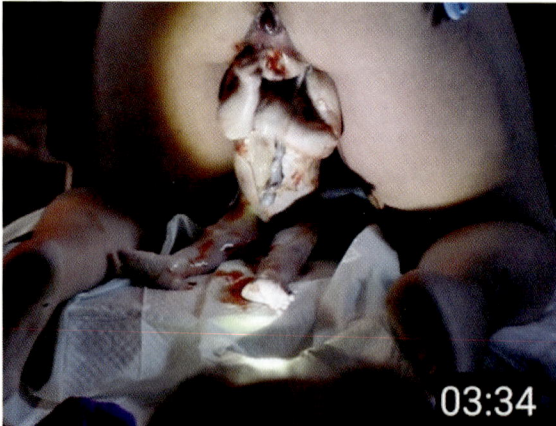
The head mouth and nose follow immediately.

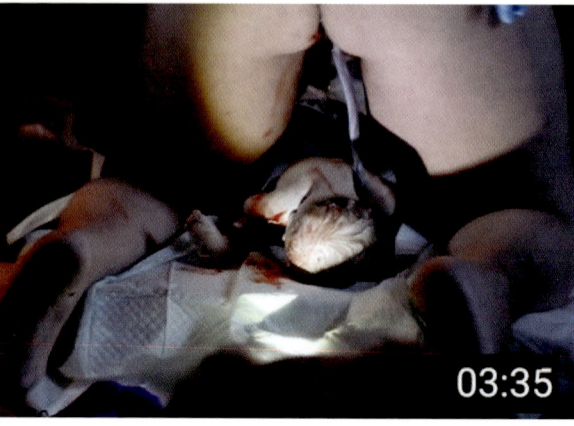
Baby plops onto the cushion. All of this (arms & head) happened in 2 seconds!

It doesn't get much smoother than that. You could have gotten into all kinds of trouble if you decided you wanted to pull on that baby. The total time, from before we started the timer for rumping to the birth, was under 4 minutes and 50 seconds. The expulsion itself took 3m35s.

Just to review your questions:

Questions

Is there a deviation?

What is causing the deviation?

Is the deviation interfering with the birth?

Do you need to intervene?

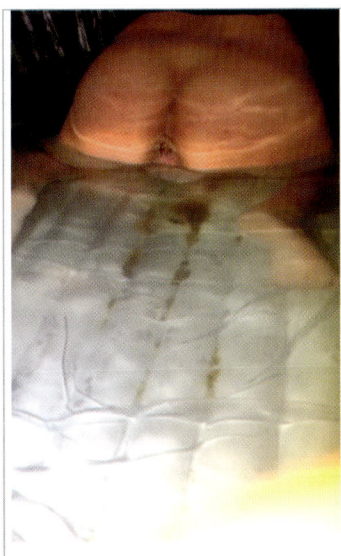 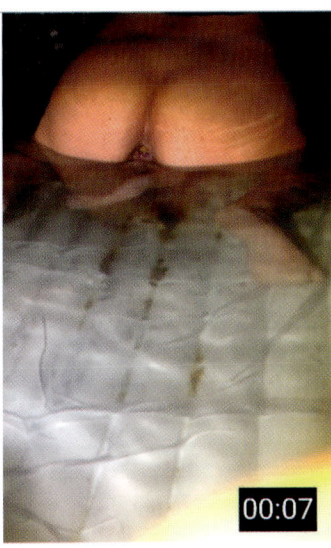 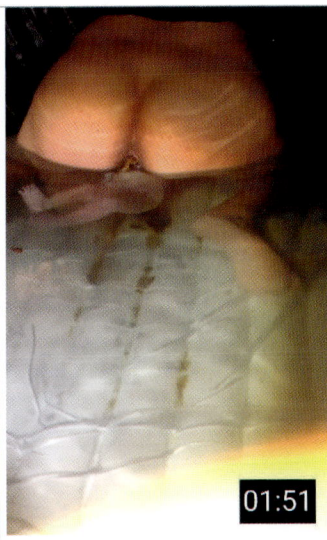 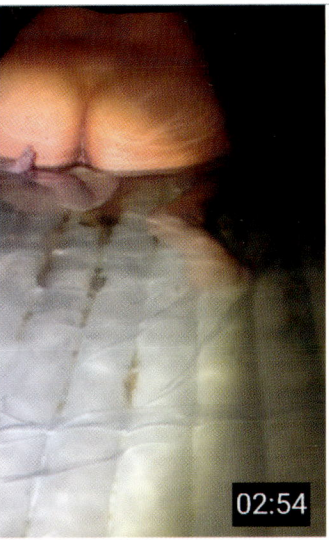

We're just now getting something that looks like rumping. I'm sorry that it's a little difficult to see.	We have the left leg out, so we have at least a complete or incomplete breech. Is there a deviation? It's probably too early to tell.	The lack of rotation we expect in a complete breech. Now the second leg has released, and the baby is still facing oblique, rather than sacrum anterior.	There appears to be good muscle tone. You could argue that's just buoyancy. But then baby kicks its feet up out of the water! The mom is telling the baby to "stop wiggling." Clearly, the baby is doing well.

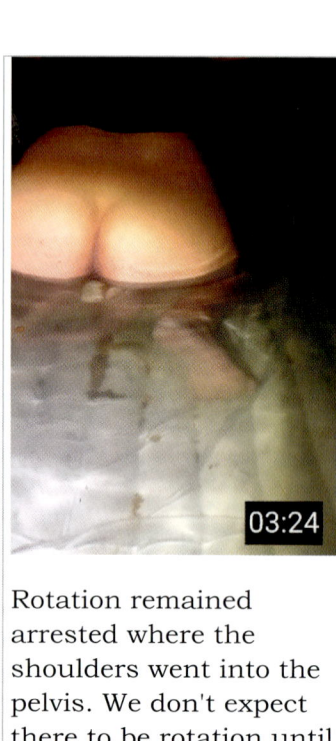

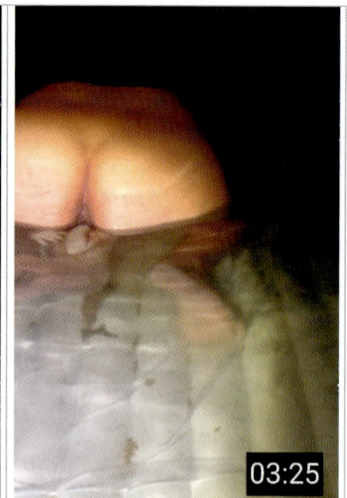

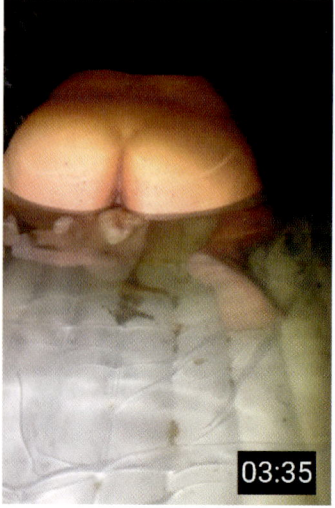

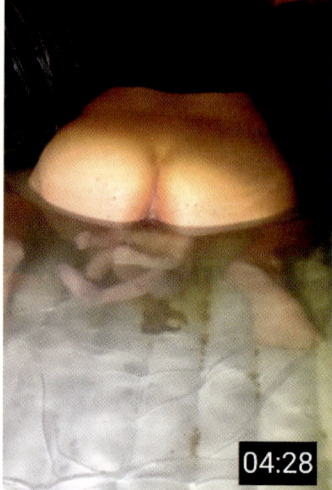

Rotation remained arrested where the shoulders went into the pelvis. We don't expect there to be rotation until the shoulders are out.

The left elbow is out.

The right arm and hand are out. The left hand is tucked underneath the perineum.

Baby continues to kick vigorously. It's having fun in a much bigger pool! Note the baby is still facing oblique and has not yet rotated to sacrum anterior.

We would now expect the baby to rotate to sacrum anterior because that's how the head will exit the pelvic outlet and perineum. It's starting to do so in this picture.

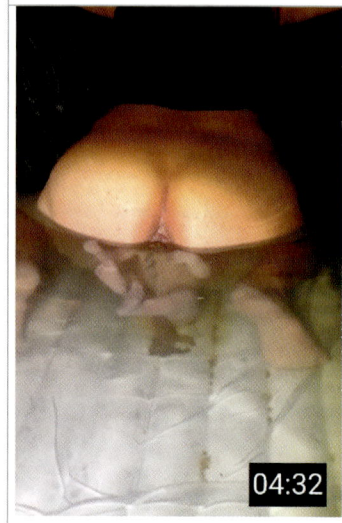

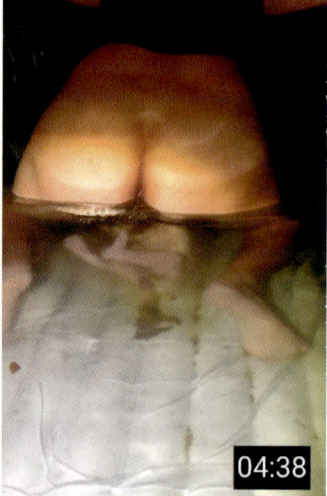

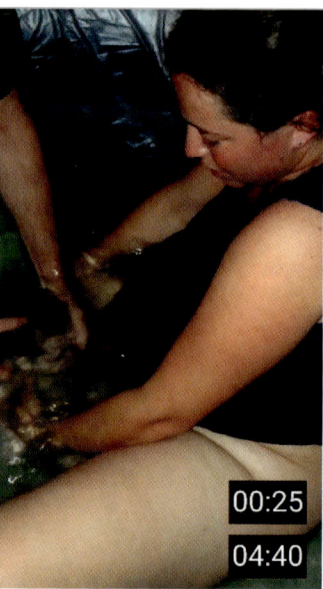

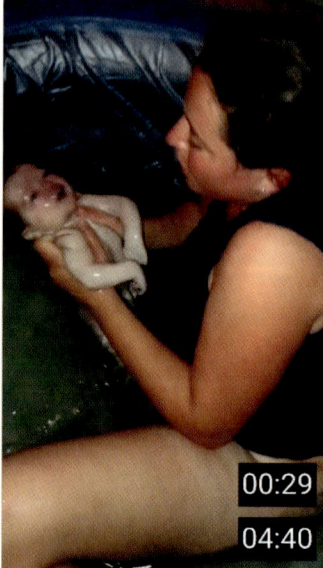

The body is mostly straight now as the head is lining up inside the pelvic outlet. One last big tummy crunch...

....and the baby's head pops out.

Unwrapping 2 loops of cord

Baby is vigorous with eyes wide open

I will also note, because I'm sure some of you are wondering what in the world I did here, that the water level is quite low. I do not normally skimp on the water so much! But this woman was discovered to be breech in labor and drove to my office from another state. I quickly set up the pool in my office and started filling it before she arrived. That's when I discovered what I thought was an on-demand hot water heater was in fact only a 10-gallon (37 liter) tank! We did the best we could without pouring cold water in there.

Obviously, you have to keep the baby under the water while untangling the cord. The receptors for the mammalian dive reflex are around the mouth and nose. When the face is submerged, that suppresses the trigger to breathe. Plus, the baby had a perfectly patent and functioning umbilical cord, so it didn't need to breathe immediately. This birth is such a nice example of leaving the cord intact and of not being too quick to cut the cord in order to resuscitate the baby. Once out of the water, the baby began breathing on its own. It was making little mewling noises when it was in its mother's arms. The whole idea that babies have to come out and scream is sadly oversold.

One side note: some people are reluctant to do physiological breech birth in a pool because of access to the mom and not being familiar with the setup. I have done several breech water births, and they have all gone extremely smoothly. The births seem to be easier from the standpoint of tissue resistance. It is my suspicion that the perineum is more pliable when it's soaked in water. I don't exactly know how to go about proving that, but I would like to. There are midwives in the world, who have done several hundred water birth breeches. A midwife I know in SW Wisconsin has done over 600 vaginal breech births, most in water. I have let go of whether I'm comfortable with waterbirth or not because a) my clients want it and b) I have reason to believe that the outcomes can be very good. I offer water births to all my breech clients (and all of my cephalic ones) and will be happy to collect more data on that as time goes forward.

What would you do?

This is a video, generously shared by one of our attendees, prior to taking our workshop.

What differences do you notice?

Happily, the birth turned out fine. What might you have done differently in the same situation?

This birth turned out fine. Do you agree with her management? What would you do differently?

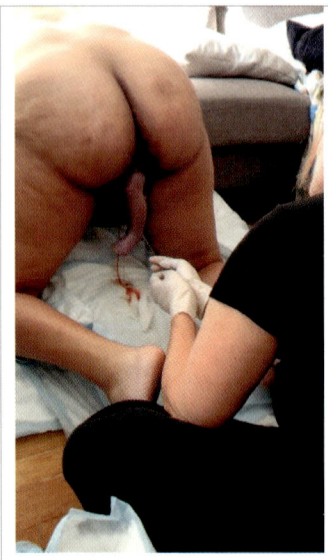

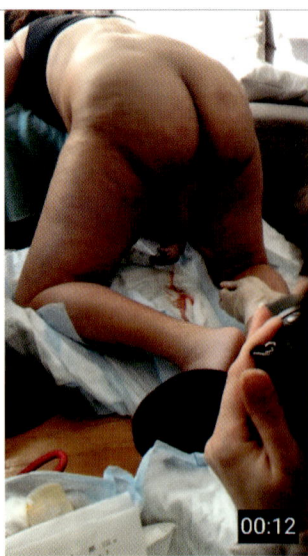

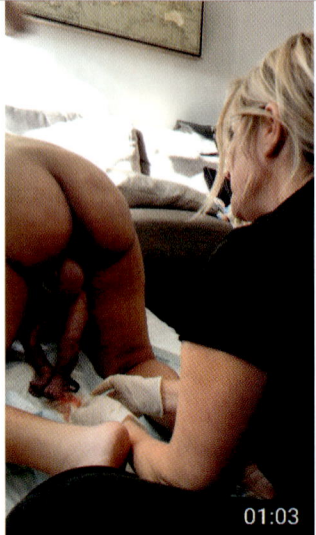

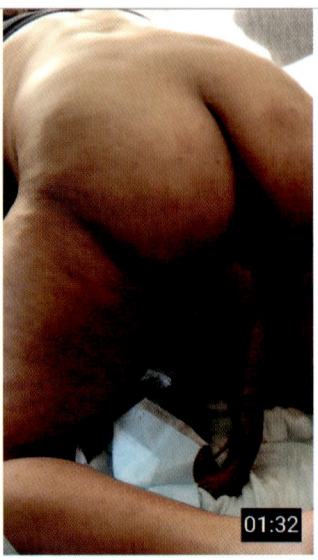

Ah, there's a foot there hanging down. Is this a footling breech?

(Remember what you learned about dropped foot breeches? This is not a footling.)

Baby is still descending very nicely. And we're out to mid-thigh there, so there's got to be buttocks nearby, and there's the other leg. The baby was a complete breech.

There is an arrest of rotation. We expect it with a complete breech, and it's fine (at this point, at least). Later on, once there is also an arrest of descent, then you know there's a problem.

See the baby tensing its legs a little against the resistance that its feet are meeting?

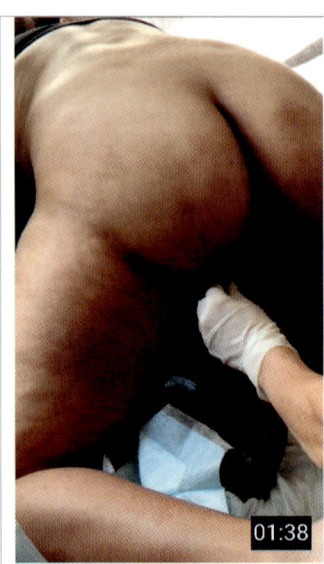

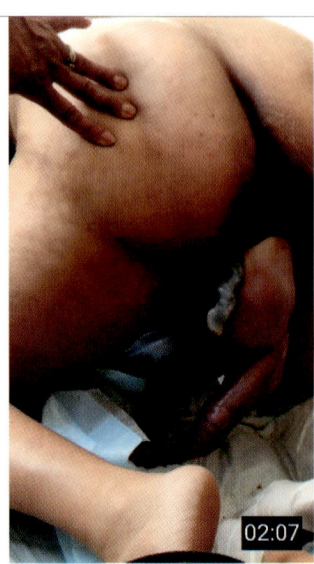

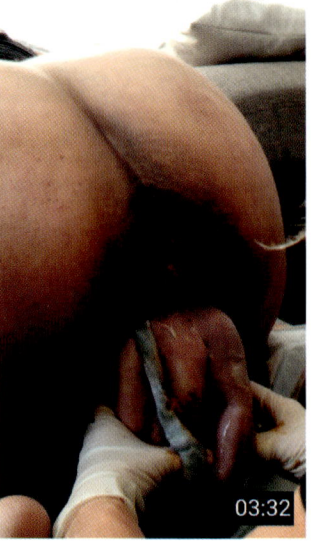

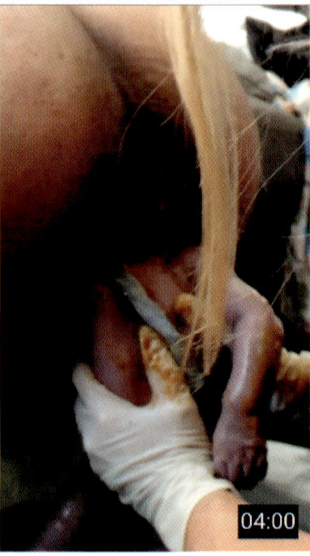

The cord looks full. She is checking it and happy with what she feels. This is before our workshop, and she was very calm and patient.

Next contraction. It's becoming more apparent that there's an obstruction. Baby is pivoting around the trapped shoulder

80 sec later. The right arm is pulled tight behind the head and clearly trapped. The cord is starting to look less full—a sign to act promptly.

The midwife is still evaluating the trapped right arm. You can see a significant amount of the scapula.

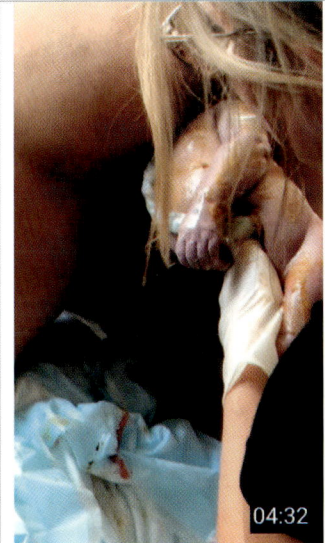

04:32

The midwife had not yet trained with us, so she starts lifting the baby laterally and trying to free the trapped arm.

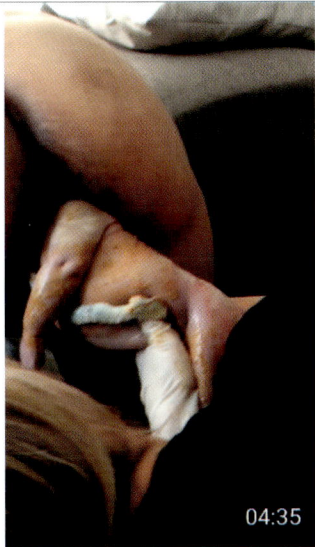

04:35

It takes her a while...

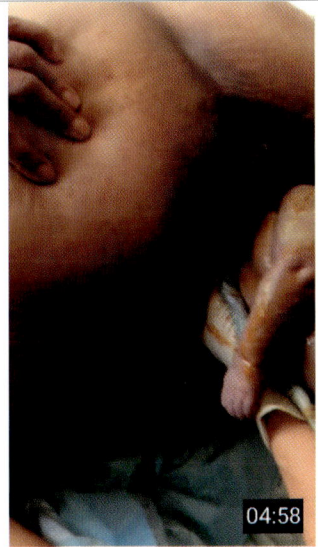

04:58

...still working...

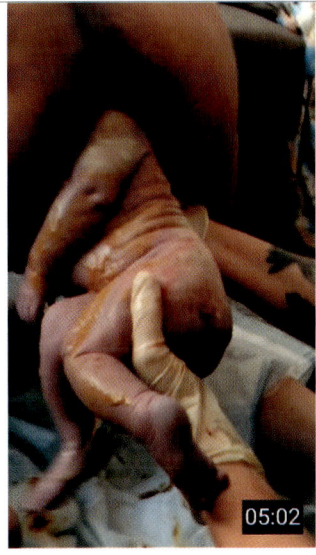

05:02

...still working...

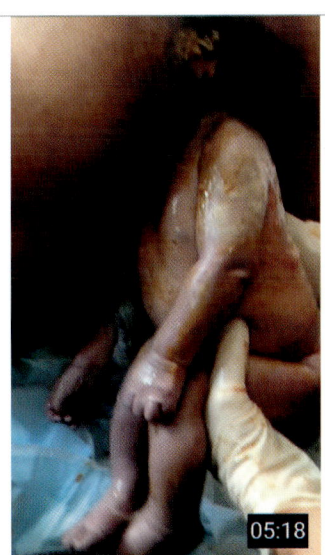

05:18

Finally, she frees the trapped anterior arm.

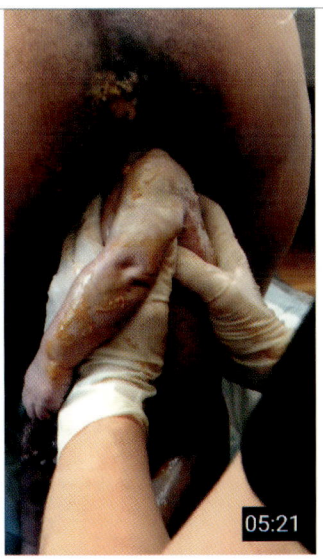

05:21

Now she gently grabs the baby's chest and helps it rotate to sacrum anterior.

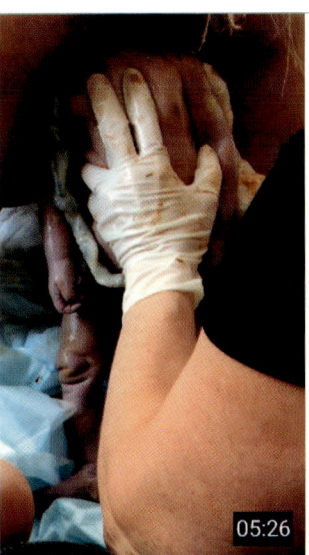

05:26

The cord is looking limp and white now—this baby needs to get out right away.

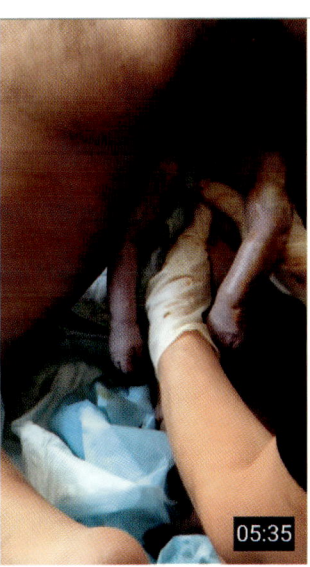

05:35

The midwife does a shoulder press.

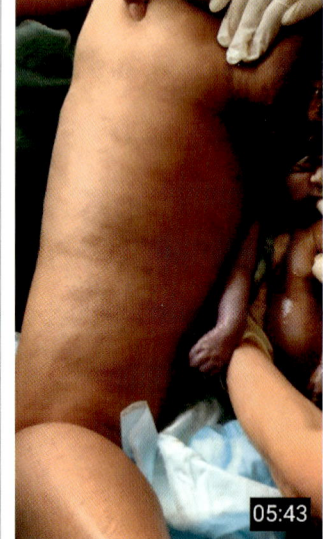

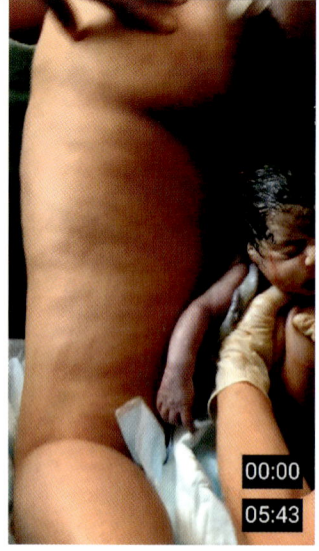

The face starts coming out after several seconds of shoulder press. (Her thumbs are poking into the chest more than I would like. Be sure to either grab the bony part of the shoulders or do a flat hand press across the entire chest.)

Baby is out and did well after some resuscitation.

What would you do?

This is a video of a primip breech, shared with the mother's permission. The midwife had not taken our workshop.

What could you have done differently?

What would you do next?

We have another birth, generously supplied by the mother whose midwives had not trained with us at the time. The breech was discovered during pushing. The mother pushed for about 5 hours with very little progress, and she was exhausted.

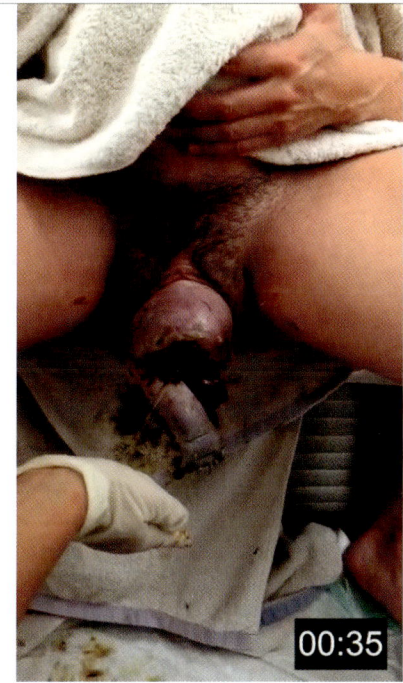

The baby is left sacrum transverse. We are seeing the baby's left leg and foot.

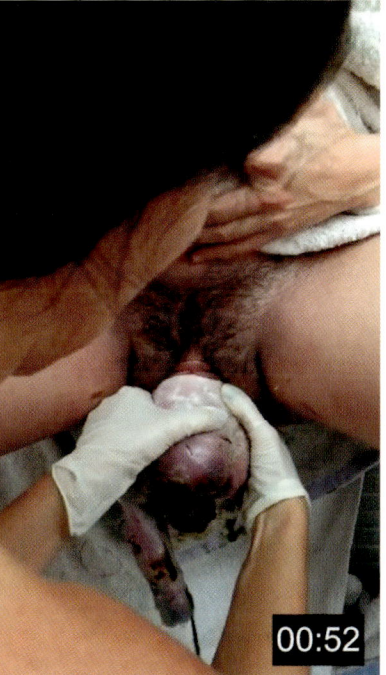

She is turning the baby to SA and pulling the baby down. Baby's legs are flexing so that means baby is doing well.

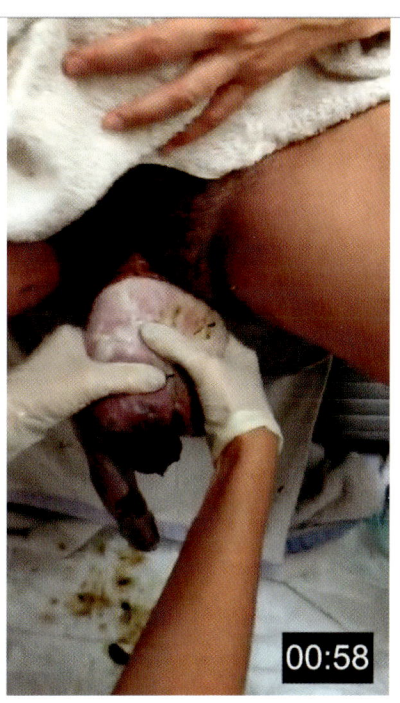

More pulling

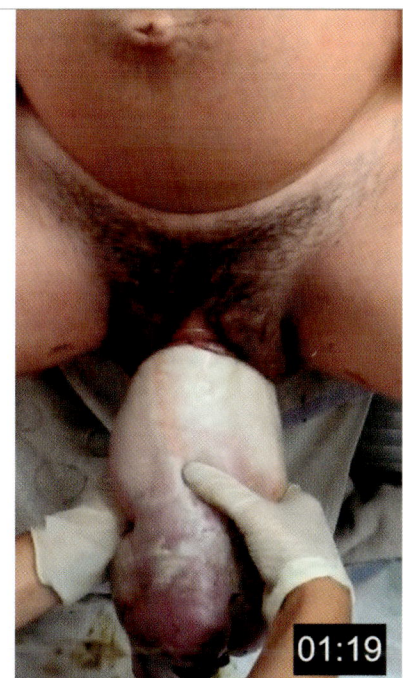

Midwife is pulling, but the mother's contraction is probably more effective than the pulling is.

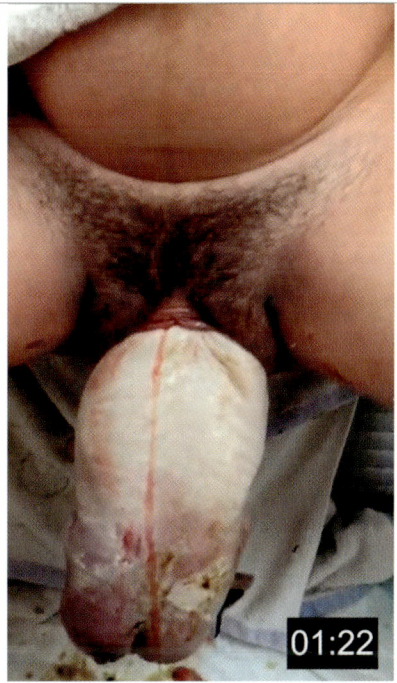

Baby is now facing sacrum anterior, which is reassuring. We don't have to worry about trapped arms.

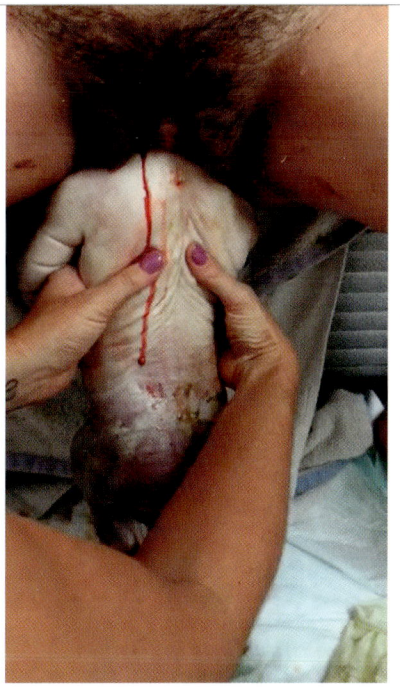

The arms delivered spontaneously shortly after, followed immediately by the head.

As a side note, this baby weighed 10.5 lbs.

Now, I am quite certain this midwife wouldn't do what she's doing right now if she had trained with us. She pulled on the baby. We know that that was risky. What could she have done differently? Imagine yourself in this scenario. What would you have done?

First off, you could encourage the mom to push and see if there was still descent happening. (In this birth, the mother was giving it maximum effort with little progress.)

Second, the mom is sitting upright on a birth stool. You could encourage the mama to get into a deep squat or a supported squat, which may have given her pushes a lot more power to flex the baby's head flexed and move it down. Or you could try kneeling or hands & knees or an asymmetrical lunge.

And a third strategy would be to try fundal pressure. If the baby is in good condition and the birth is proceeding normally, of course you wouldn't consider it. But if the baby were looking limp, or if its heart rate were concerning, or if the mother were completely exhausted and her contractions weren't doing anything and the baby stopped descending, then that would be a perfect situation for fundal pressure. You know which direction the head should be pointing because you know the baby's back is facing the mother's left. You can find the head, put pressure on the fundus and on the baby's head, and see if it comes down. My guess is it would have indeed done so in this birth.

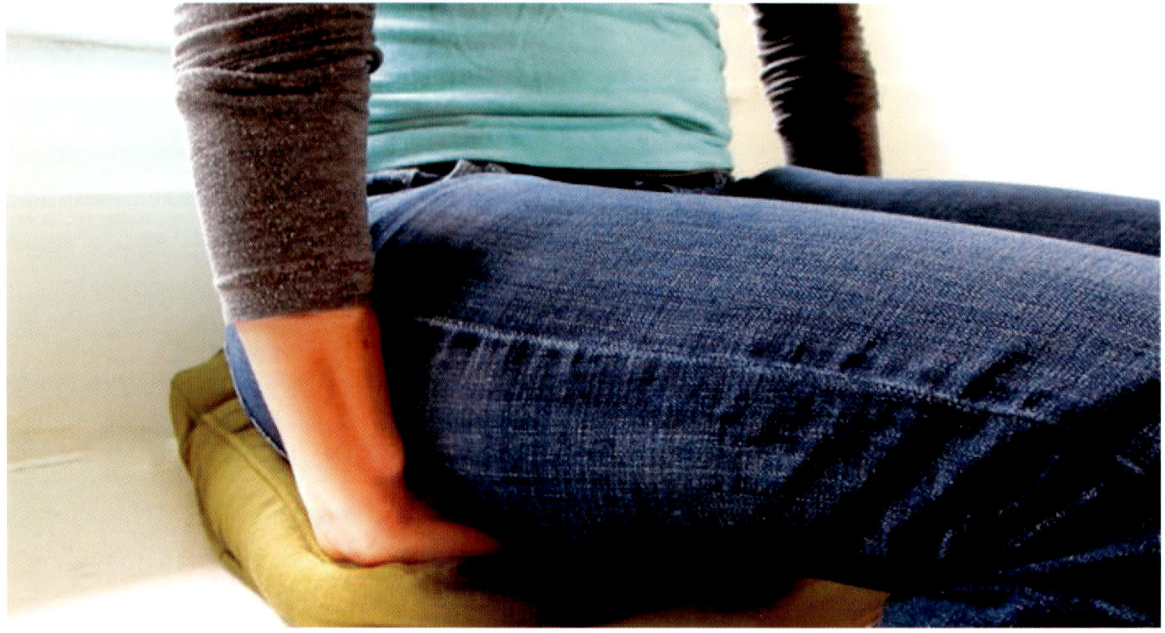

The hardest part of attending a vaginal breech birth: sitting on your hands
(image: iWitness news)

This next birth illustrates one of my favorite sayings:

If you don't know what you are doing,
don't do anything.

Intervening in a breech birth can make things worse. If you are well-trained and know when and how to intervene appropriately, then by all means assist if help is needed. But if you're not well-trained, you risk making things far worse by interfering than if you left the process alone. UK midwife Mary Cronk was well-known for saying, "Keep your hands to yourself; sit on them if necessary" (1998).

Warning: these next photos are very intense. Only turn the page if you want to proceed. This was sent to me anonymously from the public domain, and the images end before the birth completed. I don't know what the outcome was.

This birth is taking place in a hospital. There is a resident attempting a breech birth and the attending obstetrician trying to help. It is obvious that neither of them knows what they should be doing, whether physiological or otherwise. This reinforces my previous admonition: **If you don't know what you're doing, don't do anything**.

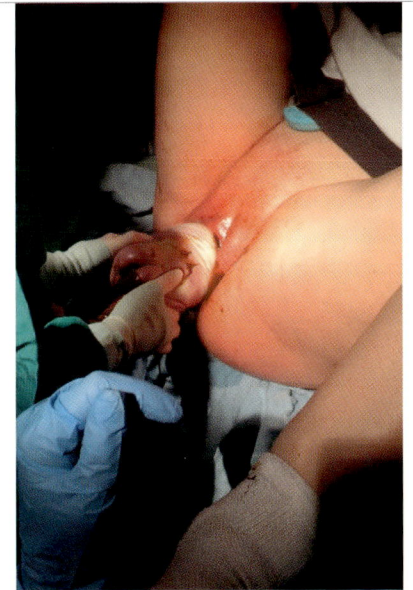 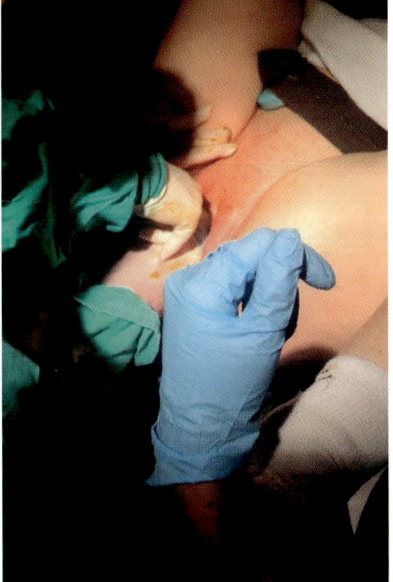 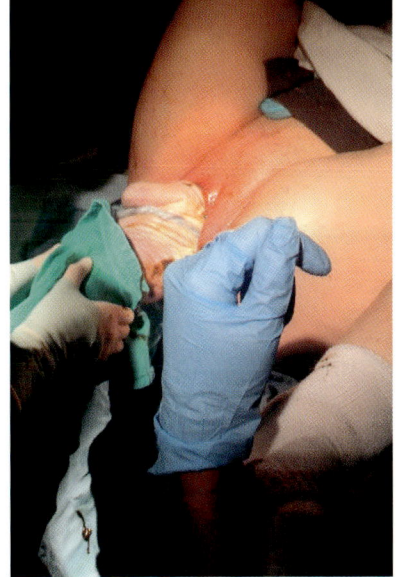

| First, we see the resident pulling and turning the baby in a manner reminiscent of a Løvset maneuver, slowly, carefully, and not going anywhere. | The OB reaches in and frees the anterior arm. | The resident tries another Løvset rotation. Notice the creases in the baby's back showing her efforts to twist. |

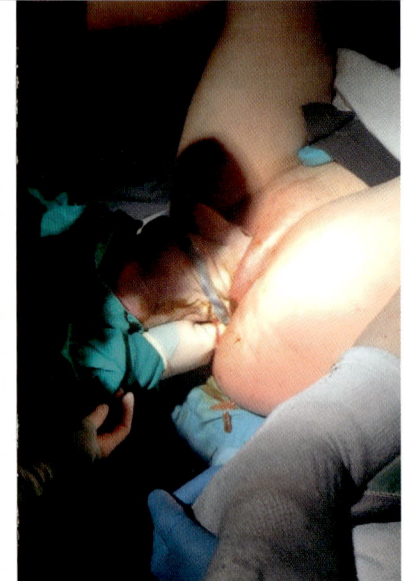

They abandon the Løvset maneuver. The attending first laterally flexes the baby because she can't figure out anything to do. She next just goes in and gets the arm.

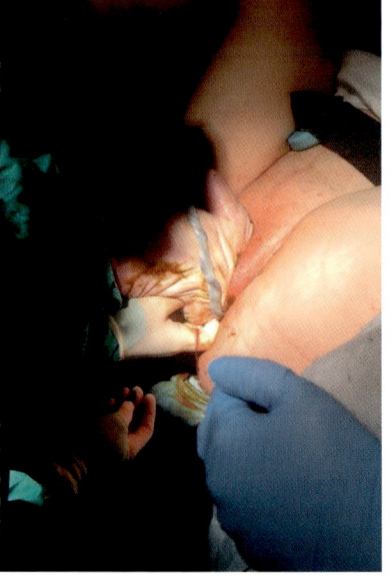

The arm releases fairly easily. Baby is still LST (back facing the mother's left). Now you've got a baby who has delivered all the way to the head. So now what do you do?

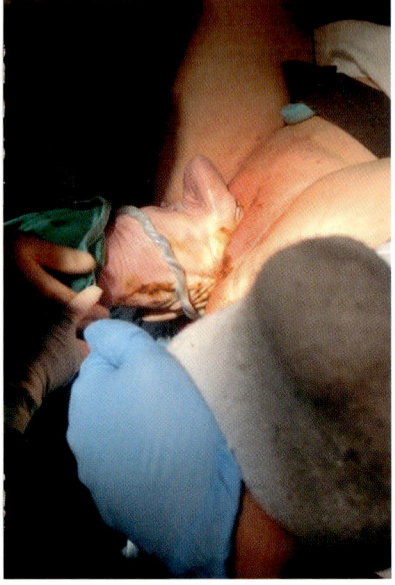

Now they attempt to deliver the head with the head still facing transverse. Obviously, this will be difficult if not impossible.

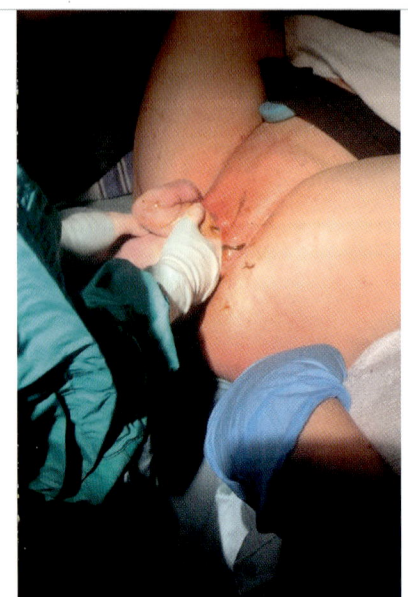

Notice that she's trying to do the MSV with the baby's head **transverse**, not sacrum anterior, which makes it a difficult maneuver, virtually impossible.

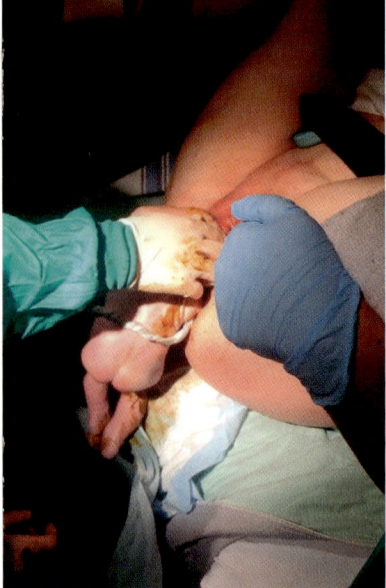

The attendant's hands are shaking violently at this point, demonstrating the level of panic in the room. The mom has an epidural and cannot assist due to being immobile.

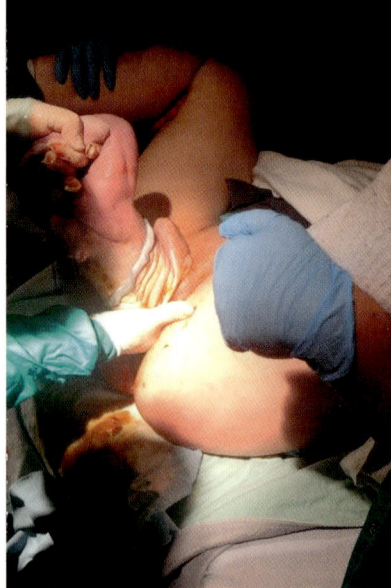

Next, they try lifting the baby's body high up and placing one hand deep in the posterior space.

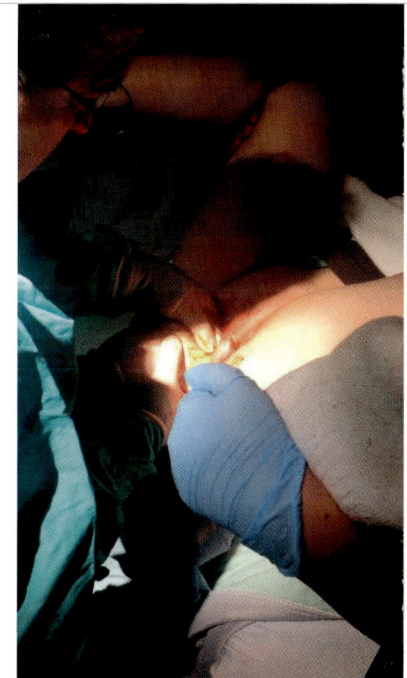

Next, they lower the baby and try releasing with a hand in the anterior space.

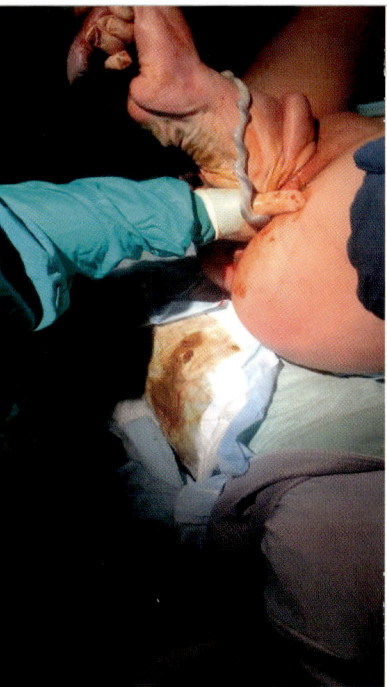

They try again by lifting the baby and inserting one hand into the posterior space.

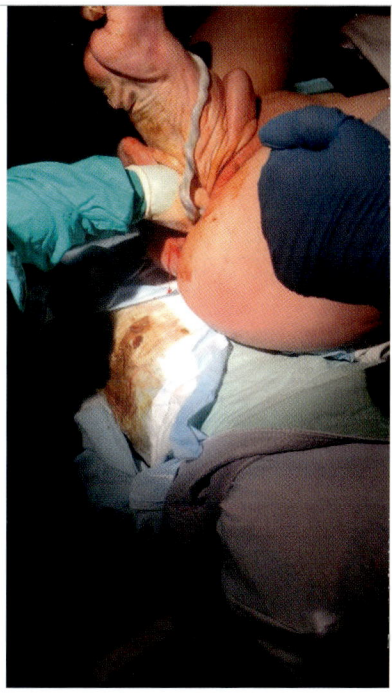

The video ends here. We have had a trapped head for 1m 45s and no sign of any progress.

Like I said, we don't know the outcome or how long this went after the video ended. Whoever took the video was obviously very concerned—and should be. Even after the mistakes, even after pulling the baby down, the birth could have been solved by reorienting the head to face sacrum anterior, then doing an appropriate maneuver to flex the head (Burns-Marshall maneuver + shoulder press, MSV, or Ritgen). This illustrates the necessity to ensure the head is oriented correctly before trying a flexion maneuver.

It's disturbing that reorienting the head never occurred to them. This kind of birth is why breech birth has gotten such a bad reputation. The techniques that we had in the past have not been the best; we have much better ones now. But even the people who were using those techniques were clearly not well-versed in what they were doing.

To end that, let me share one of my favorite quotes from Plentl & Stone, two obstetricians who studied the Bracht maneuver in the 1950s. This is not New Age

> "The art of waiting is a difficult one, and not many obstetricians have either the courage or the patience to sit idly by while the breech delivers spontaneously; this becomes even more difficult if the impatient obstetrician has a century of tradition as well as the words and writings of all contemporary teachers behind him."
>
> Plentl & Stone, 1953

information. It was known and then lost in the field of obstetrics.

That's where we find ourselves today. Our physicians and many of our midwives have lost essential knowledge and skills about breech. Our training programs do not prepare them for attending breech births. At best, obstetricians come out of residency knowing only the maneuvers for emergency extractions and recommend C-sections for everything else. There is a better way. You have now been exposed to it, and I hope you carry it forward with you.

To be sure you're not too disturbed from those previous images, here are some lovely pictures of breech births from around the world.

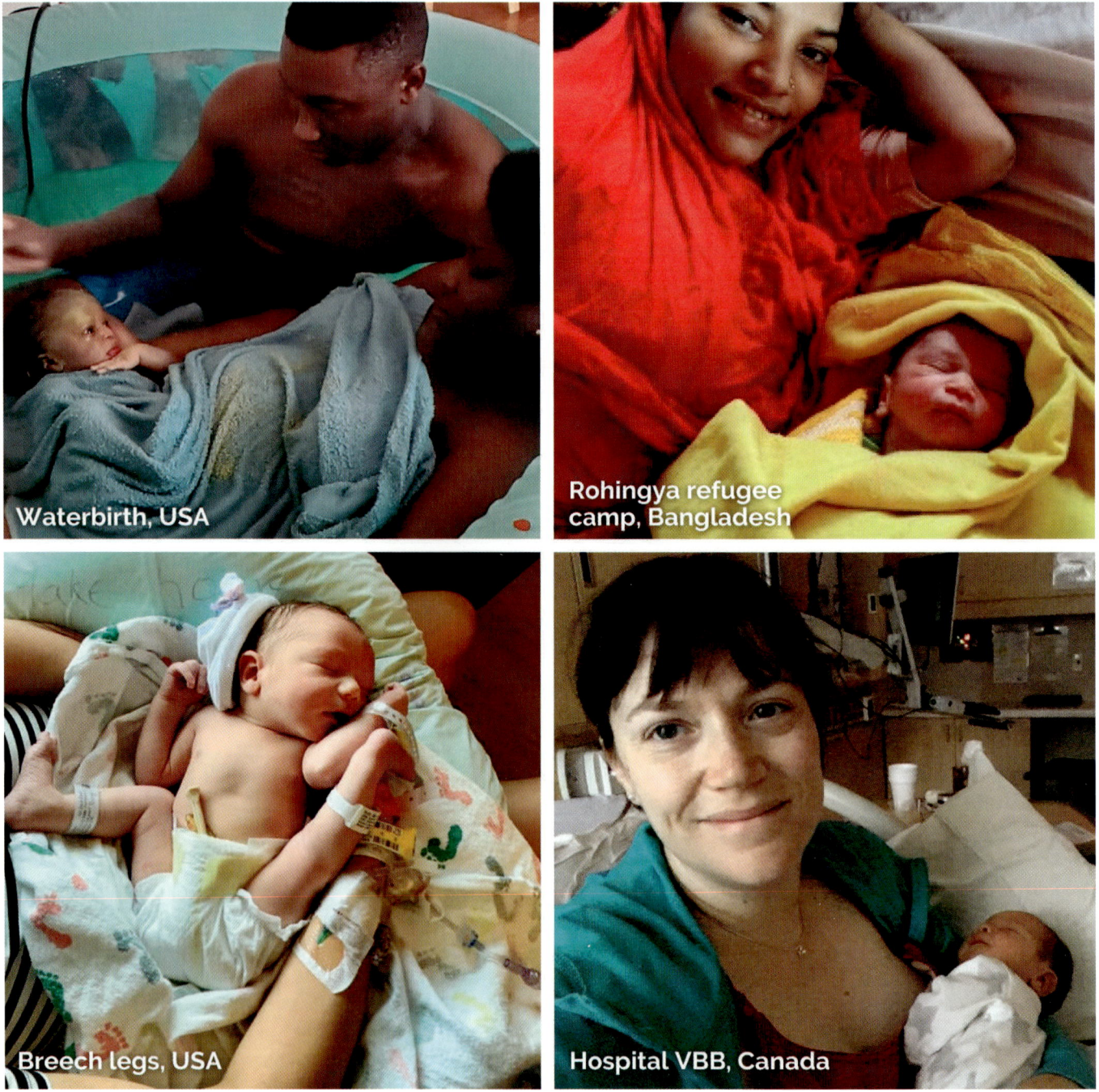

Waterbirth, USA

Rohingya refugee camp, Bangladesh

Breech legs, USA

Hospital VBB, Canada

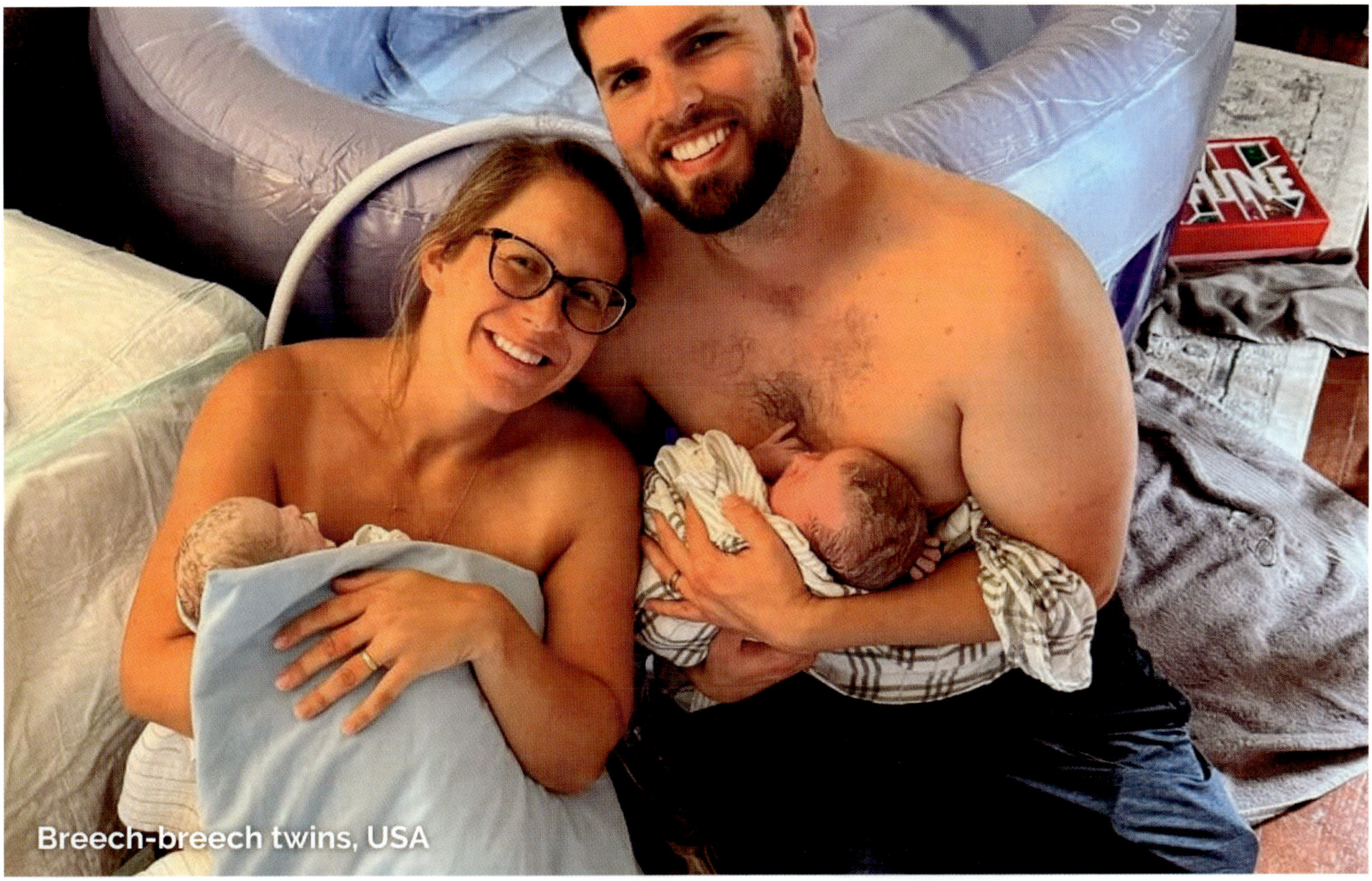

217

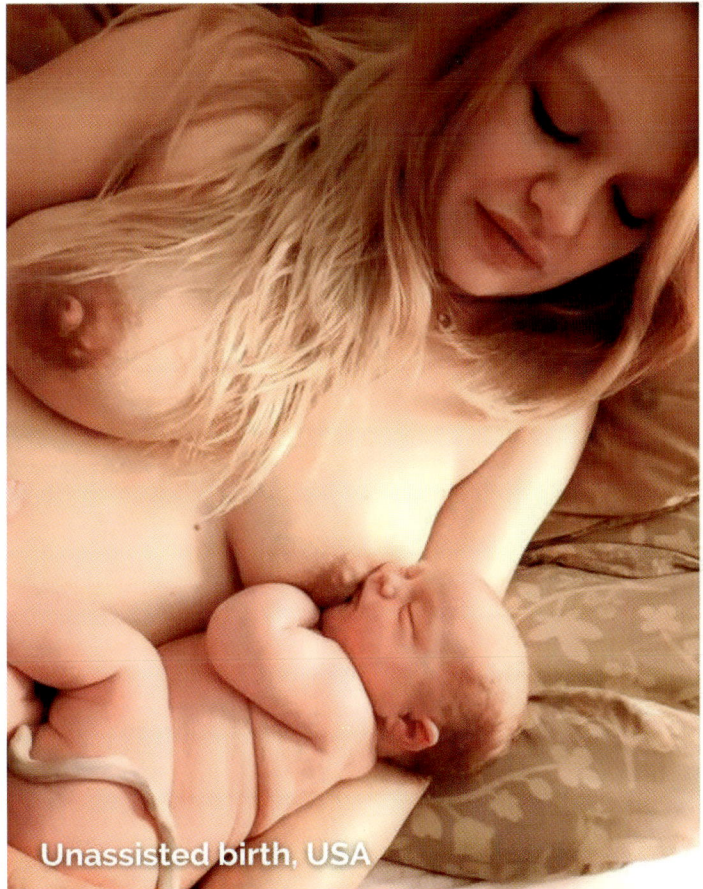

Breech-breech twins, USA

Unassisted birth, USA

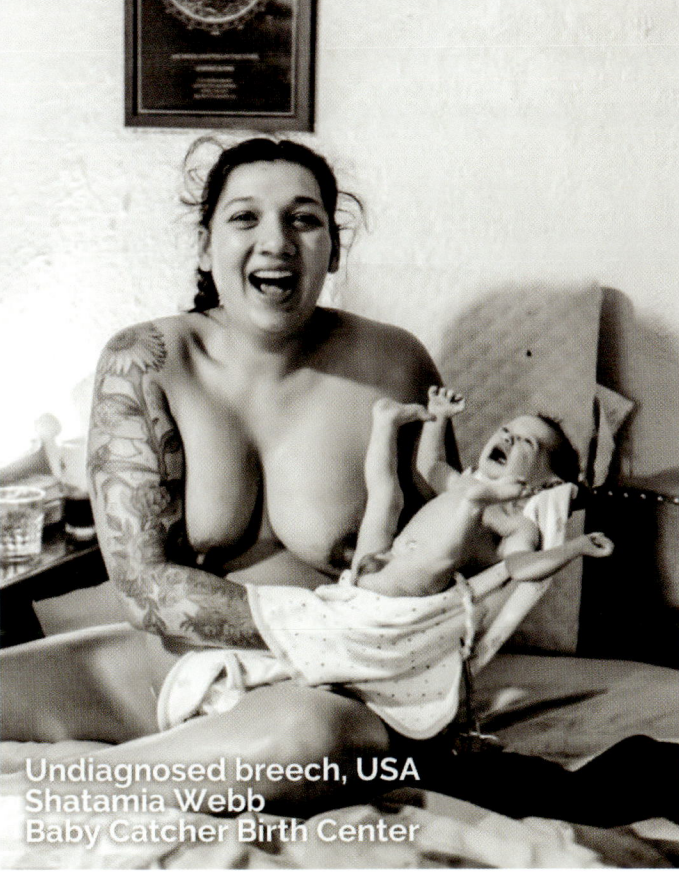

Undiagnosed breech, USA
Shatamia Webb
Baby Catcher Birth Center

© 2022 Breech Without Borders

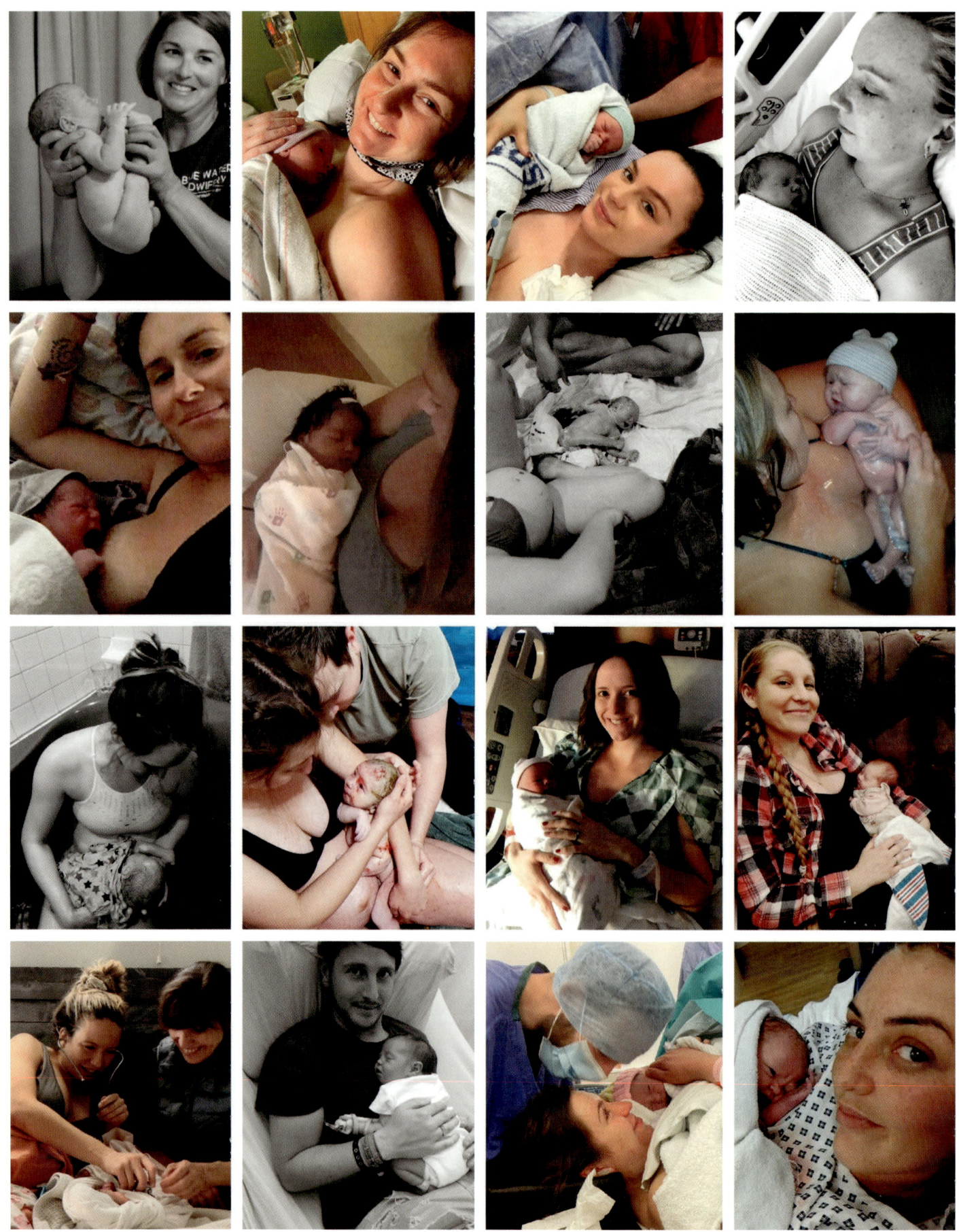

Lesson 12: Prenatal Counseling
For Known Breech Presentations

We recommend that parents take an educational breech course, such as Breech 101 or the equivalent, to become familiar with what breech birth looks like and what the risks, benefits, and alternatives are to the various choices they may have. This education may also take place via person-to-person communication where time allows.

Recommended topics to cover:

- Various care choices (ECV, pVBB, pCS before labor, pCS once labor begins)
- Mother's long-term reproductive plans: if more children are a possibility, the risk/benefit ratio of VBB vs. CS changes
- Short- and long-term risks and benefits, both maternal and neonatal, for pVBB vs pCS vs ECV, including effects on future pregnancies (this information is found in Breech 101, Breech Pro, and on the following webpage: breechwithoutborders.org/statistics).
- Risks and benefits specific to her chosen setting of birth (hospital, birth center, home). This information is found in Breech 101, Breech Pro, and on the following webpage: breechwithoutborders.org/statistics.
- Maternal values, beliefs, and needs: these could be cultural, spiritual/religious, emotional, or physical
- Importance of a skilled attendant in improving outcomes in VBB
- Family/community support and how that may influence her decision-making

Active informed consent

We recommend that parents be actively involved in creating their own informed consent document. We suggest that they write or speak (via video/audio), in their own words, why they are making a certain choice. Parents can explain the risks & benefits of the various alternatives (vaginal breech birth, C-section, ECV, etc.), what their values and preferences are, and why they would prefer to pursue a particular care path. This is a much stronger form of informed consent than having parents sign a pre-written document (which, in reality, they often do not read fully).

This process may be different for certain populations who might not prefer to express themselves in writing or via electronic recordings, such as Plain populations. Care providers should adapt the process to the needs of the population they are serving.

Lesson 13: Selection Criteria

We recommend liberal selection criteria. A large majority of women desiring a VBB are able to have one, especially with highly experienced providers and in a setting that supports undisturbed, physiological birth. Vaginal success rates tend to improve with increased provider experience. Situations that may prompt a less experienced provider to transport and/or move to C-section may be acceptable for a vaginal birth with more experienced providers.

By contrast, strict selection criteria will exclude many women who may have been able to give birth vaginally. We understand that strict criteria are established to eliminate the likelihood of an adverse outcome, but we prefer to have a liberal approach and allow the birth itself to determine the best course of action. We also recognize that less experienced providers may begin with stricter criteria and gradually expand them as they gain experience. This preference for liberal criteria is upheld in the 2020 French guidelines: "The French College of Obstetricians and Gynecologists (CNGOF) considers that planned vaginal delivery is a reasonable option in most cases." (Sentilles 2020)

The most important selection criterion is a highly motivated mother who strongly values vaginal birth, whether for cultural, medical, spiritual, and/or emotional reasons. Other recommended selection criteria:
- A fetus that is healthy and thriving
- A pregnancy with no absolute contraindications to a vaginal birth (e.g., complete placenta previa)
- Term (for home or birth center settings)

Recommended exclusion criteria:

- A fetus known to have condition incompatible with a vaginal birth generally (e.g., hydrocephalus)
- A diagnosis of asymmetric growth restriction
- A fetus showing signs of antenatal compromise (neurologic, cardiac, etc.)
- A mother who adamantly refuses a vaginal birth after being informed of the full risks of risks, benefits, and alternatives (in settings where C-section is available)

The following may be acceptable for vaginal breech birth, depending on the overall clinical picture and after counseling with the parents:

- Low AFI (absent any signs of antenatal fetal compromise)
- Cord presentation in a nonfrank breech

The following should NOT be used to systematically exclude a vaginal breech birth

- Nulliparity (first baby) or no prior vaginal births
- Type of breech presentation (frank, complete, incomplete, footling, etc.)

- Dolichocephaly
- Nuchal cord seen on ultrasound
- Estimated fetal weight, particularly EFWs in the higher ranges
- Uterine anomalies (e.g., unicornuate or bicornuate uterus)
- Post-dates pregnancies
- Medical indication for induction or augmentation
- Medical and/or obstetrical complications that, in a vertex baby, would still be compatible with a vaginal birth
- Previous C-section
- Pelvimetry (not recommended as it is not associated with improved outcomes, other than slightly reducing the in-labor CS rate)
- Maternal age
- Isolated ultrasound showing deflexed or hyperextended fetal head (babies move continually in utero, and a single ultrasound does not equal a diagnosis of persistent hyperextension)
- Ultrasonography (ultrasound can be useful but is not necessary)

Appropriate GA for a planned community breech birth

Governmental regulations may stipulate appropriate gestational ages, but generally the recommended cutoff for a planned community birth, whether breech or vertex, is around 36-37 weeks.

Prematurity

The ALARM guidelines find no benefit to routine C-section for frank or complete breech babies 1500 g and above, and/or 31+ weeks gestation. For extremely premature breech babies, there is moderate evidence that C-section may offer some protection to the baby compared to VBB, but with more short- and long-term risk to the mother and her future pregnancies. Most of the risk of a preterm breech birth still comes from the prematurity itself, not the mode of birth. Care providers should take into account the mother's values and her future reproductive plans, not just the immediate, short-term outcomes of this pregnancy and birth.

Preterm breech babies often want to come down through a partially dilated cervix, particularly at very low gestational ages due to the large discrepancy between thorax and head circumference. Our guideline team has experienced this situation in low-resource settings, sometimes leading to difficult deliveries.

Selection criteria in low-resource settings

In low-resource settings without easy access to cesarean section, there is often no breech selection criteria. A provider must be prepared for any situation. This underlines the need for breech-skilled providers particularly in low-resource areas. In such settings, a C-section may often be too dangerous to perform for anything other than life-threatening maternal complications.

Undiagnosed Breech

Learning that one's baby is breech during labor, sometimes only when birth is imminent, may be stressful or chaotic. The care provider should do everything possible to keep anxiety and stress levels low.

Counseling for undiagnosed breech

Give the mother and her partner as much information as possible, given the realities of the situation. Inform parents that, according to the research literature, outcomes are just as good with undiagnosed breeches as with known breeches. Inform the family of your skill and experience level, of the options she has available at that moment, and then–as much as possible–back away and give parents the time to process the information and make a decision of how to proceed. If this is occurring in a community setting (home or birth center), inform parents of any state regulations and of the reality of transport time and what hospital transport would entail. The better you know the woman, the better you can adapt your counseling to the situation.

We encourage discussing the possibility of a surprise breech with all clients during prenatal visits. Ask their preferences if this were to occur.

Continue to encourage the woman to follow her body and let the birth unfold. Follow the mother's lead.

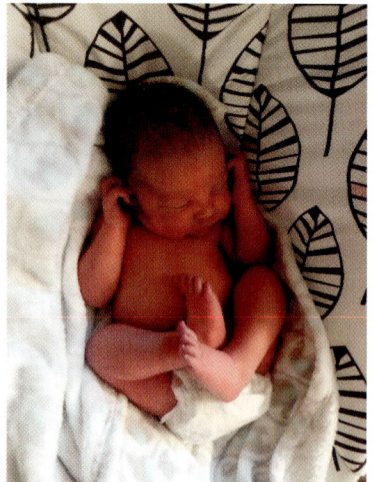 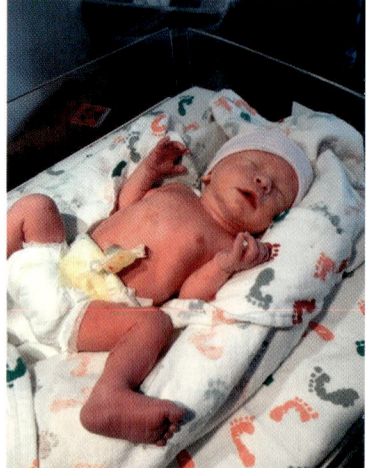 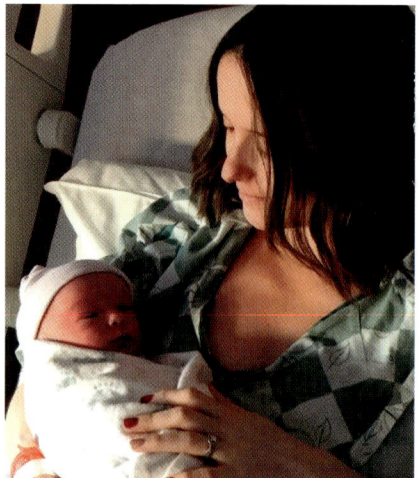

Undiagnosed breeches (left: Gab Hershman, @solagratiavita)

Lesson 14: Care During Labor

Although this topic is often termed "labor management," we cannot manage or control labor, at least not without inviting unintended consequences. The goal for the birth attendant is to quietly observe and to support the process of physiological birth. **Keep in mind the basic needs of all laboring mammals: privacy, safety, darkness, freedom from feeling observed or judged, and freedom from interruptions.** Birth attendants should *actively manage the laboring environment* to ensure the laboring woman has no disturbances.

Unless otherwise noted, our recommendations apply equally to term and preterm breech births. These recommendations are also generally applicable to *all* vaginal labors, not just breech births.

Birth teams

Clearly identify the roles of each person on the birth team ahead of time (in some birth settings, a person may take on several of these roles simultaneously):

- <u>Primary attendant responsible for any hands-on assistance</u>: Ideally the **most experienced provider** should be the one responsible for receiving the baby or directly supervising the person providing hands-on care. If the most experienced provider is outside the usual birth team, make arrangements for that person to be able to participate. There should only be one decision-maker in the room who will do the hands-on care if it becomes necessary. It can be very confusing if two people are adopting the same role.
- <u>Person responsible for assessing fetal condition, taking heart tones, charting, etc.</u>
- <u>Person responsible for resuscitation & baby care</u>: If this is someone who typically comes in during pushing/expulsion, be sure that their entrance does not disrupt the atmosphere in the room. Give them an update on the progress of events so far.
- <u>Timekeeper</u>: We recommend having someone whose only job is to keep track of time elapsed during expulsion, beginning at the birth of the bitrochanteric diameter (widest point of the fetal hips).
- <u>Videographer</u>: This could be the timekeeper, if using a tripod, or it could be someone in a non-clinical role. We strongly advise using a tripod to ensure good-quality footage without the possibility of interruption due to having to set the phone/camera down.

Having clearly defined roles can allow the rest of the birth team to relax and observe, rather than having to worry about what they are supposed to be doing.

Maternal movement and positioning

Encourage the laboring woman to move freely and change positions freely during both 1st and 2nd stage. Do NOT require the woman to stay on/in the bed. Do NOT require fixed positions at any point during the labor or birth–whether supine or upright. Ensure that the birth room has equipment that encourages movement and position changes (birth balls, squat bars, ceiling-mounted hammocks or ropes, birth stools, cushions that can be placed on the floor or other surfaces, etc.).

When left alone and encouraged to follow her body's cues, a laboring woman will instinctively move and find the positions most effective for the birth. If the woman seems "stuck," encourage her to try a different position. Sometimes the intensity of labor may freeze a woman into one position and she may feel too overwhelmed to move.

Inform the woman (ideally during prenatal counseling, if the breech is known in advance) that upright, forward-leaning positions for the birth are preferable for the following reasons:
- Shorter 2nd stage
- Fewer maternal injuries
- Fewer neonatal injuries
- Higher vaginal birth rate
- Fewer maneuvers will be required to assist the birth
- Easier for the attendant to see the baby's cardinal movements through the pelvis and to assess fetal well-being (tummy crunches, chest crease, how full the umbilical cord is, whether the perineum is hollow or bulging, etc.)

Stops, starts, and plateaus

Just as with cephalic labors, plateaus and pauses can happen with a breech labor. It is important to reframe these events with the attitude of "Rest and be thankful," rather than provoking anxiety in the mother or birth team because the labor has paused or slowed down. The most important indicator is fetal well-being, taking into account maternal well-being and energy levels as well.

Vaginal/cervical exams

We discourage routine vaginal/cervical exams, whether upon admission, to assess labor progress, or to determine if a woman is fully dilated. Routine cervical checks have no predictive value and come with several risks and inconveniences:
- Increased risk of infection
- Maternal & fetal discomfort: the intrusion and discomfort can create extended plateaus in labor due to agitating the mother; cervical exams may also disturb or irritate the baby
- Giving women false expectations and interrupting the mother's concentration

Only suggest vaginal exams for a specific indication, in which the information gathered could be useful, and only if the mother consents. If she expresses discomfort, asks the provider to stop, or says "no", withdraw immediately.

Fetal monitoring

Intermittent monitoring via a handheld doppler or fetoscope is preferred. There is no evidence to support continuous fetal monitoring for breech labors; it has never been studied in comparison with intermittent monitoring during vaginal breech births. The only information on continuous vs. intermittent monitoring comes from cephalic data, and the evidence shows that continuous monitoring comes with risks (primarily a dramatically increased cesarean section rate), inconveniences (hampering maternal movement and positioning), and few if any benefits (the only documented benefit is a very slight reduction in neonatal seizures). (See Clark 2022.) Absent data showing benefits that strongly outweigh the risks, we do not recommend continuous monitoring as the preferred method.

Continuous monitoring should only be done if all 3 conditions are present:
- A specific indication AND
- Maternal consent AND
- Wireless monitoring that does not interfere with the mother's complete freedom of movement.

Pain relief

The best pain relief methods do not interfere with maternal movement. Encourage non-pharmacological methods of pain relief. We recommend referring to SOGC Guideline "Physiological basis for pain in labour and delivery: An Evidence based approach to its management." The main recommendations are quoted below.

> - Health care providers should be familiar with the neurophysiological and hormonal mechanisms and related methods in physiological labour and birth (III-A).
> - To help women (sic) cope with normal labour, nonpharmacological approaches are recommended as a safe first-line method for pain relief and should be continued throughout labour whether or not pharmacologic methods are used (I-A).
> - To prevent suffering, health professionals should address the emotional component of pain (pain unpleasantness). This is most effectively achieved through support and nonpharmacological approaches to pain management.
> - To develop support measures consistent with the wishes of women, health professionals should work with women and listen to their needs (III-A).
> - To further reduce the need for obstetric interventions and avoid associated risks and side-effects, health professionals should provide continuous labour support with the addition of at least one other nonpharmacological pain modulating mechanism (I-A).
> - Health professionals should, where possible, promote and support the physiological progress of labour, delivery, and the postpartum period trusting the woman's ability to work with her pain and encouraging her to rely on her ability to give birth (III-A).
> - To enhance the endogenous hormone production that promotes and supports the physiologic process of labour, health care providers should reduce a woman's stress level by encouraging her and having a positive attitude where possible and by creating a calm, stress free environment (I-A).
> - Continuous labour support, as part of nonpharmacological approaches to pain management during childbirth for women should be promoted and provided for all women in labour (I-A).
> - Health professionals should encourage parents and the people assisting them to prepare for the birth by learning about birth physiology and gaining skills in working with pain (III-A).

Explain to the mother that epidurals are associated with adverse outcomes in vaginal breech birth (Macharey 2017) and that it may be more difficult to get the mother into upright positions if she has an epidural. Birthing in supine positions may then lead to other adverse outcomes (longer 2nd stage, higher rates of both maternal and neonatal injuries, higher rates of unplanned C-sections, higher need for maneuvers during the birth).

The first approach for pain relief should be non-pharmacological and should be actively encouraged and supported: water immersion, showering, movement, birth balls, hypnosis, TENS unit, sterile water injections, etc. If those methods are not adequate, the next approach should be gas & air (nitrous oxide). Injectable analgesia would come next, followed by epidural/spinal anesthesia as a last resort.

Epidurals should never be mandatory but should also not be forbidden. If the woman has exhausted all other methods of pain relief and desires additional assistance, we recommend a low-dose "walking epidural," in which the mother has enough motor control and sensation to hold herself in kneeling or standing positions. Walking epidurals and unmedicated births are both associated with good outcomes during upright vaginal breech births (Louwen 2017).

Waterbirth

Breech water birth is not well studied, but highly experienced providers report excellent outcomes. Assessing fetal well-being may be somewhat more challenging for a less experienced provider. For example, in a less-than-vigorous baby, it may be harder to ascertain fetal tone or distinguish voluntary fetal movements from maternal movements causing the baby's body to move in the water. It may also be more difficult to access the baby if maneuvers are needed. On the other hand, outcomes seem to be excellent and maternal satisfaction very high. Water immersion seems to facilitate the baby's freedom of movement, which is crucial during the expulsive stage. As you gain confidence and experience attending breech births, you may become more comfortable with breech waterbirth.

IV access

Routine IVs or IV access is not recommended. If women are encouraged to eat and drink as desired, they will rarely become dehydrated enough to require IV fluids. In addition, routine IV fluids are associated with fluid overload and decreased freedom of movement. Women report IV ports to be painfully distracting as well as symbolizing an expectation of failure. Vaginal breech births do not have significantly higher rates of in-labor CS compared to cephalic births, especially in centers or with providers who are experienced. Thus there is no need to assume failure of vaginal birth or to prepare for surgery in advance of the surgery actually happening.

Red flags during labor

Breech labors have the same red flags as cephalic labors. Ask yourself, "If this were a head-down baby, would I be concerned?" If the answer is yes, then you should be concerned and act appropriately. Certain situations will not present during breech labors, of course, such as asynclitic or OP heads.

Our team of breech experts agrees that breech labors tend to be straightforward because there is no hard, bony head that can get stuck in strange positions as it enters the pelvis. Occasionally the crisscross folded legs of a complete breech may become wedged in the pelvis and fail to descend any further. For this reason, a dropped foot breech (a complete/incomplete that drops one or both legs, usually late in labor as the cervix opens) is a reassuring sign. It is extremely rare for a dropped foot breech to become stuck in the pelvic inlet.

Second stage

Stops, starts, and plateaus

Plateaus can happen during 2nd stage, just as with cephalic labors. The most important indicator is fetal well-being, taking into account maternal well-being and energy levels as well. Put the events of 2nd stage into their larger context: overall, has the labor seemed very dysfunctional, or has it simply been slow or had occasional pauses?

Many breeches tend to have a more delayed urge to push, compared to cephalic babies. A lot of descent may occur before a significant urge to push.

Expect to see lots of meconium, especially at the point of unstoppable guttural pushing. Frank breeches tend to pass more meconium than nonfrank breeches. You may start seeing small amounts of meconium during labor but particularly during pushing. Passing meconium is normal and expected due to the mechanical squeezing of the fetal torso.

As second stage nears, the mother may exhibit more frantic behaviors and may be unable to "control" the process; she may become very vocal and more forceful in her movements, grabbing onto things. Visually/auditorily, it can feel overwhelming to people in the room. Expect that for many women, this can be a very dramatic time. We recommend preparing partners/fathers for this behavior.

Care providers should continue to sit quietly and observe, letting the mother lead the process. Follow the woman's lead and stay out of her way. Support her physically, if requested, so she can do what she has to do.

Be careful not to change the energy level in the room as the second stage begins. Keep lights dim; keep the room quiet and private. If additional staff need to enter, ask them to stay silent and unobtrusive.

To move or not to move? (to an operating room)

A vaginal breech birth should take place in the same room as the labor. We do not recommend transporting the mother to an operating room for 2nd stage. Besides the disruption that the move itself causes, which may derail the process of labor, operating rooms are often bright, cold, uncomfortable, and not equipped to support physiological birth. In addition, moving to an operating theater communicates nonconfidence in the likelihood of giving birth vaginally. If/when a cesarean section becomes necessary, that is the appropriate time to transfer to an operating room.

To push or not to push?

In a physiological birth, the woman does not decide it is time to "push." Instead, her body develops an undeniable fetal ejection reflex, and she cannot stop her body's spontaneous expulsive efforts. When is the perfect time to push? *When she can't not push*. It is not necessary to check for full dilation if the woman is experiencing this undeniable urge. (With premature births, some babies may slip down through a partially dilated cervix. This may be an indication for a vaginal exam, with the mother's consent.) Because a fetal rump is relatively soft compared to a hard, bony head, women may not feel a strong urge to bear down until the breech is on the perineum.

During a vaginal breech birth, there should be no coached pushing, breath-holding, or telling the woman "Push! Push!" The expulsive stage should be spontaneous, and the woman should follow her body's cues. (Occasionally during expulsion, the provider may see signs of decreased fetal well-being or possible mechanical disruption; this may be an indication to ask the woman to increase her expulsive efforts.)

Plateaus may occur during 2nd stage or pushing. Breech babies actively participate in finding the best way to navigate through the pelvis; pauses may occur to allow this to happen.

Why else do we recommend not pushing before the spontaneous, undeniable urge begins? One clinician consulted in creating these guidelines, who has attended around 600 physiological breech births, has only seen cervical head entrapment twice in her career. Both times, it occurred at term when the woman started forcefully pushing long before she felt any urge to bear down and despite the midwife asking her to stop pushing.

For women laboring with epidurals, a "laboring down" passive phase is recommended. The SOGC guidelines allow for up to 90 minutes of passive 2nd stage plus up to 60 minutes of active pushing.

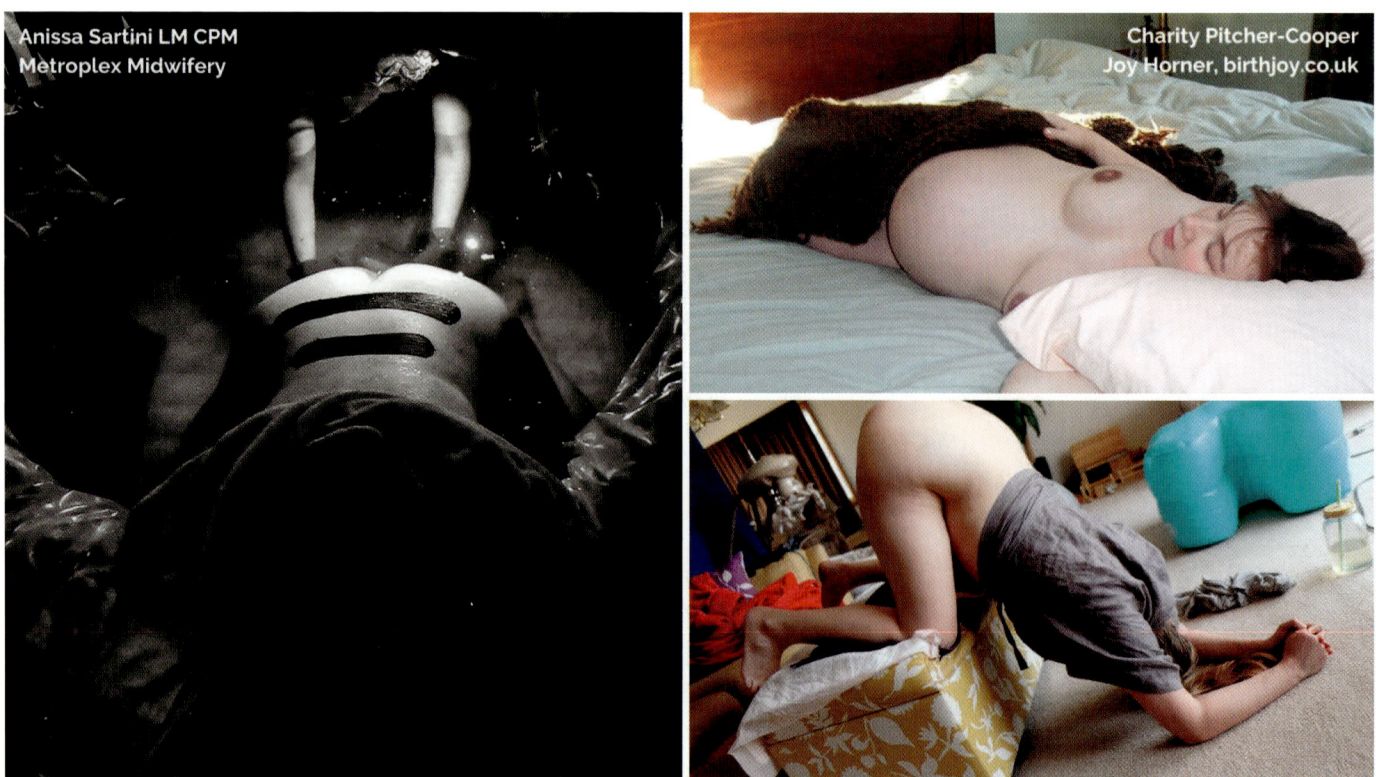

Freedom of movement & position changes are crucial

Expulsive stage (from rumping to birth)

Breech experience and being present continually during the birth are key to interpreting the events of expulsion. If a provider has been present throughout the entire labor, they can interpret deviations more easily.

Water immersion may be helpful in this process because it allows the baby to move freely in a comfortable, familiar environment and keeps the baby relaxed.

Timing is one element to be aware of, particularly time from bitrochanteric diameter, but a comprehensive assessment of baby's well-being is key (FHR, tone, color, capillary filling, presence/absence of tummy crunches, fullness of umbilical cord). Also pay careful attention to the last several FHRs prior to rumping and the presence or absence of decelerations.

Contraction patterns

Pay close attention to the contractions leading up to the expulsive stage. Are they short or long? Spaced far apart or close together? Do they seem powerful or relatively ineffective? Consider intervening sooner if contractions are short, weak, and/or spaced farther apart.

Timing

There is a vigorous debate in the breech literature about whether we should set time limits on the expulsive stage and how long those limits should be. The highly experienced providers who created these guidelines feel that time limits or time-based algorithms are not advisable; instead, care providers should look at the whole clinical picture and rely upon fetal well-being (in combination with factors such as frequency/intensity of contractions, descent/rotation, and signs of mechanism disruption) for deciding when to intervene or not.

The baby's well-being is a key indicator during the expulsive stage. Timing is one element to consider, and we recommend that one member of the birth team be in charge of keeping time once the rump is born (bitrochanteric diameter, or widest point of the hips). However, we discourage intervening based solely upon time elapsed. Applying interventions based on a clock can interfere with good decision-making and distract providers from reacting to what the baby is showing them.

Trust that the baby will communicate what is happening and whether you need to assist: what is the FHR? How vigorous is the baby? Is it losing tone? Is it navigating the pelvis as expected? How full is the cord? Some babies may tolerate longer expulsion stages and come out completely vigorous, while others might need assistance nearly immediately after rumping.

Maneuvers and when to intervene

Providers should *never touch the baby in any way* unless they have gone through our vaginal breech decision tree and answered all 4 decision tree questions first (see lesson 11 and the handout on p. 4).

Providers should fully understand the 10 mechanisms of physiological breech birth as well as the deviations. Note that half of these mechanisms are not visible when viewing the birth from the mother's front (mother is supine or sitting upright on a birth stool). This is another reason why being able to view the birth from behind the mother is preferable.

If there are signs of significant mechanism disruption and/or fetal compromise, it may be time to intervene. **The first-line intervention is maternal movement and positioning**. Often movement will shift the pelvic dimensions and allow the baby to continue navigating the pelvis.

The next line of intervention is to apply the appropriate maneuver to the situation. See the "Problems and Solutions" handout on pg. 5 for a list of maneuvers care providers should be familiar with.

Wait for the next contraction? Not necessarily

If the baby has made significant descent in one contraction, the next contraction may not come for a very long time, if at all. This is especially true once the baby is born to the armpits or to the neck. At this point, the fundus will remain quite high, near the mother's belly button, and any further progress will come mainly from maternal efforts. Do not hesitate to encourage maternal pushing.

Listen to the baby—literally

Once the baby is out past the umbilicus, you can listen to the baby's heart directly with a doppler or fetoscope, or you can palpate the cord for a pulse (you may not always be able to feel a pulse via the cord). Do not hesitate to get this additional information if you are at all concerned about the baby's condition.

Cord prolapse/cord presentation

In nonfrank breeches, a cord prolapse or presenting cord is generally non-concerning. Research indicates the cord prolapse in nonfrank breeches is relatively common (~ 5-6%) but not as dangerous. In contrast, cord prolapse in frank breeches is relatively rare (< 0.7%) but more dangerous. A frank breech cord prolapse should be treated similarly to a cephalic cord prolapse due to the higher likelihood of cord compression. Due to the looser fit of a nonfrank breech in the lower uterine segment, the cord is generally not compromised. In term breeches, cord prolapse tends to happen towards the end of the labor–a compelling reason not to rupture membranes.

If cord prolapse occurs, listen carefully to the fetal heart tones. If birth is imminent and if the baby shows no signs of compromise, proceed with a vaginal birth. If cord prolapse occurs early in labor, and in settings where C-section is widely available, moving to surgery may be a good option. However, cord prolapse may not equal a compromised cord, even early in labor. Another clinician consulted for these guidelines, who has attended over 500 vaginal breech births in both developed and developing settings, has never had a complete/incomplete cord prolapse leading to poor outcomes or a compromised baby.

Footling/dropped foot breech

For complete, incomplete, and footling breeches, the foot or feet might drop down in advance of the rest of the baby. It may take minutes or hours before the rest of the baby descends into the pelvis and spontaneous pushing begins. Do NOT tell the mother to begin to push when you see feet or legs. Do NOT reach in and try to feel the cervix. Do NOT touch the feet or wrap them in a towel or try to keep them warm—remember, the feet don't breathe! Expect bruising, discoloration, and/or swelling in the legs. It can be very uncomfortable for providers or parents to see feet long in advance of the rest of the body; proper preparation is key.

What not to do during expulsion

- Do not touch the baby without a specific indication (e.g., the need to do a maneuver).
- Do not pull on the baby; power from above is better than pulling from below.
- Do not wrap the baby in a warm towel or otherwise handle the baby unnecessarily.
- Do not pull down a loop of umbilical cord.
- Do not routinely release frank breech legs; they rarely inhibit descent. The legs will release with additional uterine power (i.e., contractions or fundal pressure).
- Do not rupture membranes; allow the baby to be born in the caul if membranes do not release spontaneously.
- Do not wipe meconium or maternal feces.
- Do not inhibit the mother's spontaneous movements during expulsion; she may crouch down lower, wiggle her hips, etc. (Occasionally she may be so close to the bed or ground when in a kneeling crouch that you may need to ask if she can lift herself up slightly, to give the baby enough room to emerge.)

Episiotomy & perineal care

There is good evidence that perineal outcomes are better after vaginal breech births compared to vertex births. Do not touch the perineum as the mother is pushing or as the baby is emerging (no touching, stretching, or counter-pressure) unless the mother actively requests it. No routine episiotomies. Experienced breech providers rarely perform episiotomies during vaginal breech births and speculate the episiotomy may interfere with the baby's movements through the pelvis and soft tissues.

Transfer from community to hospital settings

We recommend following the Best Practice Transfer Guidelines developed by the Home Birth Consensus Summit (https://www.homebirthsummit.org/best-practice-transfer-guidelines/). The guidelines note: "Good communication and coordination between providers during these transfers minimizes the potential for negative impact on outcomes. As the safety of the mother and infant is always of the highest priority, it is important to have detailed guidelines used by all health care providers involved in such transfers." Below are model practices quoted from the Home Birth Summit Transfer Guidelines.

Model practices for the midwife

- In the prenatal period, the midwife provides information to the woman about hospital care and procedures that may be necessary and documents that a plan has been developed with the woman for hospital transfer should the need arise.
- The midwife assesses the status of the woman, fetus, and newborn throughout the maternity care cycle to determine if a transfer will be necessary.
- The midwife notifies the receiving provider or hospital of the incoming transfer, reason for transfer, brief relevant clinical history, planned mode of transport, and expected time of arrival.
- The midwife continues to provide routine or urgent care en route in coordination with any emergency services personnel and addresses the psychosocial needs of the woman during the change of birth setting.
- Upon arrival at the hospital, the midwife provides a verbal report, including details on current health status and need for urgent care. The midwife also provides a legible copy of relevant prenatal and labor medical records.
- The midwife may continue in a primary role as appropriate to her scope of practice and privileges at the hospital. Otherwise the midwife transfers clinical responsibility to the hospital provider.
- The midwife promotes good communication by ensuring that the woman understands the hospital provider's plan of care and the hospital provider understands the woman's need for information regarding care options.
- If the woman chooses, the midwife may remain to provide continuity and support.

Model practices for the hospital provider and staff

- Hospital providers and staff are sensitive to the psychosocial needs of the woman that result from the change of birth setting.
- Hospital providers and staff communicate directly with the midwife to obtain clinical information in addition to the information provided by the woman.
- Timely access to maternity and newborn care providers may be best accomplished by direct admission to the labor and delivery or pediatric unit.
- Whenever possible, the woman and her newborn are kept together during the transfer and after admission to the hospital.
- Hospital providers and staff participate in a shared decision-making process with the woman to create an ongoing plan of care that incorporates the values, beliefs, and preferences of the woman.
- If the woman chooses, hospital personnel will accommodate the presence of the midwife as well as the woman's primary support person during assessments and procedures.
- The hospital provider and the midwife coordinate follow up care for the woman and newborn, and care may revert to the midwife upon discharge.
- Relevant medical records, such as a discharge summary, are sent to the referring midwife.

Videoing births

We strongly recommend videoing all breech births where possible (some populations, such as Plain communities, may not allow photos or videos to be taken). Watching videos is an essential learning tool; videos often reveal things that attendants missed during the actual birth.

Assure the parents that the video belongs to them and will only be shared with the immediate birth team, unless they give specific permission to share beyond that circle. We highly recommend putting the phone/camera on a tripod to avoid losing important footage if the phone/camera gets set aside.

Resuscitation, cord clamping, and neonatal transitions

Local or national guidelines may vary on when and how to initiate resuscitation.

Stunned or "shocky" babies are normal after a vaginal breech birth. If the baby's heart rate is not overly concerning, you can give the baby 1 minute to transition before initiating resuscitation. **NEVER cut or clamp the cord before or during resuscitation.** Ensure that the birth team (or pediatric team, if applicable) is prepared for bedside resuscitation with the cord intact. If the baby appears compromised, cutting the cord is the worst thing a provider can do as it removes the baby's oxygen supply. A recent randomized controlled trial by Andersson et al., comparing resuscitation with the cord intact vs. clamped and cut, found improved SpO2 and higher Apgar scores in the intact group. Below are key points about the importance of keeping the cord intact before and during resuscitation, from an article by Gruneberg and Crozier, 2015.

- Early cord clamping before initiation of respiration may create the need for resuscitative measures by causing a reflex bradycardia
- Maintaining cord integrity allows the placenta to fulfil its respiratory function, providing a continued source of oxygen to a non-breathing baby
- The prevention of hypovolaemia, achieved through delayed cord clamping is especially important for preterm babies
- The increased volume from delayed cord clamping leads to decreased need for drug therapy and volume expanders, reversing bradycardia and restoring blood pressure
- It is practical to initiate the first resuscitative measures while maintaining cord integrity

Gruneberg F & Crozier K. Delayed cord clamping in the compromised baby. *BJOG* 23(2). Feb 2015: 102-108.

Differences in neonatal transitions

During cephalic births, the baby's head is molded (often tied to a reduction of FHR) as it moves through the pelvis, followed by the head flushing with blood and the chest being squeezed. When the abdomen comes out and the lungs are decompressed, it forces the baby to take a breath. These processes provoke a need for the baby to express itself dramatically after the birth.

In comparison, during a vaginal breech birth, the baby's head does not go through the same stimulation, and the baby's chest is compressed before the head is compressed. Together, this can lead to a temporarily stunned or shocked baby and delayed respirations. It is common to see or hear some shallow breathing, but the deep breath or cry may be somewhat delayed. We recommend counseling parents and staff about this ahead of time. Keep in mind that this is the baby's first experience outside the uterus and that we need to be observant and ready to act, but not overly aggressively.

A note about populations with high rates of seizure disorders

In many Amish/Plain communities, genetic seizure disorders are relatively common. A long gap between the birth and the baby taking its first breath may be an indication for hospital transport due to suspected genetic disorders.

After the birth: Debriefing and processing

Once the mother and baby are stable and settled in, the birth team should do some immediate processing (not in the mother's presence, of course).

We recommend debriefing with the parents several days or weeks after the birth. Ask them to be honest with their experiences, both positive and negative, so you can adapt and improve your care.

The birth team should also do a full debrief about the birth, especially in cases of difficult/complex cases. Ongoing debriefs of every breech birth, inviting other staff when possible, is good practice. It helps keep the entire team unified, avoids gossiping or hearsay, and enables learning opportunities.

Lesson 15: Transient Neonatal Trauma after Vaginal Breech Birth

By Kristine Lauria, CPM

In the normal course of breech birth, it is not at all uncommon—and in fact it can be expected—that there is going to be some bruising and/or swelling of the presenting part of the baby that comes through the pelvis, particularly when the birth has been long and descent has been slow. The longer the baby is in the pelvis, the more likely we are to see the effects of that slow descent.

It is not uncommon to see bruising and swelling on the side of the buttock that presented—the labia, the testicles, the feet, whatever the presenting part was—can have bruising, swelling and sometimes blistering of that part. The effects can sometimes be quite extreme.

Case #1: Bruising and contusions on hip	Case #2: Bruising on buttock and swollen scrotum

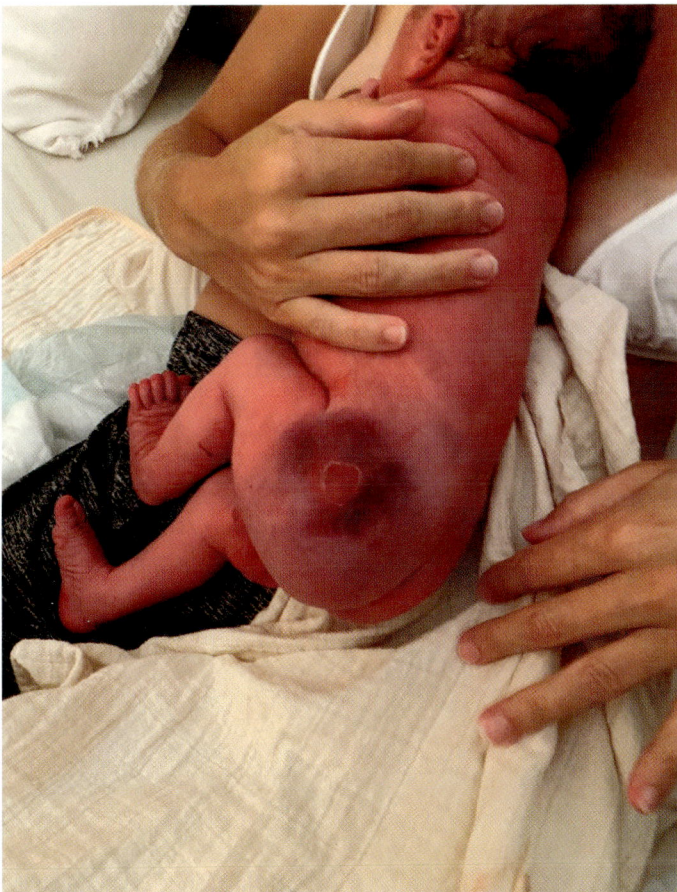 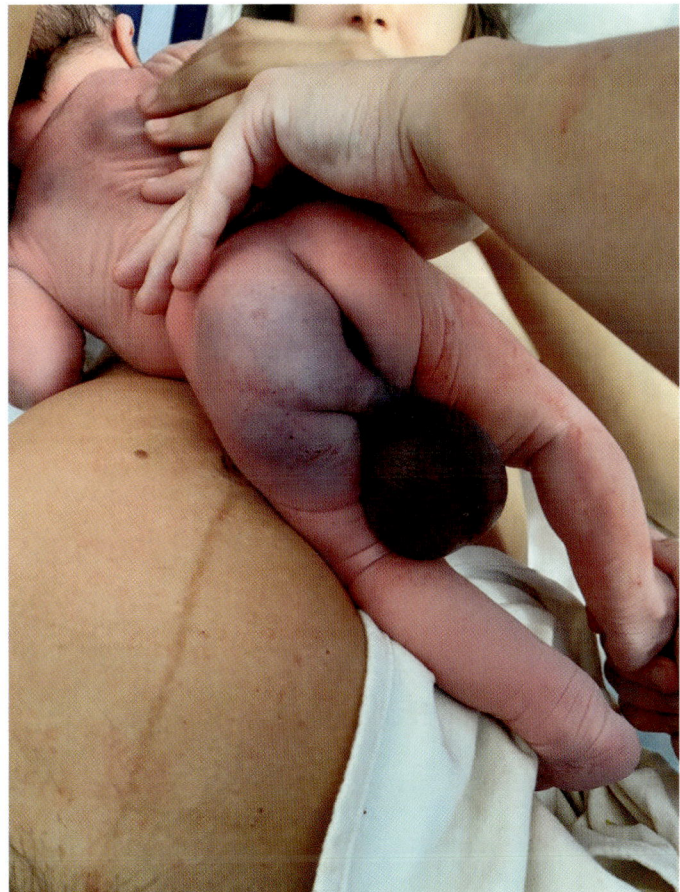

Case #3: Bruising on buttock and labial swelling

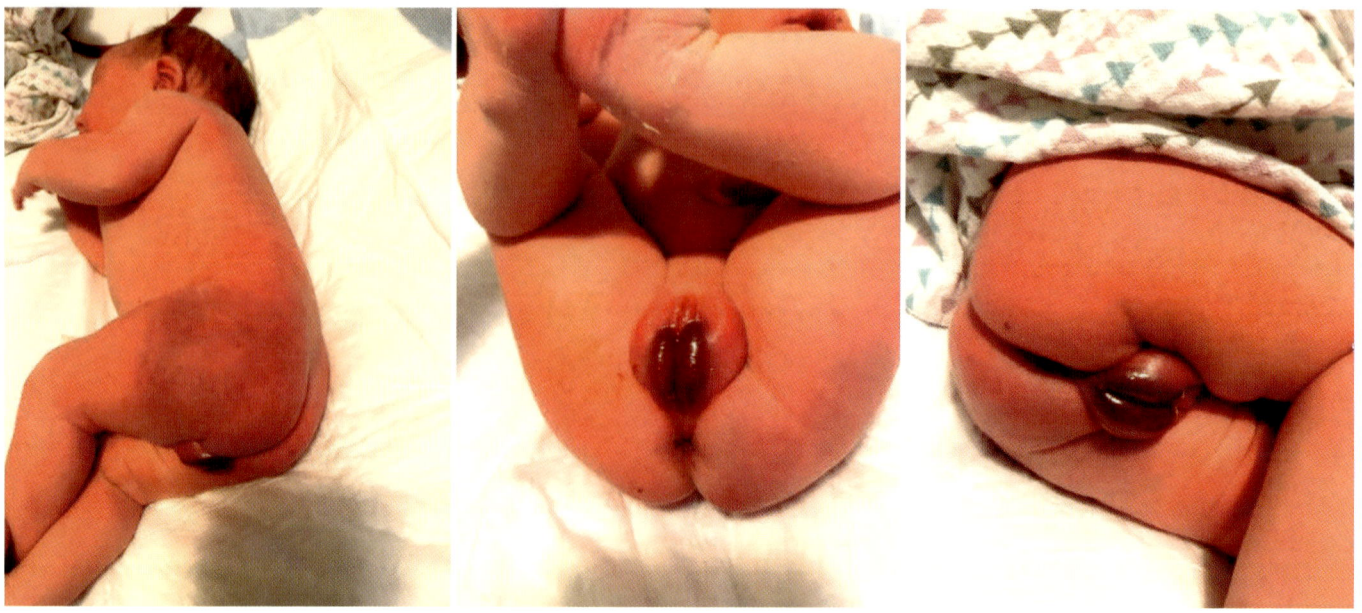

Case #4: Bruising on buttock

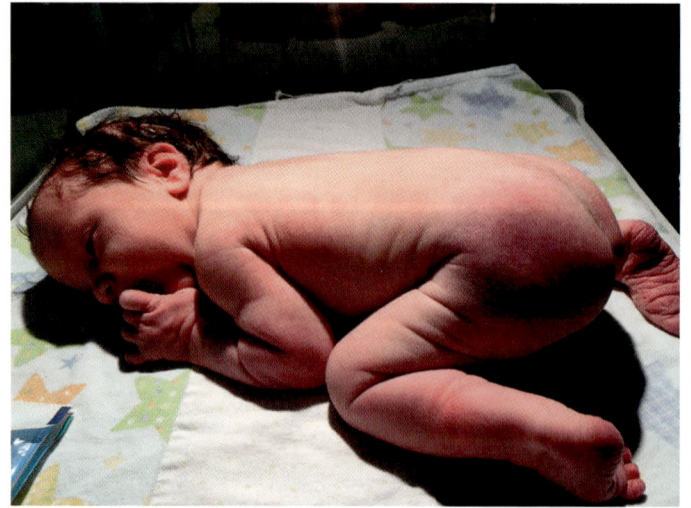

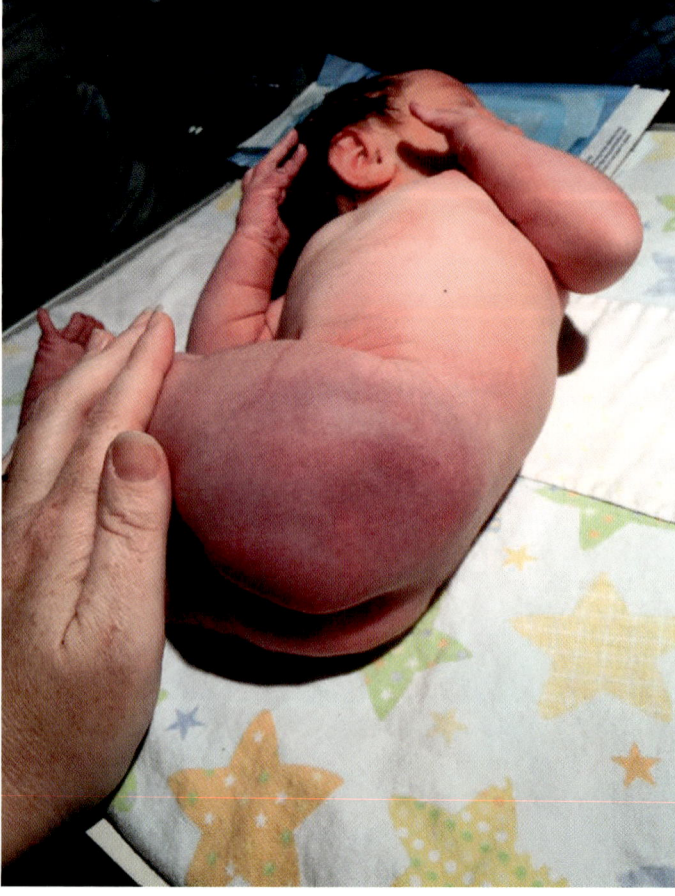

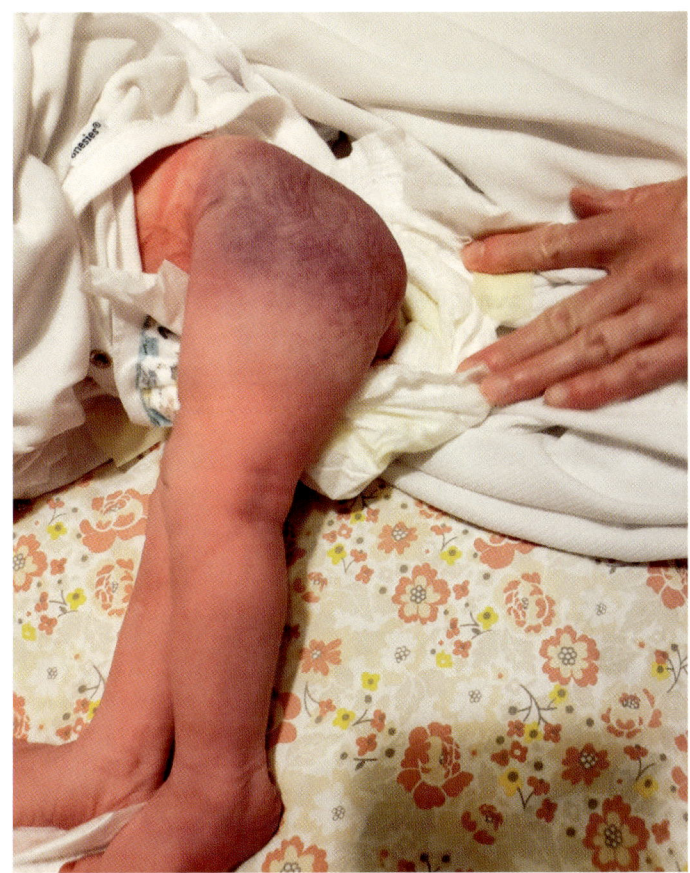

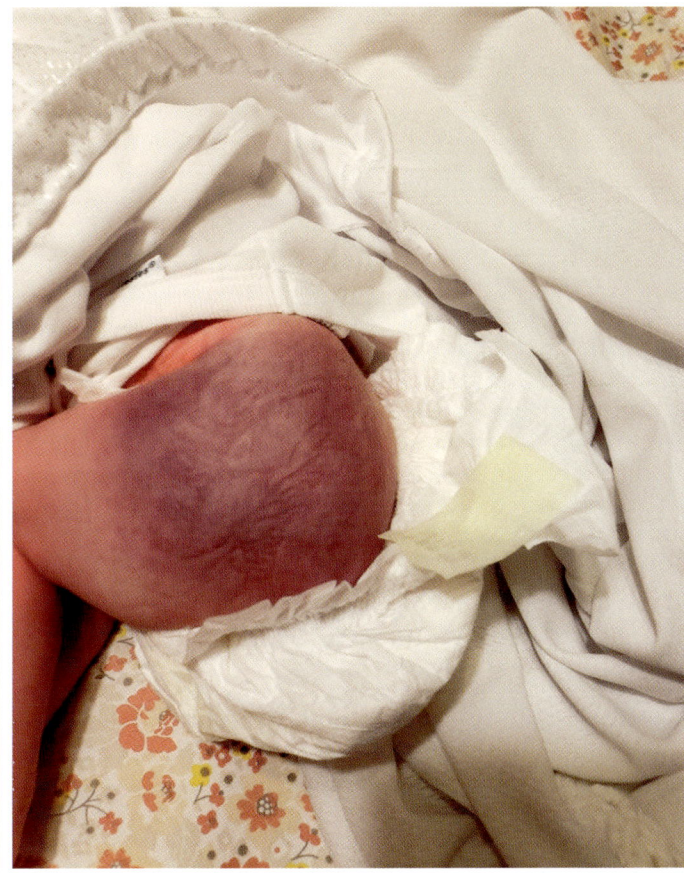

Case #5: Bruising on buttock

Above: These two pictures were taken shortly after the birth.

Left: Healing process 2 days postpartum.

Case #6: Contusions and peeling skin on buttock and labia (a few days after birth)

This was an undiagnosed breech at a birth center. The baby was transported a few hours after the birth due to some respiratory concerns. Staff at the admitting hospital were unfamiliar with vaginal breech birth and assumed these injuries were due to parental sexual abuse, despite the trauma being well-documented in the baby's chart as a birth injury due to VBB. This baby was removed from the family by Child Protective Services, and the family had to hire an attorney and engage in a lengthy process to recover their baby. BWB clinicians submitted testimony and the baby was released to the family soon thereafter.

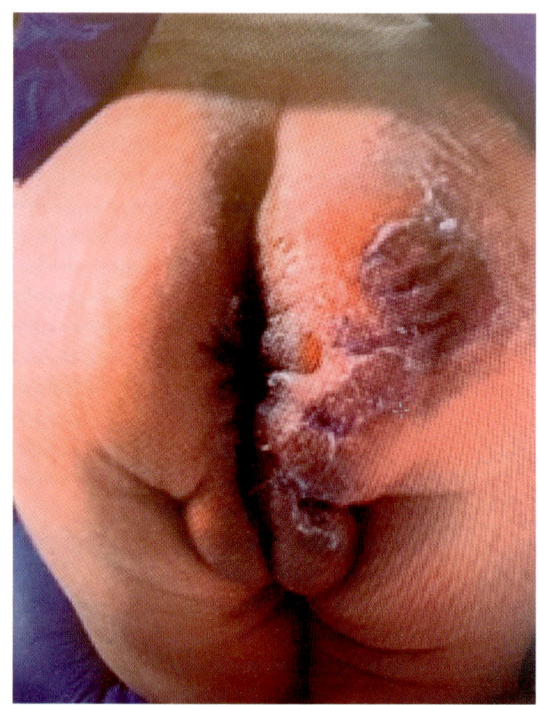

Jaime Rose

Case #7: Dropped foot breech with bruising and swelling on the presenting leg

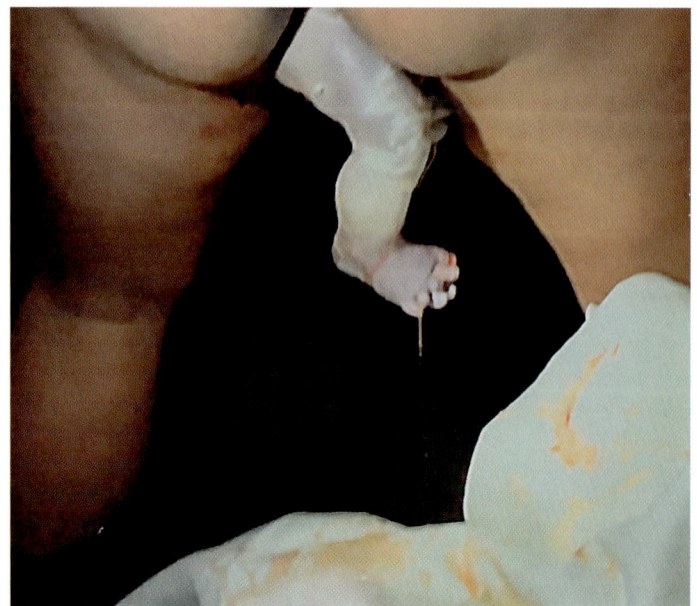

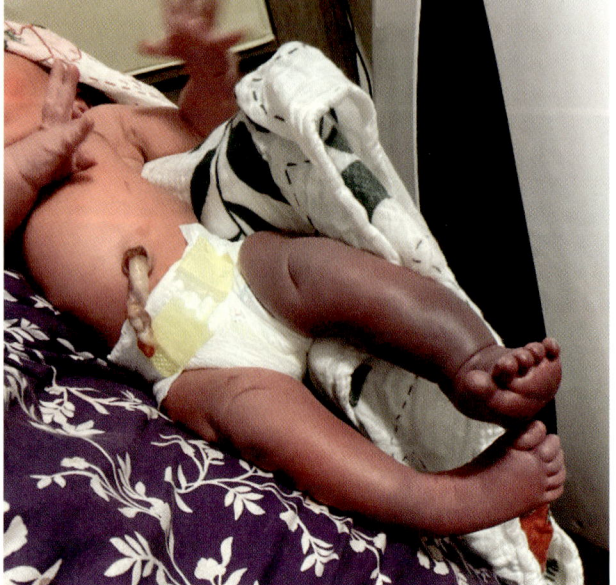

When possible prior to the birth, explain to the parents that sometimes bruising and swelling of the presenting part of the baby can occur; this is normal and they need not be alarmed. Once the baby is born, if indeed there is some bruising and swelling, point it out to the parents and explain to them exactly what is being seen and that all limbs are moving bilaterally and there is no cause for concern. It is important they have a good understanding in the event they are questioned by well-meaning family or another care provider.

In the case of swollen genitals, if the baby is nursing and passing urine/meconium, let them know this is all within normal range. Like any other bruise, we can expect it will start to dissipate over the next few days. In the absence of any other issues or concerns, it is perfectly acceptable to hold off on any consult.

If you are unsure whether the amount of bruising swelling or peeling skin that you're seeing is normal, consult someone who has a lot of experience with breech birth to help you determine if there is cause for concern.

It is extremely important that you document on the chart exactly what you are seeing and what you have explained to the parents. If possible, ask permission from the parents to take photos of the affected area so you have photo documentation. Also try to take photos that follow the progression of the healing. If the parents do not agree, then just document extensively in the chart.

Why is documentation of these birth injuries very important? If the family follows up with a pediatrician or family physician in the days following the birth, and that provider has some concern because they are not used to seeing vaginally born breech babies and don't know the extent to which they can have swelling and bruising, it can be problematic, not just for you but also for the parents.

In some cases, Child Protective Services (or equivalent) has taken children away from their parents because of trauma sustained in the normal course of a vaginal breech birth. This is why documentation is so crucially important. Until vaginal breech birth comes more into the mainstream and more physicians are used to seeing the normal consequences of vaginal breech birth, we need to keep documenting and educating.

If you have a baby with swelling and bruising and you can take photos, get permission to share them with other providers in an effort to educate. We need to continue to share resources of these kinds of things so that we're all aware of what can be expected.

Case #8: Peripheral cyanosis in the limbs

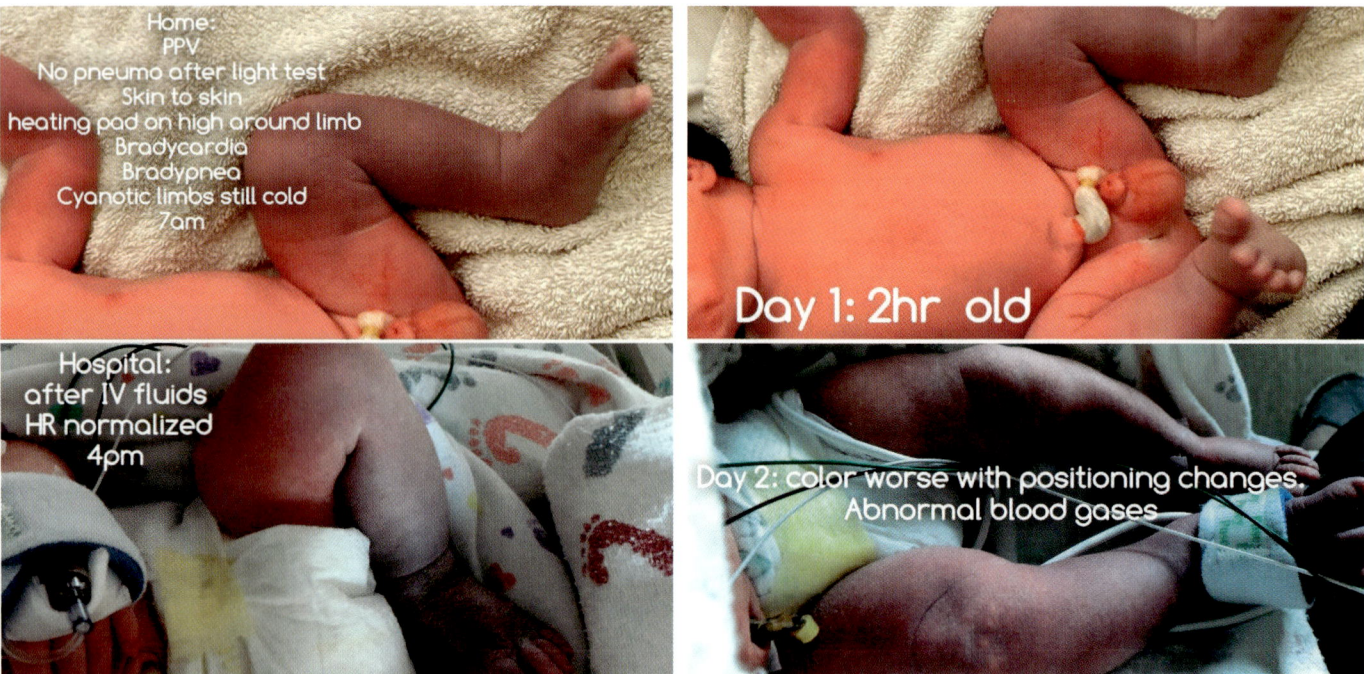

Case #9: Bruising on left wrist where it was hung up on the pubic bone.

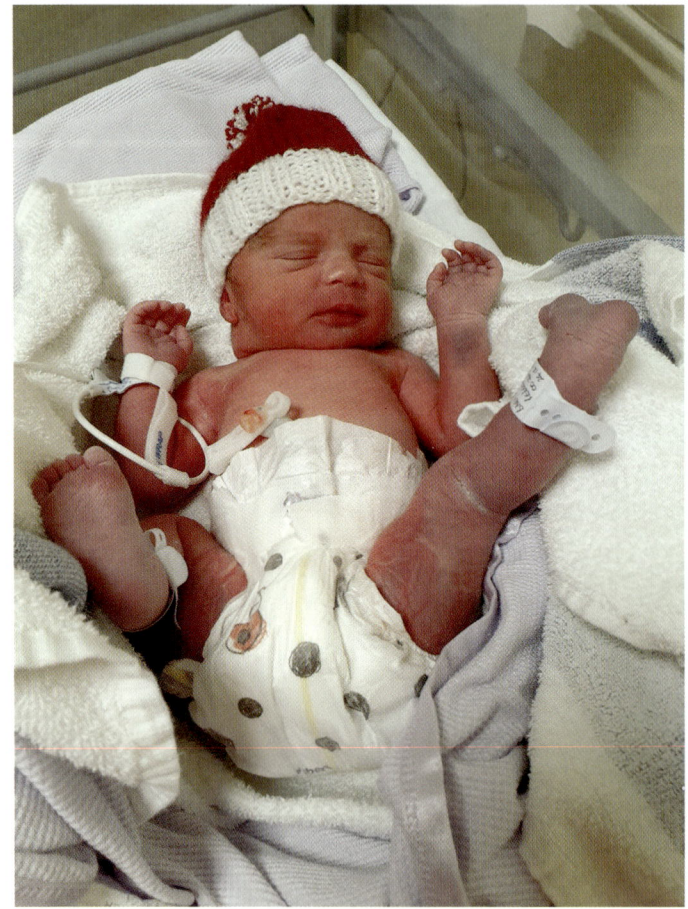

This illustrates how various parts of the baby can become obstructed.

We want to honor the brave women who undergo major surgery to bring their children into the world. Some of these surgeries are wanted and welcomed; others are done under duress. We envision a world in which every woman has support for the birth of her choice, including physiological vaginal breech birth.

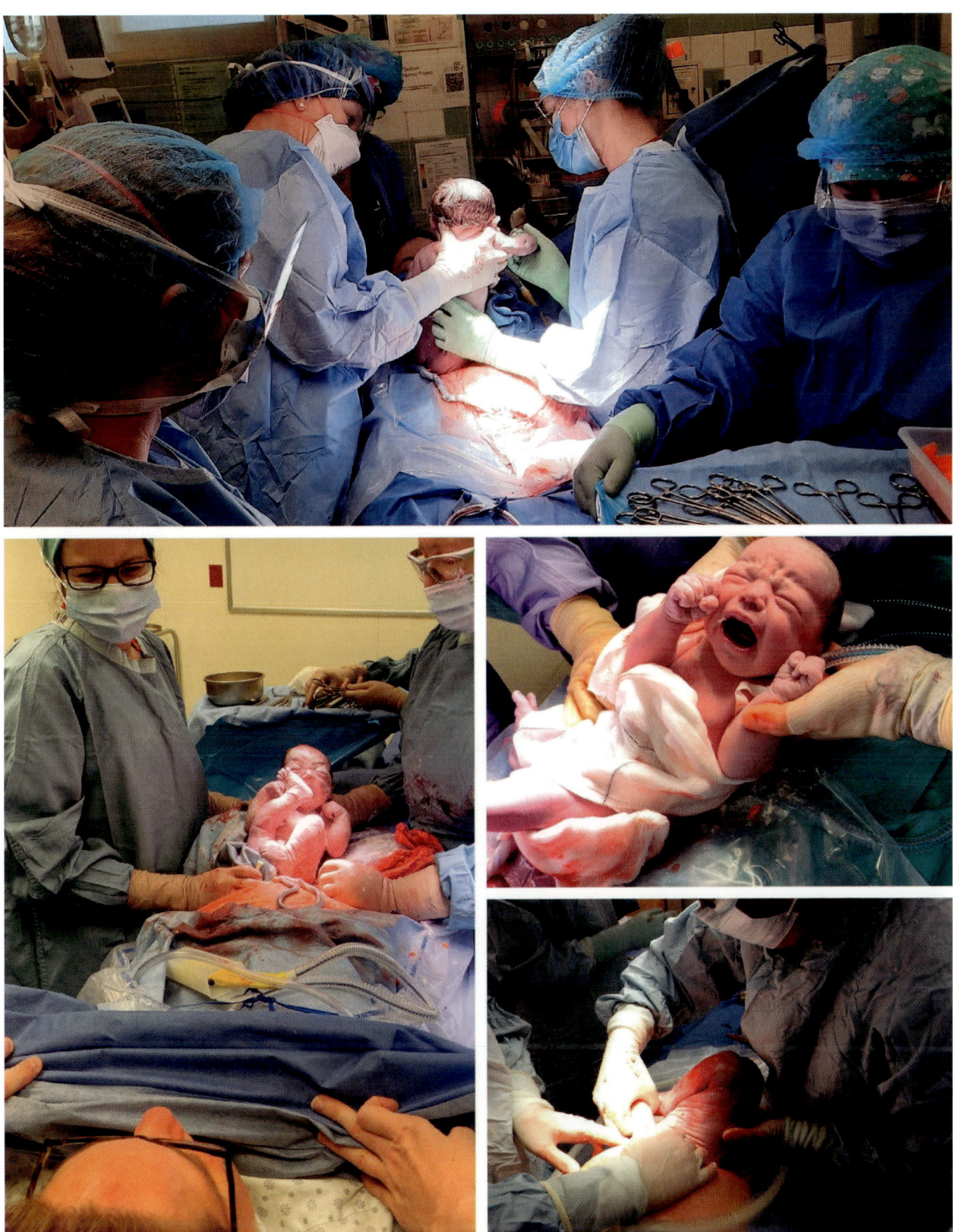

Image credits

We thank the parents, midwives, and doctors for allowing us to use these images to help educate maternity care providers. Unless otherwise noted, all photos and videos were submitted to Breech Without Borders for educational purposes. When we were unable to contact the image's owner, we have listed where the image appeared online. The following image contributors have requested to be named as follows:

Abby with @mamasmidwives
Alex
Alexis
Amanda
Angela Joanne Williams
Anissa Sartini LM CPM
    Metroplex Midwifery
    metroplexmidwifery.com
Ashley Winter
Bridget Brimacombe
Cassidy Piney
Charity Pitcher-Cooper
Cherry with Laura Latina
Christiane Miller, CPM
Cora Williams
Eirini, ΜΑΜούσκες (@mamouskes)
Ellis Walsh
Eveny & Baby Jeremy Medeiros
Fabiana Beracochea,
    @fabianaberacocheafotografia
    fabiberacochea.wixsite.com/
    fabianaphotography
Gab Hershman, @solagratiavita
Georgie Riley

Jaime Rose
Jamilah Pemberton
    Midwife: Sunshine Tomlin
    Photographer: Jesse Malley
Jemma Holmes, @freya.in.norfolk
Jennifer Sherriff
Jordan Shaw
Joy Horner, birthjoy.co.uk
Katie
Kiana N Johnson
Laura Siddons, @thenestingplaceli
Lesa Zenauskas with traditional
    midwife ZenDoula
Maria Forozidou
Mary Beliz, marybelizphotos.com
    @marybeliz_birthphotography
    Midwife: Fadwah Halaby
    midwife360.com
    Educator/doula: Barbara
    Harper, waterbirth.org
Megan Toulouse
Melissa Espey-Mueller of North
    Dallas Doula Associates
Nikita Richardson

Olivia Danielson-Veed
Pavla Salvetová
Rachel C
Rachel M
Rebecca Heaps
Rebecca Wanosik
    Midwife: Robin Massey CPM
    Birth Works LLC
    Photos.: Jerrica Rosenauer
    Willow + Rose Birth Services
    www.willowrosebirth.com
    @willowrosebirth
Shannon
Sharaya Gunst
    Midwife Heather Lemanski
    Photographer Grace Baker
Shatamia Webb, Baby Catcher
    Birth Center
Shelby Reed
Stephanie Crunk, midwife
Stephanie French
Victoria

The pelvis & fetus drawings come from *Introduction à l'étude clinique et à la pratique des accouchements,* 1909 edition by Louis Hubert Farabeuf and Dr. Henri V (gallica.bnf.fr).

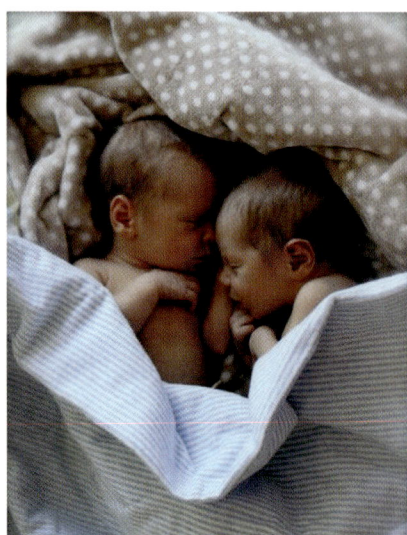

Twins attended by a BWB clinician

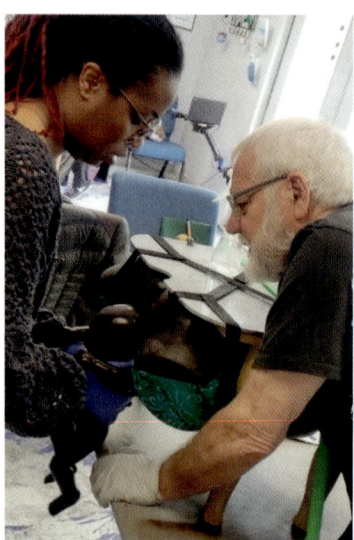

Dr. David Hayes and a workshop participant

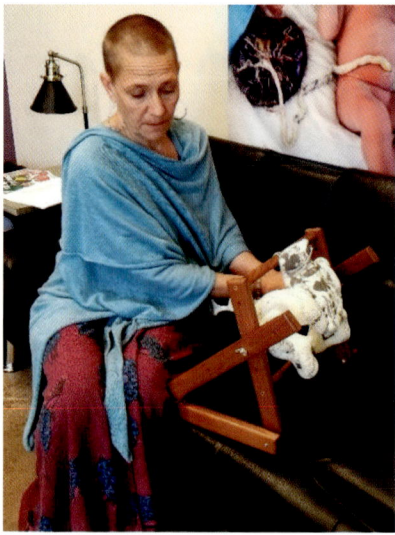

Kristine Lauria, CPM with a foldable simulator

Selected References

Abasiattai AM, Bassey EA, Etuk SJ, Udoma EJ, Ekanem AD. Caesarean section in the management of singleton breech delivery in Calabar, Nigeria. Niger J Clin Pract. 2006 Jun;9(1):22-5.

Adegbola O, Akindele OM. Outcome of term singleton breech deliveries at a University Teaching Hospital in Lagos, Nigeria. Niger Postgrad Med J. 2009 Jun;16(2):154-7.

Adjaoud S, Demailly R, Michel-Semail S, Rakza T, Storme L, Deruelle P, Garabedian C, Subtil D. Is trial of labor harmful in breech delivery? A cohort comparison for breech and vertex presentations. J Gynecol Obstet Hum Reprod. 2017 May;46(5):445-448.

Akinola SE, Archibong EI, Bhawani KP, Sobande AA. Assisted breech delivery, is the art fading? Saudi Med J. 2002 Apr;23(4):423-6.

Alarab M, Regan C, O'Connell MP, Keane DP, O'Herlihy C, Foley ME. Singleton vaginal breech delivery at term: still a safe option. Obstet Gynecol. 2004 Mar;103(3):407-12.

Albrechtsen S, Dalaker K. Seteleie--klassifikasjon og nomenklatur [Breech presentation--classification and nomenclature]. Tidsskr Nor Laegeforen. 1994 Jun 20;114(16):1845-6. Norwegian.

Albrechtsen S, Rasmussen S, Irgens LM. Secular trends in peri- and neonatal mortality in breech presentation; Norway 1967-1994. Acta Obstet Gynecol Scand. 2000 Jun;79(6):508-12.

Alexandersson O, Bixo M, Högberg U. Evidence-based changes in term breech delivery practice in Sweden. Acta Obstet Gynecol Scand. 2005 Jun;84(6):584-7.

Al-lakkany NS, Badawy AM, Bassiouni BA. Can the fetal-pelvic index predict fetal-pelvic disproportion during vaginal breech delivery? J Obstet Gynaecol. 2002 Mar;22(2):140-2.

Almgren M, Schlinzig T, Gomez-Cabrero D, Gunnar A, Sundin M, Johansson S, et al. Cesarean delivery and hematopoietic stem cell epigenetics in the newborn infant: implications for future health? Am J Obstet Gynecol. 2014 Nov;211(5):502.e1,502.e8.

Al-Najjar FS, Al-Shafiai AM. Safety of vaginal breech delivery. Saudi Med J. 2004 Oct;25(10):1517-8.

Alshaheen H, Abd Al-Karim A. Perinatal outcomes of singleton term breech deliveries in Basra. East Mediterr Health J. 2010 Jan;16(1):34-9.

Amoa AB, Sapuri M, Klufio CA. Perinatal outcome and associated factors of persistent breech presentation at the Port Moresby General Hospital, Papua New Guinea. P N G Med J. 2001 Mar-Jun;44(1-2):48-56.

Andersen GL, Irgens LM, Skranes J, Salvesen KA, Meberg A, Vik T. Is breech presentation a risk factor for cerebral palsy? A Norwegian birth cohort study. Dev Med Child Neurol. 2009 Nov;51(11):860-5.

Anderssen O et al. Intact cord resuscitation versus early cord clamping in the treatment of depressed newborn infants during the first 10 minutes of birth (Nepcord III) – a randomized clinical trial. Maternal Health, Neonatology, and Perinatology. 2019; 5(15):1-11.

Andreasen S, Nielsen EW, Øian P. Delivery of a breech presentation. Tidsskr Nor Laegeforen. 2010 Mar 25;130(6):605-8.

Ardier E, Sibony O, Depret-Mosser S, Puech F. La présentation du siège. In: Lansac J, Marret H, Oury J, editors. Pratique de l'accouchement. 4th ed. Paris: Elsevier Masson; 2006. p. 125-44.

Babay ZA, Al-Nuaim LA, Addar MH, Abdulkarim AA. Undiagnosed term breech: management and outcome. Saudi Med J. 2000 May;21(5):478-81.

Babović I, Arandjelovic M, Plesinac S, Sparic R. Vaginal delivery or cesarean section at term breech delivery--chance or risk? J Matern Fetal Neonatal Med. 2016;29(12):1930-4.

Babović I, Plesiinac S, Radojicic Z, Opalic J, Argirovic R, Mladenovic-Bogdanovic Z, et al. Vaginal delivery versus cesarean section for term breech delivery. Vojnosanit Pregl. 2010 Oct;67(10):807-11.

Banks M. Active breech birth: The point of least resistance. New Zealand College of Midwives Journal. 2007;36:6.

Banks M. Breech, posterior and a deflexed head! An active birth solution? Midwifery Today Int Midwife. 2009 Autumn;(91)(91):22-4.

Bassaw B, Rampersad N, Roopnarinesingh S, Sirjusingh A. Correlation of fetal outcome with mode of delivery for breech presentation. J Obstet Gynaecol. 2004 Apr;24(3):254-8.

Belfrage P, Gjessing L. The term breech presentation. A retrospective study with regard to the planned mode of delivery. Acta Obstet Gynecol Scand. 2002 Jun;81(6):544-50.

Ben Aissia N, Youssef A, Said MC, Gara MF. Breech presentation: vaginal delivery or planned caesarean section? Tunis Med. 2004 May;82(5):425-30.

Berhan Y, Berhan A. A meta-analysis of reverse breech extraction to deliver a deeply impacted head during cesarean delivery. Int J Gynaecol Obstet. 2014 Feb;124(2):99-105.

Berhan Y, Haileamlak A. The risks of planned vaginal breech delivery versus planned caesarean section for term breech birth: a meta-analysis including observational studies. BJOG. 2016 Jan;123(1):49-57.

Bin YS, Roberts CL, Ford JB, Nicholl MC. Outcomes of breech birth by mode of delivery: a population linkage study. Aust N Z J Obstet Gynaecol. 2016 Oct;56(5):453-9.

Bisits A. The value of imaging pelvimetry in the management of the breech presentation at term. Aust N Z J Obstet Gynaecol. 2015 Feb;55(1):99-100.

Bogner G, Strobl M, Schausberger C, Fischer T, Reisenberger K, Jacobs VR. Breech delivery in the all fours position: a prospective observational comparative study with classic assistance. J Perinat Med. 2015 Nov;43(6):707-13.

Borbolla Foster A, Bagust A, Bisits A, Holland M, Welsh A. Lessons to be learnt in managing the breech presentation at term: an 11-year single-centre retrospective study. Aust N Z J Obstet Gynaecol. 2014 Aug;54(4):333-9.

Bottcher B, Radley SC. Pelvimetry: changing trends and attitudes. J Obstet Gynaecol. 2001 Sep;21(5):459-62.

Bourtembourg A, Ramanah R, Martin A, Pugin-Vivot A, Maillet R, Riethmuller D. Fetal heart rate patterns of breech presentations during expulsion. A comparative study with cephalic presentations. J Gynecol Obstet Biol Reprod (Paris). 2015 Jun;44(6):577-86.

Broche DE, Riethmuller D, Vidal C, Sautiere JL, Schaal JP, Maillet R. Obstetric and perinatal outcomes of a disreputable presentation: the nonfrank breech. J Gynecol Obstet Biol Reprod (Paris). 2005 Dec;34(8):781-8.

Brouwer WK, Veenstra van Nieuwenhoven AL, Santema JG. Neonatal outcome after a planned vaginal breech birth: no association with parity or birth weight, but more birth injuries than in planned cesarean section. Ned Tijdschr Geneeskd. 2001 Aug 11;145(32):1554-7.

Buerkle B, Rueter K, Hefler LA, Tempfer-Bentz EK, Tempfer CB. Objective Structured Assessment of Technical Skills (OSATS) evaluation of theoretical versus hands-on training of vaginal breech delivery management: a randomized trial. Eur J Obstet Gynecol Reprod Biol. 2013 Dec;171(2):252-6.

Burgos J, Rodriguez L, Cobos P, Osuna C, Del Mar Centeno M, Larrieta R, et al. Management of breech presentation at term: a retrospective cohort study of 10 years of experience. J Perinatol. 2015 Oct;35(10):803-8.

Cardwell CR, Stene LC, Joner G, Cinek O, Svensson J, Goldacre MJ, et al. Caesarean section is associated with an increased risk of childhood-onset type 1 diabetes mellitus: a meta-analysis of observational studies. Diabetologia. 2008 May;51(5):726-35.

Clark SL. Category II Intrapartum Fetal Heart Rate Patterns Unassociated With Recognized Sentinel Events: Castles in the Air. Obstet Gynecol. 2022 Jun 1;139(6):1003-1008.

Collea JV, Chein C, Quilligan EJ. The randomized management of term frank breech presentation: a study of 208 cases. Am J Obstet Gynecol. 1980 May 15;137(2):235-44.

Cronk M. Keep your hands off the breech. MBE AIMS Journal. 1998 Autumn;10(3).

Cuppen I, Eggink AJ, Lotgering FK, Rotteveel JJ, Mullaart RA, Roeleveld N. Influence of birth mode on early neurological outcome in infants with myelomeningocele. Eur J Obstet Gynecol Reprod Biol. 2011 May;156(1):18-22.

Daskalakis G, Anastasakis E, Papantoniou N, Mesogitis S, Thomakos N, Antsaklis A. Cesarean vs. vaginal birth for term breech presentation in 2 different study periods. Int J Gynaecol Obstet. 2007 Mar;96(3):162-6.

Daviss BA, Moll E, Hedditch A, Hermsen B, The Montfort Hospital and the Ottawa Hospital, Canada, OLVG Hospital Amsterdam, Oxford Radcliffe Hospitals NHS Foundation Trust, UK. Can forceps be eliminated in vaginal breech with upright postiion manoeuvres & the

"Crowning Touch"? Poster presentation, FIGO. October 2021.

Daviss BA, Johnson KC, Lalonde AB. Evolving evidence since the term breech trial: Canadian response, European dissent, and potential solutions. J Obstet Gynaecol Can. 2010 Mar;32(3):217-24.

Daviss BA. Rethinking The Physiology of Vaginal Breech Birth: Manual of Best Evidence-Based Manoeuvres, 11th Edition February 2021.

Daviss BA, Johnson KC. Upright breech birth: New video research risks reviving Friedman's curse. Birth. 2022 Mar;49(1):11-15.

de Leeuw JP, de Haan J, Derom R, Thiery M, Martens G, van Maele G. Mortality and early neonatal morbidity in vaginal and abdominal deliveries in breech presentation. J Obstet Gynaecol. 2002 Mar;22(2):127-39.

Deering S, Brown J, Hodor J, Satin AJ. Simulation training and resident performance of singleton vaginal breech delivery. Obstet Gynecol. 2006 Jan;107(1):86-9.

Delotte J, Schumacker-Blay C, Bafghi A, Lehmann P, Bongain A. Medical information and patients' choices. Influences on term singleton breech deliveries. Gynecol Obstet Fertil. 2007 Sep;35(9):747-50.

Delotte J, Trastour C, Bafghi A, Boucoiran I, D'Angelo L, Bongain A. Influence of mode of delivery in term breech presentation on the Apgar score and transfer in neonatal care unit. Results of the management of 568 singleton pregnancies in a level III French maternity. J Gynecol Obstet Biol Reprod (Paris). 2008 Apr;37(2):149-53.

Demirci O, Tugrul AS, Turgut A, Ceylan S, Eren S. Pregnancy outcomes by mode of delivery among breech births. Arch Gynecol Obstet. 2012 Feb;285(2):297-303.

Descargues G, Doucet S, Mauger-Tinlot F, Gravier A, Lemoine JP, Marpeau L. Influence of the type of breech presentation on delivery in selected primiparous women at term. J Gynecol Obstet Biol Reprod (Paris). 2001 Nov;30(7 Pt 1):664-73.

Diab AE. Uterine ruptures in Yemen. Saudi Med J. 2005 Feb;26(2):264-9.

Djurić J, Arsenijevic S, Bankovic D, Protrka Z, Sorak M, Dimitrijevic A, et al. Breech presentation at term: caesarean section or vaginal delivery? Srp Arh Celok Lek. 2011 Mar-Apr;139(3-4):155-60.

Dubois J. Aspects actuels des problèmes que pose l'accouchement en préésentation du siège [Some present aspects of the problems of breech presentation and delivery (author's transl)]. J Gynecol Obstet Biol Reprod (Paris). 1981;10(5):479-92. French.

Easter SR, Gardner R, Barrett J, Robinson JN, Carusi D. Simulation to Improve Trainee Knowledge and Comfort About Twin Vaginal Birth. Obstet Gynecol. 2016 Oct;128 Suppl 1:34S-9S.

Eide MG, Oyen N, Skjaerven R, Irgens LM, Bjerkedal T, Nilsen ST. Breech delivery and intelligence: a population-based study of 8,738 breech infants. Obstet Gynecol. 2005 Jan;105(1):4-11.

Evans J. Breech birth: abnormal or unusual? Midwifery Today Int Midwife. 2013 Summer;(106):16-8.

Evans J. Stepping into the breech...and the the midwife's story. Pract Midwife. 2006 Jun;9(6):19-20.

Evans J. Understanding physiological breech birth. Essentially MIDIRS. 2012 Feb;3(2):17-21.

Fahy K. Do the findings of the Term Breech Trial apply to spontaneous breech birth? Women Birth. 2011 Mar;24(1):1-2.

Fawole AO, Adeyemi AS, Adewole IF, Omigbodun AO. A ten-year review of breech deliveries at Ibadan. Afr J Med Med Sci. 2001 Mar-Jun;30(1-2):87-90.

Ferreira JC, Borowski D, Czuba B, Cnota W, Wloch A, Sodowski K, et al. The evolution of fetal presentation during pregnancy: a retrospective, descriptive cross-sectional study. Acta Obstet Gynecol Scand. 2015 Jun;94(6):660-3.

Fischbein SJ, Freeze R. Breech birth at home: outcomes of 60 breech and 109 cephalic planned home and birth center births. BMC Pregnancy Childbirth. 2018 Oct 11;18(1):397.

Fischbein SJ. A maneuver for head entanglement in term breech/vertex twin labor. J Case Rep Images Obstet Gynecol 2018;4:100042Z08SF2018.

Franz M, von Bismarck A, Delius M, Ertl-Wagner B, Deppe C, Mahner S, et al. MR pelvimetry: prognosis for successful vaginal delivery in patients with suspected fetopelvic disproportion or breech presentation at term. Arch Gynecol Obstet. 2017 Feb;295(2):351-9.

Frye A. Holistic Midwifery: A Comprehensive Textbook for Midwives in Homebirth Practice. Vol. II: Care of the Mother and Baby From the Onset of Labor Through the First Hours After Birth. Portland, OR: Labrys Press; 2004.

Gannard-Pechin E, Ramanah R, Desmarets M, Maillet R, Riethmuller D. Term breech presentations in singleton pregnancies: a continuous series of 418 cases. J Gynecol Obstet Biol Reprod (Paris). 2013 Nov;42(7):685-92.

Gilbert WM, Hicks SM, Boe NM, Danielsen B. Vaginal versus cesarean delivery for breech presentation in California: a population-based study. Obstet Gynecol. 2003 Nov;102(5 Pt 1):911-7.

Gimovsky ML, Wallace RL, Schifrin BS, Paul RH. Randomized management of the nonfrank breech presentation at term: a preliminary report. Am J Obstet Gynecol. 1983 May 1;146(1):34-40.

Giuliani A, Scholl WM, Basver A, Tamussino KF. Mode of delivery and outcome of 699 term singleton breech deliveries at a single center. Am J Obstet Gynecol. 2002 Dec;187(6):1694-8.

Glezerman M. Five years to the term breech trial: the rise and fall of a randomized controlled trial. Am J Obstet Gynecol. 2006 Jan;194(1):20-5.

Goffinet F, Carayol M, Foidart JM, Alexander S, Uzan S, Subtil D, et al. Is planned vaginal delivery for breech presentation at term still an option? Results of an observational prospective survey in France and Belgium. Am J Obstet Gynecol. 2006 Apr;194(4):1002-11.

Golfier F, Vaudoyer F, Ecochard R, Champion F, Audra P, Raudrant D. Planned vaginal delivery versus elective caesarean section in singleton term breech presentation: a study of 1116 cases. Eur J Obstet Gynecol Reprod Biol. 2001 Oct;98(2):186-92.

Gruneberg F, Crozier K. Delayed cord clamping in the compromised baby. BJOG. 2015 Feb;23(2):102-108.

Gultekin IB, Altinboga O, Karahanoglu E, Dogan NG, Icer B, Alkan A, et al. To what extent do the presentation of fetus, amniotic fluid index and fetal weight at term affect the cardiac axis? J Electrocardiol. 2016 Jul-Aug;49(4):560-3.

Habib S, Riaz S, Abbasi N, Ayaz A, Bibi A, Parveen Z. Vaginal breech delivery: still a safe option. J Ayub Med Coll Abbottabad. 2013 Jul-Dec;25(3-4):38-40.

Haheim LL, Albrechtsen S, Berge LN, Bordahl PE, Egeland T, Henriksen T, et al. Breech birth at term: vaginal delivery or elective cesarean section? A systematic review of the literature by a Norwegian review team. Acta Obstet Gynecol Scand. 2004 Feb;83(2):126-30.

Halmesmaki E. Vaginal term breech delivery--a time for reappraisal? Acta Obstet Gynecol Scand. 2001 Mar;80(3):187-90.

Hannah ME, Hannah WJ, Hewson SA, Hodnett ED, Saigal S, Willan AR. Planned caesarean section versus planned vaginal birth for breech presentation at term: a randomised multicentre trial. Term Breech Trial Collaborative Group. Lancet. 2000 Oct 21;356(9239):1375-83.

Hannah ME, Hannah WJ, Hodnett ED, Chalmers B, Kung R, Willan A, et al. Outcomes at 3 months after planned cesarean vs planned vaginal delivery for breech presentation at term: the international randomized Term Breech Trial. JAMA. 2002 Apr 10;287(14):1822-31.

Hannah ME, Whyte H, Hannah WJ, Hewson S, Amankwah K, Cheng M, et al. Maternal outcomes at 2 years after planned cesarean section versus planned vaginal birth for breech presentation at term: the international randomized Term Breech Trial. Am J Obstet Gynecol. 2004 Sep;191(3):917-27.

Hartnack Tharin JE, Rasmussen S, Krebs L. Consequences of the Term Breech Trial in Denmark. Acta Obstet Gynecol Scand. 2011 Jul;90(7):767-71.

Hellsten C, Lindqvist PG, Olofsson P. Vaginal breech delivery: is it still an option? Eur J Obstet Gynecol Reprod Biol. 2003 Dec 10;111(2):122-8.

Herbst A, Thorngren-Jerneck K. Mode of delivery in breech presentation at term: increased neonatal morbidity with vaginal delivery. Acta Obstet Gynecol Scand. 2001 Aug;80(8):731-7.

Hibbard JU, Ismail MA, Wang Y, Te C, Karrison T, Ismail MA. Failed vaginal birth after a cesarean section: how risky is it? I. Maternal morbidity. Am J Obstet Gynecol. 2001 Jun;184(7):1365,71; discussion 1371-3.

Hoehner C, Kelsey A, El-Beltagy N, Artal R, Leet T. Cesarean section in term breech presentations: do rates of adverse neonatal outcomes differ by hospital birth volume? J Perinat Med. 2006;34(3):196-202.

Hoffmann J, Thomassen K, Stumpp P, Grothoff M, Engel C, Kahn T, et al. New MRI Criteria for Successful Vaginal Breech Delivery in Primiparae. PLoS One. 2016 Aug 17;11(8):e0161028.

Hofmeyr GJ, Hannah M, Lawrie TA. Planned caesarean section for term breech delivery. Cochrane Database Syst Rev. 2015 Jul 21;(7):CD000166. doi(7):CD000166.

Hofmeyr GJ, Hannah ME. Planned caesarean section for term breech delivery. Cochrane Database Syst Rev. 2000;(2)(2):CD000166.

Hofmeyr GJ, Hannah ME. Planned Caesarean section for term breech delivery. Cochrane Database Syst Rev. 2001;(1)(1):CD000166.

Högberg U, Claeson C, Krebs L, Svanberg AS, Kidanto H. Breech delivery at a University Hospital in Tanzania. BMC Pregnancy Childbirth. 2016 Nov 8;16(1):342.

Hopkins LM, Esakoff T, Noah MS, Moore DH, Sawaya GF, Laros RK,Jr. Outcomes associated with cesarean section versus vaginal breech delivery at a university hospital. J Perinatol. 2007 Mar;27(3):141-6.

Hruban L, Janku P, Ventruba P, Oskrdalova L, Skorkovska K, Hodicka Z, et al. Vaginal breech delivery after 36 week of pregnancy in a selected group of pregnancy - analysis of perinatal results in years 2008-2011. Ceska Gynekol. 2014 Nov;79(5):343-9.

Iankov M, Katsulov A, Gruncharov I. The place of the planned cesarean section in women with breech presentation. Akush Ginekol (Sofiia). 2005;44(2):10-2.

Impey L. Literature on the management of term breech pregnancy including the RCOG 2017 guideline update. North of England Breech Conference; March 31, 2017; Sheffield, England.

Izetbegović S. Procedure of breech presentation delivery in correlation with newborns vitality during period 2002-2005. Med Arh. 2006;60(6 Suppl 1):41-2.

Jadoon S, Khan Jadoon SM, Shah R. Maternal and neonatal complications in term breech delivered vaginally. J Coll Physicians Surg Pak. 2008 Sep;18(9):555-8.

Jain A, Pandey S, Kumar R, Sethi C, Sharma S. A retrospective study to correlate breech presentation and enhanced risk of postspinal hypotension during cesarean delivery. Local Reg Anesth. 2015 Dec 16;8:129-34.

Jennewein L, Allert R, Möllmann CJ, Paul B, Kielland-Kaisen U, Raimann FJ, Brüggmann D, Louwen F. The influence of the fetal leg position on the outcome in vaginally intended deliveries out of breech presentation at term - A FRABAT prospective cohort study. PLoS One. 2019 Dec 2;14(12):e0225546.

Jennewein L, Brüggmann D, Fischer K, Raimann FJ, Pfeifenberger HR, Agel L, Zander N, Eichbaum C, Louwen F. Learning Breech Birth in an Upright Position Is Influenced by Preexisting Experience-A FRABAT Prospective Cohort Study. J Clin Med. 2021 May 14;10(10):2117.

Jennewein L, Kielland-Kaisen U, Paul B, Möllmann CJ, Klemt AS, Schulze S, Bock N, Schaarschmidt W, Brüggmann D, Louwen F. Maternal and neonatal outcome after vaginal breech delivery at term of children weighing more or less than 3.8 kg: A FRABAT prospective cohort study. PLoS One. 2018 Aug 23;13(8):e0202760.

Jensen VM, Wust M. Can Caesarean section improve child and maternal health? The case of breech babies. J Health Econ. 2015 Jan;39:289-302.

Jeve YB, Navti OB, Konje JC. Comparison of techniques used to deliver a deeply impacted fetal head at full dilation: a systematic review and meta-analysis. BJOG. 2016 Feb;123(3):337-45.

Jeyabalan A, Larkin RW, Landers DV. Vaginal breech deliveries selected using computed tomographic pelvimetry may be associated with fewer adverse outcomes. J Matern Fetal Neonatal Med. 2005 Jun;17(6):381-5.

Jordan A, Antomarchi J, Bongain A, Tran A, Delotte J. Development and validation of an objective structured assessment of technical skill tool for the practice of breech presentation delivery. Arch Gynecol Obstet. 2016 Aug;294(2):327-32.

Jordan A, El Haloui O, Breaud J, Chevalier D, Antomarchi J, Bongain A, et al. Training of residents in obstetrics and gynecology: Assessment of an educational program including formal lectures and practical sessions using simulators. Gynecol Obstet Fertil. 2015 Jul-Aug;43(7-8):560-7.

Kalumbi C, Tadesse E. An audit of deliveries and outcome at Queen Elizabeth Central Hospital, Blantyre, in 1999. Malawi Med J. 2001 Sep;13(3):34-5.

Kayem G, Goffinet F, Clement D, Hessabi M, Cabrol D. Breech presentation at term: morbidity and mortality according to the type of delivery at Port Royal Maternity hospital from 1993 through 1999. Eur J Obstet Gynecol Reprod Biol. 2002 May 10;102(2):137-42.

Keirse MJ. Evidence-based childbirth only for breech babies? Birth. 2002 Mar;29(1):55-9.

Kessler J, Moster D, Albrechtsen S. Intrapartum monitoring with cardiotocography and ST-waveform analysis in breech presentation: an observational study. BJOG. 2015 Mar;122(4):528-35.

Kew N, DuPlessis J, La Paglia D, Williams K. Predictors of Cephalic Vaginal Delivery Following External Cephalic Version: An Eight-Year Single-Centre Study of 447 Cases. Obstet Gynecol Int. 2017;2017:3028398.

Kielland-Kaisen U, Paul B, Jennewein L, Klemt A, Möllmann CJ, Bock N, Schaarschmidt W, Brüggmann D, Louwen F. Maternal and neonatal outcome after vaginal breech delivery of nulliparous versus multiparous women of singletons at term-A prospective evaluation of the Frankfurt breech at term cohort (FRABAT). Eur J Obstet Gynecol Reprod Biol. 2020 Sep;252:583-587.

Kimbala J, Mukuku O, Kinenkinda X, Kizonde J. Transverse presentation and modalities of delivery: caesarean section versus large internal cephalic version and breech extraction; about 162 births at the maternity Jason Sendwe of Lubumbashi, DR Congo. Pan Afr Med J. 2014 Nov 18;19:300.

Klemt AS, Schulze S, Brüggmann D, Louwen F. MRI-based pelvimetric measurements as predictors for a successful vaginal breech delivery in the Frankfurt Breech at term cohort (FRABAT). Eur J Obstet Gynecol Reprod Biol. 2019 Jan;232:10-17. doi: 10.1016/j.ejogrb.2018.09.033. Epub 2018 Oct 22.

Kodama Y, Sameshima H, Yamashita R, Oohashi M, Ikenoue T. Intrapartum fetal heart rate patterns preceding terminal bradycardia in infants (>34 weeks) with poor neurological outcome: A regional population-based study in Japan. J Obstet Gynaecol Res. 2015 Nov;41(11):1738-43.

Kotaska A. Inappropriate use of randomised trials to evaluate complex phenomena: case study of vaginal breech delivery. BMJ. 2004 Oct 30;329(7473):1039-42.

Kouam L, Miller EC. Einige neue Aspekte zum Nabelschnurvorfall [Prolapse of umbilical cord - new aspects (author's transl)]. Zentralbl Gynakol. 1980;102(13):724-33. German.

Krause M, Fischer T, Feige A. Welchen Einfluss hat die Stellung der Beine bei der Beckenendlage auf den Entbindungsmodus und die neonatale Frühmorbidität? [What effect does leg position in breech presentation have on mode of delivery and early neonatal morbidity?]. Z Geburtshilfe Neonatol. 1997 Jul-Aug;201(4):128-35. German.

Krebs L. Breech at term. Early and late consequences of mode of delivery. Dan Med Bull. 2005 Dec;52(4):234-52.

Krebs L, Langhoff-Roos J. Elective cesarean delivery for term breech. Obstet Gynecol. 2003 Apr;101(4):690-6.

Krupitz H, Arzt W, Ebner T, Sommergruber M, Steininger E, Tews G. Assisted vaginal delivery versus caesarean section in breech presentation. Acta Obstet Gynecol Scand. 2005 Jun;84(6):588-92.

Kumari AS, Grundsell H. Mode of delivery for breech presentation in grandmultiparous women. Int J Gynaecol Obstet. 2004 Jun;85(3):234-9.

Lansac J, Crenn-Hebert C, Riviere O, Vendittelli F. How singleton breech babies at term are born in France: a survey of data from the AUDIPOG network. Eur J Obstet Gynecol Reprod Biol. 2015 May;188:79-82.

Larsson C, Saltvedt S, Wiklund I, Andolf E. Planned vaginal delivery versus planned caesarean section: short-term medical outcome analyzed according to intended mode of delivery. J Obstet Gynaecol Can. 2011 Aug;33(8):796-802.

Lashen H, Fear K, Sturdee D. Trends in the management of the breech presentation at term; experience in a District General hospital over a 10-year period. Acta Obstet Gynecol Scand. 2002 Dec;81(12):1116-22.

Lazarov N, Lazarov L. Fetal mortality of children in breech presentation for the period 1990-2001 (12 years). Akush Ginekol (Sofiia). 2008;47 Suppl 3:48-50.

Lee HC, El-Sayed YY, Gould JB. Population trends in cesarean delivery for breech presentation in the United States, 1997-2003. Am J Obstet Gynecol. 2008 Jul;199(1):59.e1,59.e8.

Leung WC, Pun TC, Wong WM. Undiagnosed breech revisited. Br J Obstet Gynaecol. 1999 Jul;106(7):638-41.

Liu S, Liston RM, Joseph KS, Heaman M, Sauve R, Kramer MS, et al. Maternal mortality and severe morbidity associated with low-risk planned cesarean delivery versus planned vaginal delivery at term. CMAJ. 2007 Feb 13;176(4):455-60.

Louwen F, Daviss BA, Johnson KC, Reitter A. Does breech delivery in an upright position instead of on the back improve outcomes and avoid cesareans? Int J Gynaecol Obstet. 2017 Feb;136(2):151-61.

Lumbiganon P, Laopaiboon M, Gulmezoglu AM, Souza JP, Taneepanichskul S, Ruyan P, et al. Method of delivery and pregnancy outcomes in Asia: the WHO global survey on maternal and perinatal health 2007-08. Lancet. 2010 Feb 6;375(9713):490-9.

Lyons J, Pressey T, Bartholomew S, Liu S, Liston RM, Joseph KS, et al. Delivery of breech presentation at term gestation in Canada, 2003-2011. Obstet Gynecol. 2015 May;125(5):1153-61.

Macharey G, Ulander VM, Heinonen S, Kostev K, Nuutila M, Vaisanen-Tommiska M. Risk factors and outcomes in "well-selected" vaginal breech deliveries: a retrospective observational study. J Perinat Med. 2017 Apr 1;45(3):291-7.

Maier B, Georgoulopoulos A, Zajc M, Jaeger T, Zuchna C, Hasenoehrl G. Fetal outcome for infants in breech by method of delivery: experiences with a stand-by service system of senior obstetricians and women's choices of mode of delivery. J Perinat Med. 2011 Jul;39(4):385-90.

Mailath-Pokorny M, Preyer O, Dadak C, Lischka A, Mittlbock M, Wagenbichler P, et al. Breech presentation: a retrospective analysis of 12-years' experience at a single center. Wien Klin Wochenschr. 2009;121(5-6):209-15.

Martínez Galiano JM, Herrera Gomez A, Pacheco Adamuz MJ. Childbirth via the vagina birth canal. Breech presentation through the cervix uteri. Rev Enferm. 2008 Jun;31(6):9-12.

Maslovitz S, Barkai G, Lessing JB, Ziv A, Many A. Recurrent obstetric management mistakes identified by simulation. Obstet Gynecol. 2007 Jun;109(6):1295-300.

Mattila M, Rautkorpi J, Heikkinen T. Pregnancy outcomes in breech presentation analyzed according to intended mode of delivery. Acta Obstet Gynecol Scand. 2015 Oct;94(10):1102-4.

Mattiolo S, Spillane E, Walker S. Physiological breech birth training: An evaluation of clinical practice changes after a one-day training program. Birth. 2021 Dec;48(4):558-565.

Mazhar SB, Kausar S. Outcome of singleton breech deliveries beyond 28 weeks gestation: the experience at MCH Centre, PIMS. Mother and Child Health. Pakistan Institute of Medical Sciences. J Pak Med Assoc. 2002 Oct;52(10):471-5.

McMaster-Fay RA. Managing the breech presentation at term: the place of pelvimetry. Aust N Z J Obstet Gynaecol. 2015 Feb;55(1):99.

Meye JF, Mayi S, Zue AS, Engongah-Beka T, Kendjo E, Ole BS. Neonatal prognosis for breech infants delivered vaginally at the Josephine Bongo Maternity Hospital in Libreville, Gabon. Sante. 2003 Apr-Jun;13(2):81-4.

Michel S, Drain A, Closset E, Deruelle P, Ego A, Subtil D, et al. Evaluation of a decision protocol for type of delivery of infants in breech presentation at term. Eur J Obstet Gynecol Reprod Biol. 2011 Oct;158(2):194-8.

Mishra M, Sinha P. Does caesarean section provide the best outcome for mother and baby in breech presentation? A perspective from the developing world. J Obstet Gynaecol. 2011 Aug;31(6):495-8.

Mohammed NB, NoorAli R, Anandakumar C, Qureshi RN, Luby S. Management trend and safety of vaginal delivery for term breech fetuses in a tertiary care hospital of Karachi, Pakistan. J Perinat Med. 2001;29(3):250-9.

Möllmann CJ, Kielland-Kaisen U, Paul B, Schulze S, Jennewein L, Louwen F, Brüggmann D. Vaginal breech delivery of pregnancy before and after the estimated due date-A prospective cohort study. Eur J Obstet Gynecol Reprod Biol. 2020 Sep;252:588-593.

Molkenboer JF, Debie S, Roumen FJ, Smits LJ, Nijhuis JG. Maternal health outcomes two years after term breech delivery. J Matern Fetal Neonatal Med. 2007 Apr;20(4):319-24.

Molkenboer JF, Reijners EP, Nijhuis JG, Roumen FJ. Moderate neonatal morbidity after vaginal term breech delivery. J Matern Fetal Neonatal Med. 2004 Dec;16(6):357-61.

Molkenboer JF, Vencken PM, Sonnemans LG, Roumen FJ, Smits F, Buitendijk SE, et al. Conservative management in breech deliveries leads to similar results compared with cephalic deliveries. J Matern Fetal Neonatal Med. 2007 Aug;20(8):599-603.

Moore WT, Steptoe PP. The experience of the Johns Hopkins Hospital with breech presentation: an analysis of 1,444 cases. Southern Medical Journal. 1943 Apr;36(4):295-303.

Morken NH, Albrechtsen S, Backe B, Iversen OE. Caesarean section does not prevent cerebral palsy in singleton term breech infants. Dev Med Child Neurol. 2010 Jul;52(7):684,5; author reply 685-6.

Mourali M, Kawali A, Fitouhi L, Hadroug L, Gharsa A, Hmila F, et al. Delivery in breech presentation: what way should we choose? Tunis Med. 2013 Jan;91(1):21-6.

Mukuku O, Kimbala J, Kizonde J. Breech vaginal delivery: a study of maternal and neonatal morbidity and mortality. Pan Afr Med J. 2014 Jan 17;17:27.

Münstedt K, von Georgi R, Reucher S, Zygmunt M, Lang U. Term breech and long-term morbidity -- cesarean section versus vaginal breech delivery. Eur J Obstet Gynecol Reprod Biol. 2001 Jun;96(2):163-7.

Nahid F. Outcome of singleton term breech cases in the pretext of mode of delivery. J Pak Med Assoc. 2000 Mar;50(3):81-5.

Nalliah S, Loh KY, Japaraj RP, Mukudan K. Is there a place for selective vaginal breech delivery in Malaysian hospitals: experiences from the Ipoh Hospital. J Matern Fetal Neonatal Med. 2009 Feb;22(2):129-36.

National Accreta Foundation [Internet].: National Accreta Foundation; 2017 [cited Oct 17, 2017]. Available from: https://preventaccreta.org/.

Neu J, Rushing J. Cesarean versus vaginal delivery: long-term infant outcomes and the hygiene hypothesis. Clin Perinatol. 2011 Jun;38(2):321-31.

Nkata M. Perinatal mortality in breech delivery. Trop Doct. 2001 Oct;31(4):222-3. Nkwabong E, Fomulu JN, Kouam L, Ngassa PC. Outcome of breech deliveries in cameroonian nulliparous women. J Obstet Gynaecol India. 2012 Oct;62(5):531-5.

Noblot E, Raia-Barjat T, Lajeunesse C, Trombert B, Weiss S, Colombie M, et al. Training program for the management of

two obstetric emergencies within a French perinatal care network. Eur J Obstet Gynecol Reprod Biol. 2015 Jun;189:101-5.

Nordin NM. An audit of singleton breech deliveries in a hospital with a high rate of vaginal delivery. Malays J Med Sci. 2007 Jan;14(1):28-37.

Oboro VO, Dare FO, Ogunniyi SO. Outcome of term breech by intended mode of delivery. Niger J Med. 2004 Apr-Jun;13(2):106-9.

Odent, Michel, Doris Haire, Sheila Kitzinger, Jane Pincus, and Juliette Levin. 1984. Birth reborn. New York: Pantheon.

Øian P, Albrechtsen S, Berge LN, Børdal PE, Egeland T, Henriksen T: Fødsel av barn i seteleie til termin: assistert vaginal fødsel eller keisersnitt. SMM-report 3/2003. Oslo: The Norwegian Knowledge Centre for the Health Services (NOKC); 2003.

Orji EO, Ajenifuja KO. Planned vaginal delivery versus Caesarean section for breech presentation in Ile-Ife, Nigeria. East Afr Med J. 2003 Nov;80(11):589-91.

Ouattara A, Some AD, Ouattara H, Lankoande J. Prognosis for term breech presentations in Africa (Bobo Dioulasso, Burkina Faso). Med Sante Trop. 2016 May 1;26(2):155-8.

Park YS, Ryu KY, Shim SS, Hoh JK, Park MI. Comparison of fetal heart rate patterns using nonlinear dynamics in breech versus cephalic presentation at term. Early Hum Dev. 2013 Feb;89(2):101-6.

Pasupathy D, Wood AM, Pell JP, Fleming M, Smith GC. Time trend in the risk of delivery-related perinatal and neonatal death associated with breech presentation at term. Int J Epidemiol. 2009 Apr;38(2):490-8.

Paul B, Möllmann CJ, Kielland-Kaisen U, Schulze S, Schaarschmidt W, Bock N, Brüggmann D, Louwen F, Jennewein L; FRABAT FRAnkfurt Breech At Term study group. Maternal and neonatal outcome after vaginal breech delivery at term after cesarean section - a prospective cohort study of the Frankfurt breech at term cohort (FRABAT). Eur J Obstet Gynecol Reprod Biol. 2020 Sep;252:594-598.

Phipps H, Roberts CL, Nassar N, Raynes-Greenow CH, Peat B, Hutton EK. The management of breech pregnancies in Australia and New Zealand. Aust N Z J Obstet Gynaecol. 2003 Aug;43(4):294,7; discussion 261.

Powell R, Walker S, Barrett A. Informed consent to breech birth in New Zealand. N Z Med J. 2015 Aug 7;128(1418):85-92.

Pradhan P, Mohajer M, Deshpande S. Outcome of term breech births: 10-year experience at a district general hospital. BJOG. 2005 Feb;112(2):218-22.

Reijners EP, Roumen FJ. More moderate neonatal morbidity in the case of non-randomized vaginal delivery of term breech pregnancies. Ned Tijdschr Geneeskd. 2001 Aug 11;145(32):1558-61.

Reitter A, Daviss BA, Bisits A, Schollenberger A, Vogl T, Herrmann E, et al. Does pregnancy and/or shifting positions create more room in a woman's pelvis? Am J Obstet Gynecol. 2014 Dec;211(6):662.e1,662.e9.

Reitter A, Halliday A, Walker S. Practical insight into upright breech birth from birth videos: A structured analysis. Birth. 2020 Jun;47(2):211-219.

Rietberg CC, Elferink-Stinkens PM, Brand R, van Loon AJ, Van Hemel OJ, Visser GH. Term breech presentation in The Netherlands from 1995 to 1999: mortality and morbidity in relation to the mode of delivery of 33824 infants. BJOG. 2003 Jun;110(6):604-9.

Rietberg CC, Elferink-Stinkens PM, Visser GH. The effect of the Term Breech Trial on medical intervention behaviour and neonatal outcome in The Netherlands: an analysis of 35,453 term breech infants. BJOG. 2005 Feb;112(2):205-9.

Roberts CL, Peat B, Algert CS, Henderson-Smart D. Term breech birth in New South Wales, 1990-1997. Aust N Z J Obstet Gynaecol. 2000 Feb;40(1):23-9.

Royal College of Obstetricians and Gynaecologists. Management of Breech Presentation: Green-top Guideline No. 20b. BJOG. 2017 Jun;124(7):e151-77.

Rozenberg P. Is there a role for X-ray pelvimetry in the twenty-first century? Gynecol Obstet Fertil. 2007 Jan;35(1):6-12.

Rutgers RA, Van Eygen L. Mortality related to caesarean section in rural Matebeleland North Province, Zimbabwe. Cent Afr J Med. 2008 May-Aug;54(5-8):24-7.

Sanchez-Ramos L, Wells TL, Adair CD, Arcelin G, Kaunitz AM, Wells DS. Route of breech delivery and maternal and neonatal outcomes. Int J Gynaecol Obstet. 2001 Apr;73(1):7-14.

Sänger N, Louwen F, Reinhard J, Yuan J, Hanker L. Signal quality of non-invasive fetal electrocardiogram in vaginal breech delivery: a case-controlled study. Arch Gynecol Obstet. 2013 Nov;288(5):1017-20.

Scamell M. Can all-fours breech birth ever be a reality within the NHS? Pract Midwife. 2010 Jul-Aug;13(7):29-30.

Schiff E, Friedman SA, Mashiach S, Hart O, Barkai G, Sibai BM. Maternal and neonatal outcome of 846 term singleton breech deliveries: seven-year experience at a single center. Am J Obstet Gynecol. 1996 Jul;175(1):18-23.

Schutte JM, Steegers EA, Santema JG, Schuitemaker NW, van Roosmalen J, Maternal Mortality Committee Of The Netherlands Society Of Obstetrics. Maternal deaths after elective cesarean section for breech presentation in the Netherlands. Acta Obstet Gynecol Scand. 2007;86(2):240-3.

Sibony O, Touitou S, Luton D, Oury JF, Blot PH. A comparison of the neonatal morbidity of second twins to that of a low-risk population. Eur J Obstet Gynecol Reprod Biol. 2003 Jun 10;108(2):157-63.

Singh A, Mishra N, Dewangan R. Delivery in breech presentation: the decision making. J Obstet Gynaecol India. 2012 Aug;62(4):401-5.

Siváková J, Biringer K, Hrtankova M, Sumichrastova P, Kudela E, Sivak S, et al. Breech presentation - an analysis of results in one perinatal center. Ceska Gynekol. 2014 Apr;79(2):107-14.

Sletten J, Kessler J. QRS abnormalities of the fetal electrocardiogram, and their implications for ST-interval analysis during labor. Acta Obstet Gynecol Scand. 2015 Oct;94(10):1128-35.

Sobande A, Yousuf F, Eskandar M, Almushait MA. Breech delivery before and after the term breech trial recommendation. Saudi Med J. 2007 Aug;28(8):1213-7.

Sobande AA. Pregnancy outcome in singleton term breeches from a referral hospital in Saudi Arabia. West Afr J Med. 2003 Jan-Mar;22(1):38-41.

Sobande A, Archibong EI, Abdelmoneim I, Albar HM. Changing patterns in the management and outcome of breech presentation over a 7-year period. Review from a referral hospital in Saudi Arabia. J Obstet Gynaecol. 2003 Jan;23(1):34-7.

Sorensen HT, Steffensen FH, Olsen J, Sabroe S, Gillman MW, Fischer P, et al. Long-term follow-up of cognitive outcome after breech presentation at birth. Epidemiology. 1999 Sep;10(5):554-6.

Steer PJ. Breech labour is not a particular indication for STAN monitoring. BJOG. 2015 Mar;122(4):535,0528.13038. Epub 2014 Aug 12.

Stefanović M, Lukic B, Kutlešić R, Vukomanović P. Vaginal birth in breech presentation in morbidly obese woman. J Obstet Gynaecol. 2018 Aug;38(6):876-877. doi: 10.1080/01443615.2017.1394991. Epub 2018 Mar 20.

Sullivan EA, Moran K, Chapman M. Term breech singletons and caesarean section: a population study, Australia 1991-2005. Aust N Z J Obstet Gynaecol. 2009 Oct;49(5):456-60.

Swedish Collaborative Breech Study Group. Term breech delivery in Sweden: mortality relative to fetal presentation and planned mode of delivery. Acta Obstet Gynecol Scand. 2005 Jun;84(6):593-601.

Sy T, Diallo Y, Diallo A, Soumah A, Diallo FB, Hyjazi Y, et al. Breech presentation: mode of delivery and maternal and fetal outcomes at the Dean Clinic of Gynecology and Obstetrics, Conakry University Hospital. Mali Med. 2011;26(2):41-4.

Takai IU, Kwayabura AS, Bukar M, Idrissa A, Obed JY. A 5-year retrospective review of singleton term breech deliveries seen at a tertiary hospital in northern Nigeria. Arch Int Surg. 2016;6:7-11.

Thavagnanam S, Fleming J, Bromley A, Shields MD, Cardwell CR. A meta-analysis of the association between Caesarean section and childhood asthma. Clin Exp Allergy. 2008 Apr;38(4):629-33.

Toijonen A, Palomaki O, Huhtala H, Uotila J. Selective vaginal breech delivery at term - still an option. Acta Obstet Gynecol Scand. 2012 Oct;91(10):1177-83.

Toijonen A, Palomaki O, Huhtala H, Uotila J. Maternal experiences of vaginal breech delivery. Birth. 2014 Dec;41(4):316-22.

Toijonen A, Palomaki O, Huhtala H, Uotila J. Cardiotocography in breech versus vertex delivery: an examiner-blinded, cross-sectional nested case-control study. BMC Pregnancy Childbirth. 2016 Oct 21;16(1):319.

Trolle D. Considerations on breech presentation as an indication for caesarean section. Dan Med Bull: 1960 Jul;7:117-20.

Turner MJ. The Term Breech Trial: are the clinical guidelines justified by the evidence? J Obstet Gynaecol. 2006 Aug;26(6):491-4.

Ulander VM, Gissler M, Nuutila M, Ylikorkala O. Are health expectations of term breech infants unrealistically high? Acta Obstet Gynecol Scand. 2004 Feb;83(2):180-6.

Uotila J, Tuimala R, Kirkinen P. Good perinatal outcome in selective vaginal breech delivery at term. Acta Obstet Gynecol Scand. 2005 Jun;84(6):578-83.

Usta IM, Nassar AH, Khabbaz AY, Abu Musa AA. Undiagnosed term breech: impact on mode of delivery and neonatal outcome. Acta Obstet Gynecol Scand. 2003 Sep;82(9):841-4.

van Bogaert LJ, Misra A. Neonatal outcomes after vaginal and caesarean breech delivery. S Afr Med J. 2007 Oct;97(10):949.

van den Akker T. Who pays the price? (Foreign) women and future siblings. 1st Amsterdam Breech Conference; June 30, 2016; Amsterdam, The Netherlands.

van Dillen J, Zwart JJ, Schutte J, Bloemenkamp KW, van Roosmalen J. Severe acute maternal morbidity and mode of delivery in the Netherlands. Acta Obstet Gynecol Scand. 2010 Nov;89(11):1460-5.

van Eygen L, Rutgers S. Caesarean section as preferred mode of delivery in term breech presentations is not a realistic option in rural Zimbabwe. Trop Doct. 2008 Jan;38(1):36-9.

van Roosmalen J, van den Akker T. Safety concerns for caesarean section. BJOG. 2014 Jun;121(7):909-10.

Vázquez JA, Villanueva LA, Lara-Figueroa G, Martínez-Ayala H, Garcia-Lara E. Association between gestational age, weight, and Apgar score in newborns extracted in pelvic presentation. Ginecol Obstet Mex. 2001 Mar;69:122-5.

Vendittelli F, Pons JC, Lemery D, Mamelle N, Obstetricians of the AUDIPOG Sentinel Network. The term breech presentation: Neonatal results and obstetric practices in France. Eur J Obstet Gynecol Reprod Biol. 2006 Apr 1;125(2):176-84.

Vendittelli F, Riviere O, Pons JC, Mamelle N, Obstetriciens du Reseau Sentinelle AUDIPOG. Breech presentation at term: evolution of French practices and an analysis of neonatal results in regards to obstetrical management of breech presentation, from AUDIPOG Database. J Gynecol Obstet Biol Reprod (Paris). 2002 May;31(3):261-72.

Verhoeven AT, de Leeuw JP, Bruinse HW. Breech presentation at term: elective caesarean section is the wrong choice as a standard treatment because of too high risks for the mother and her future children. Ned Tijdschr Geneeskd. 2005 Oct 1;149(40):2207-10.

Vidaeff AC. Breech delivery before and after the term breech trial. Clin Obstet Gynecol. 2006 Mar;49(1):198-210.

Villar J, Carroli G, Zavaleta N, Donner A, Wojdyla D, Faundes A, et al. Maternal and neonatal individual risks and benefits associated with caesarean delivery: multicentre prospective study. BMJ. 2007 Nov 17;335(7628):1025.

Visser GH, Rietberg CC, Oepkes D, Vandenbussche FP. Breech presentation: infant versus mother. Ned Tijdschr Geneeskd. 2005 Oct 1;149(40):2211-4.

Vistad I, Cvancarova M, Hustad BL, Henriksen T. Vaginal breech delivery: results of a prospective registration study. BMC Pregnancy Childbirth. 2013 Jul 24;13:153,2393-13-153.

Vistad I, Klungsoyr K, Albrechtsen S, Skjeldestad FE. Neonatal outcome of singleton term breech deliveries in Norway from 1991 to 2011. Acta Obstet Gynecol Scand. 2015 Sep;94(9):997-1004.

Vlemmix F, Bergenhenegouwen L, Schaaf JM, Ensing S, Rosman AN, Ravelli AC, et al. Term breech deliveries in the Netherlands: did the increased cesarean rate affect neonatal outcome? A population-based cohort study. Acta Obstet Gynecol Scand. 2014 Sep;93(9):888-96.

Walker S. Breech birth: an unusual normal. Pract Midwife. 2012 Mar;15(3):18, 20-1.

Walker S, Dasgupta T, Shennan A, Sandall J, Bunce C, Roberts P. Development of a core outcome set for effectiveness studies of breech birth at term (Breech-COS)-an international multi-stakeholder Delphi study: study protocol. Trials. 2022 Apr 4;23(1):249.

Walker S, Dasgupta T, Halliday A, Reitter A. Development of a core outcome set for effectiveness studies of breech birth at term (Breech-COS): A systematic review on variations in outcome reporting. Eur J Obstet Gynecol Reprod Biol. 2021 Aug;263:117-126.

Walker S, Breslin E, Scamell M, Parker P. Effectiveness of vaginal breech birth training strategies: An integrative review of the literature. Birth. 2017 Jun;44(2):101-9.

Walker S, Parker P, Scamell M. Expertise in physiological breech birth: A mixed-methods study. Birth. 2018 Jun;45(2):202-209.

Walker S, Spillane E. Face-to-pubes rotational maneuver for bilateral nuchal arms in a vaginal breech birth, resolved in an upright maternal position: A case report. Birth. 2020 Jun;47(2):246-252.

Walker S, Powell RL. Low overall mortality and morbidity for breech babies in the Netherlands. Acta Obstet Gynecol Scand. 2014 Dec;93(12):1329.

Walker S, Reading C, Silverwood-Cope O, Cochrane V. Physiological breech birth. Evaluation of a training programme for birth professionals. Pract Midwife. 2017 Feb;20(2):25-8.

Walker S, Scamell M, Parker P. Principles of physiological breech birth practice: A Delphi study. Midwifery. 2016 Dec;43:1-6.

Walker S, Scamell M, Parker P. Standards for maternity care professionals attending planned upright breech births: A Delphi study. Midwifery. 2016 Mar;34:7-14.

Walker S. Response to: vaginal birth in breech presentation in morbidly obese woman. J Obstet Gynaecol. 2019 Apr;39(3):437-438.

Walker S, Reitter A. The structure of breech revolutions, a response to: "Upright breech birth: New video research risks reviving Friedman's curse". Birth. 2022 Mar;49(1):16-18.

Walker S. Turning breech upside down: upright breech birth. MIDIRS Midwifery Digest. 2015;25(30:325-330.

Walker S, Cochrane V. Unexpected breech: what can midwives do? Pract Midwife. 2015 Nov;18(10):26-9.

Whyte H, Hannah ME, Saigal S, Hannah WJ, Hewson S, Amankwah K, et al. Outcomes of children at 2 years after planned cesarean birth versus planned vaginal birth for breech presentation at term: the International Randomized Term Breech Trial. Am J Obstet Gynecol. 2004 Sep;191(3):864-71.

Wildschut HI, van Belzen-Slappendel H, Jans S. The art of vaginal breech birth at term on all fours. Clin Case Rep. 2017 Jan 23;5(2):182-6.

Wright RC. Reduction of perinatal mortality and morbidity in breech delivery through routine use of cesarean section. Obstet Gynecol. 1959 Dec;14:758-63.

Zander N, Raimann FJ, Al Naimi A, Brüggmann D, Louwen F, Jennewein L. Combined Assessment of the Obstetrical Conjugate and Fetal Birth Weight Predicts Birth Mode Outcome in Vaginally Intended Breech Deliveries of Primiparous Women-A Frabat Study. J Clin Med. 2022 Jun 3;11(11):3201.

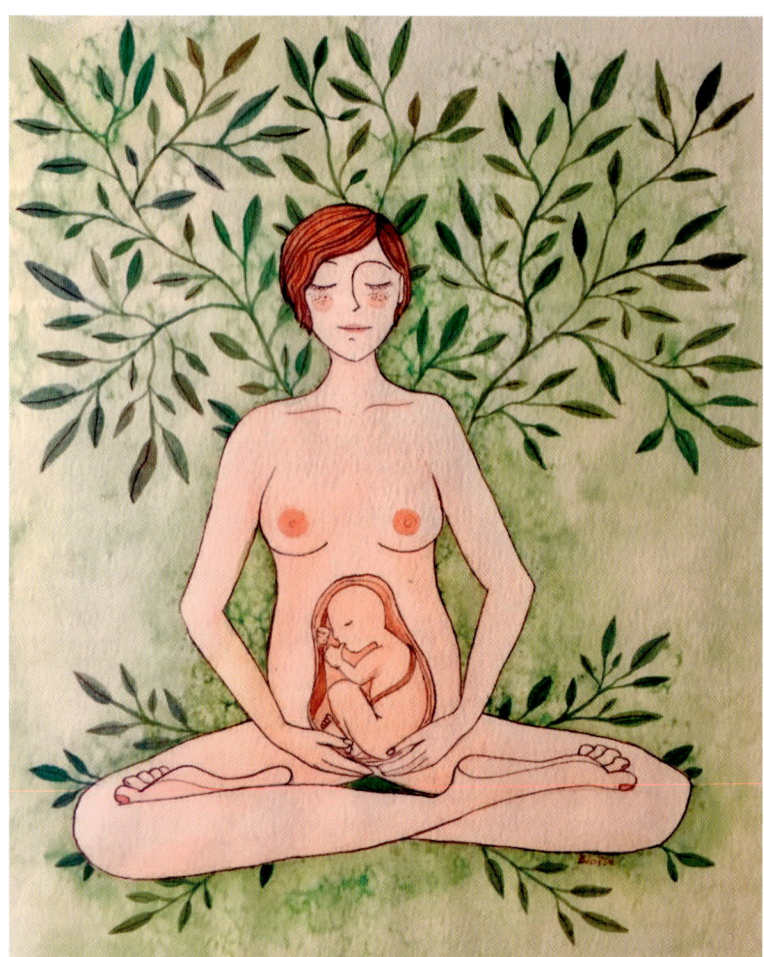

Artwork by a mother of two breech babies: the first born by C-section, the second vaginally (VBAC in a Canadian hospital)

249

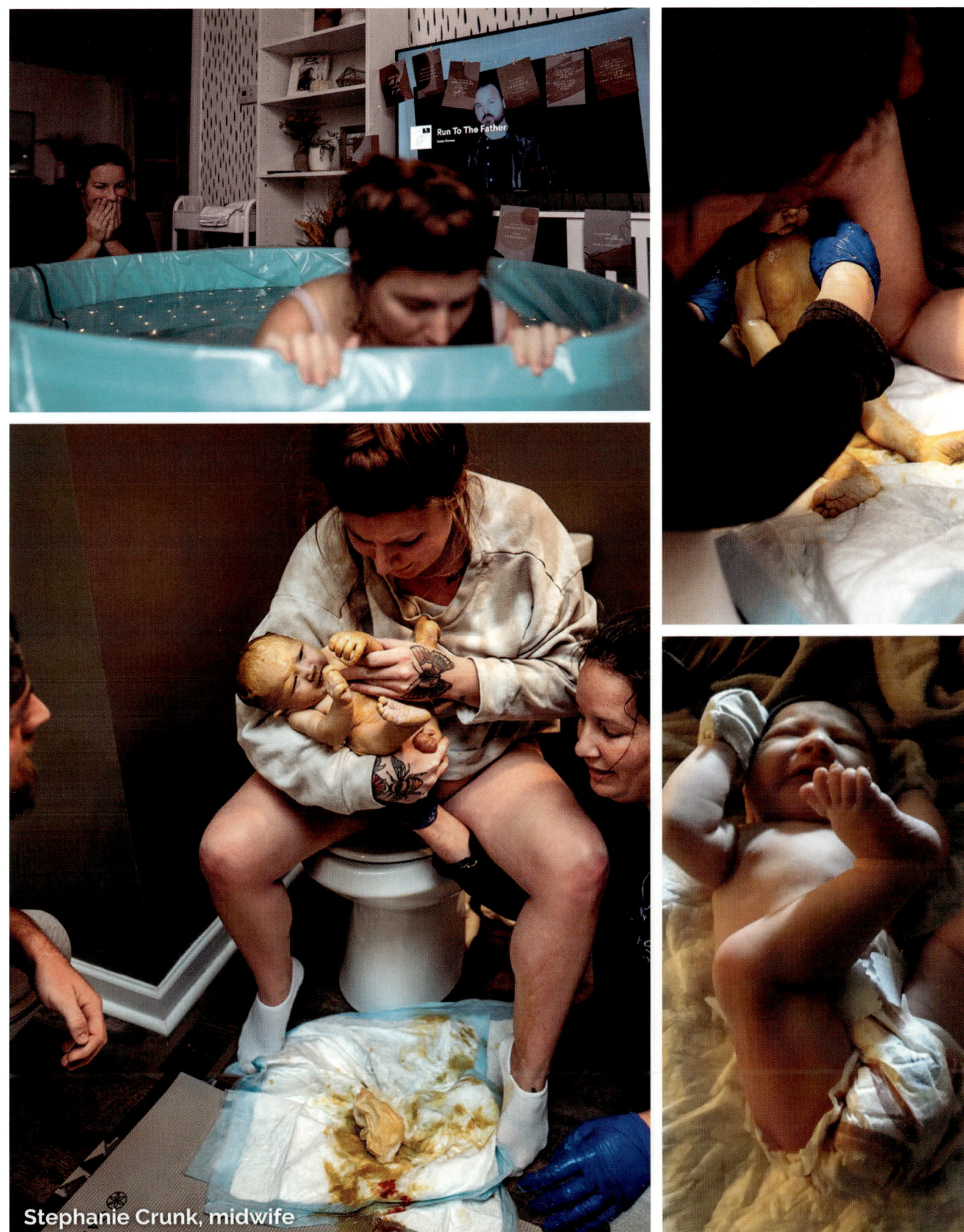

Stephanie Crunk, midwife

© 2022 Breech Without Borders

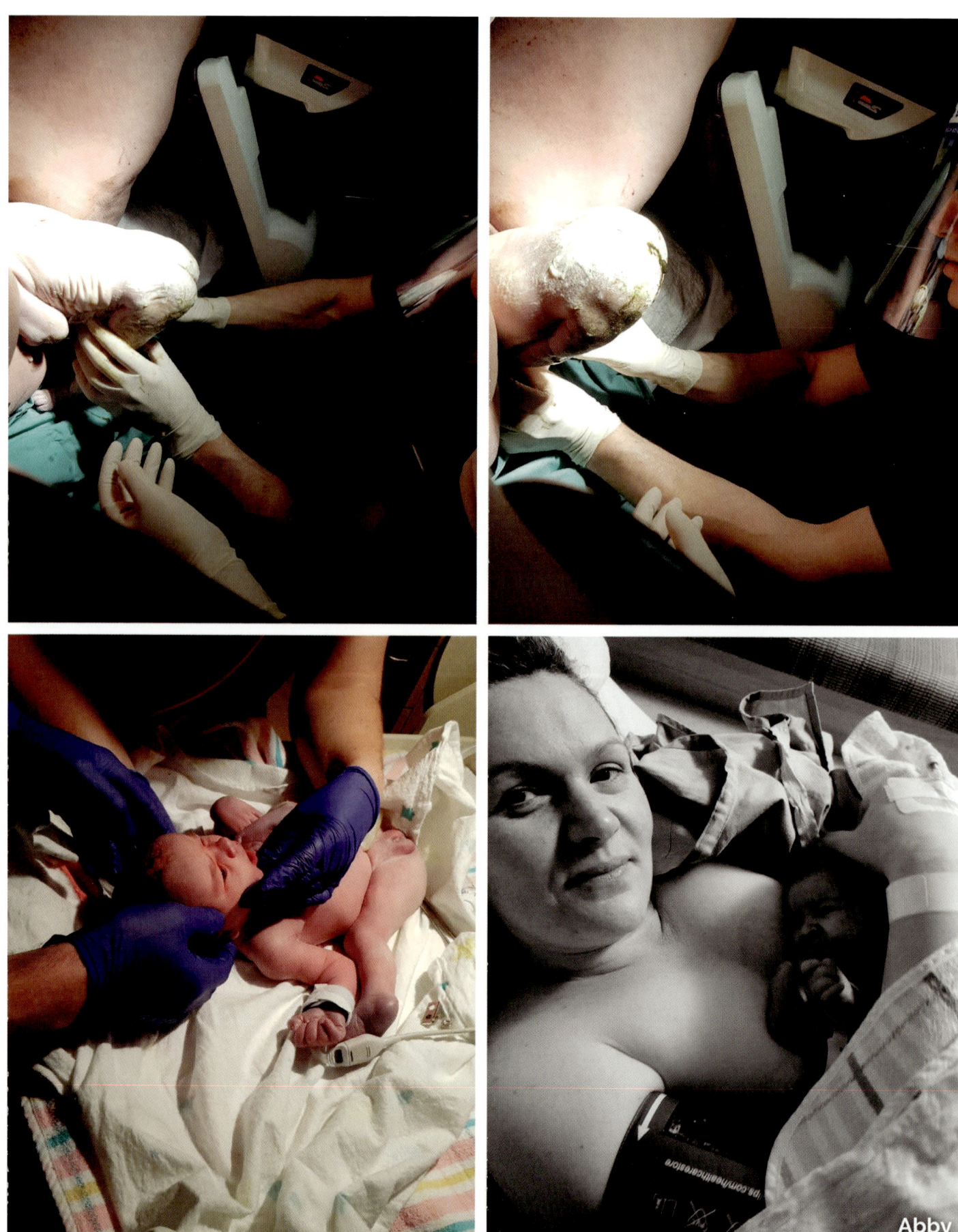

Abby

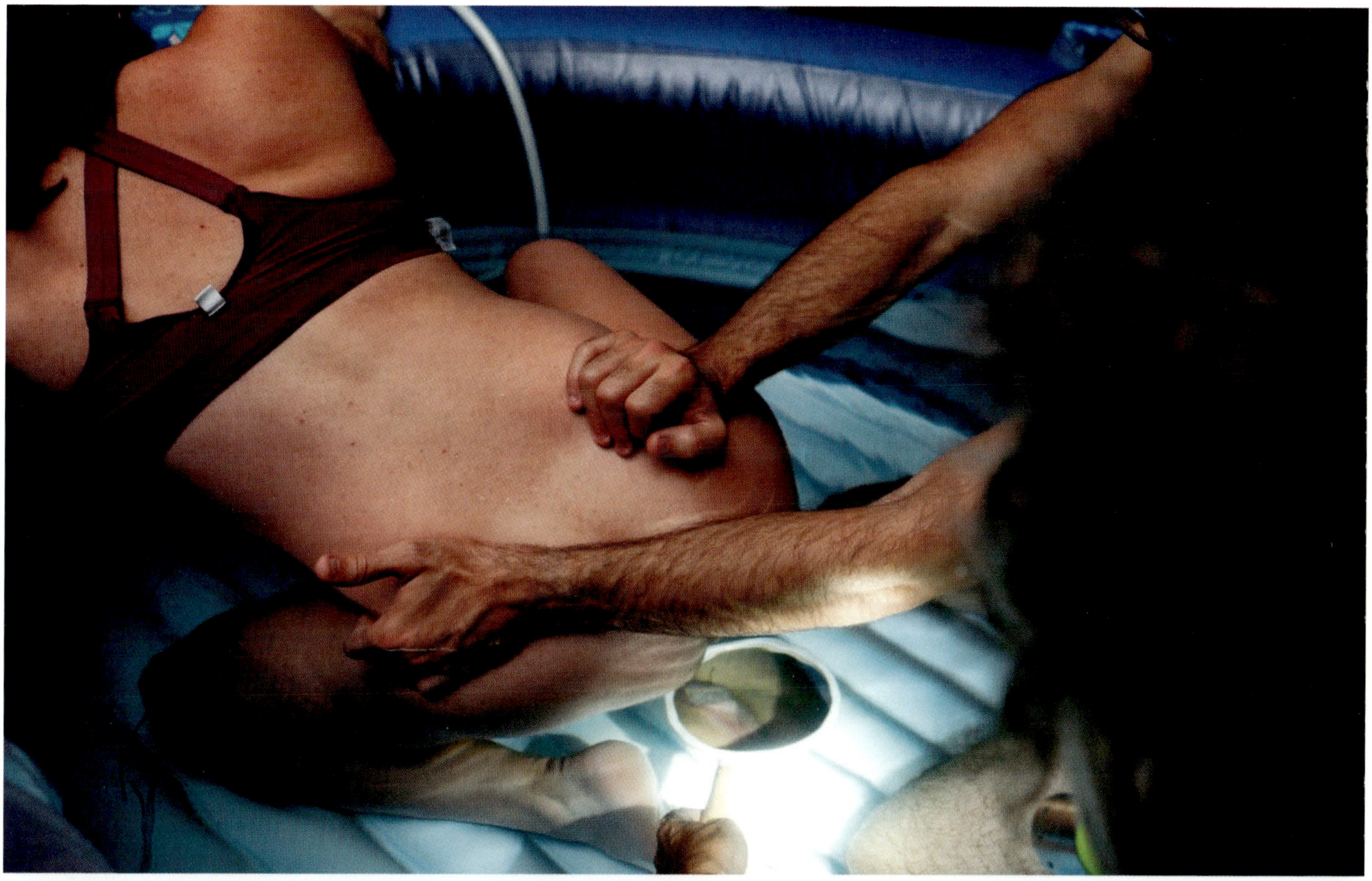

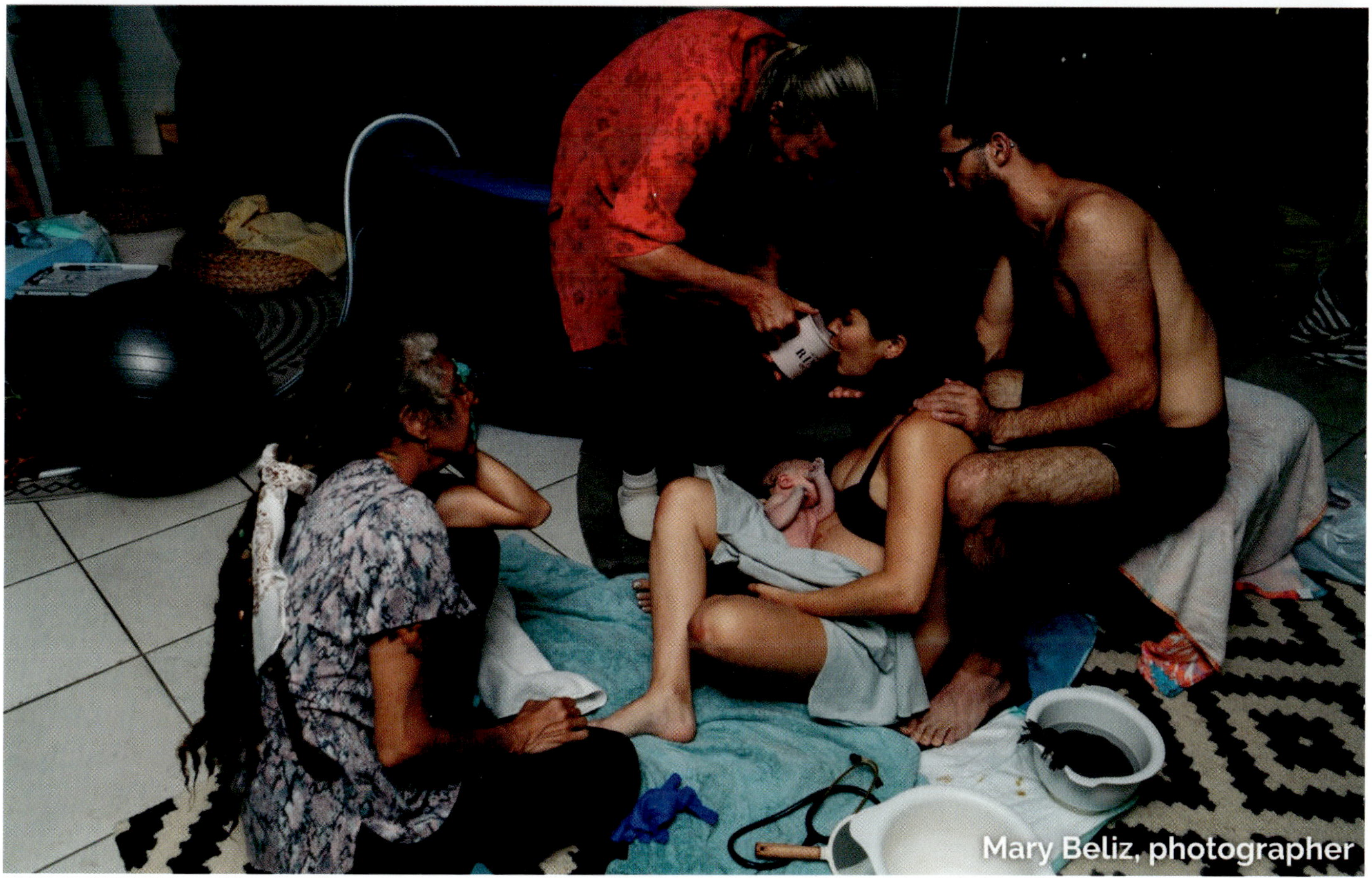

Mary Beliz, photographer

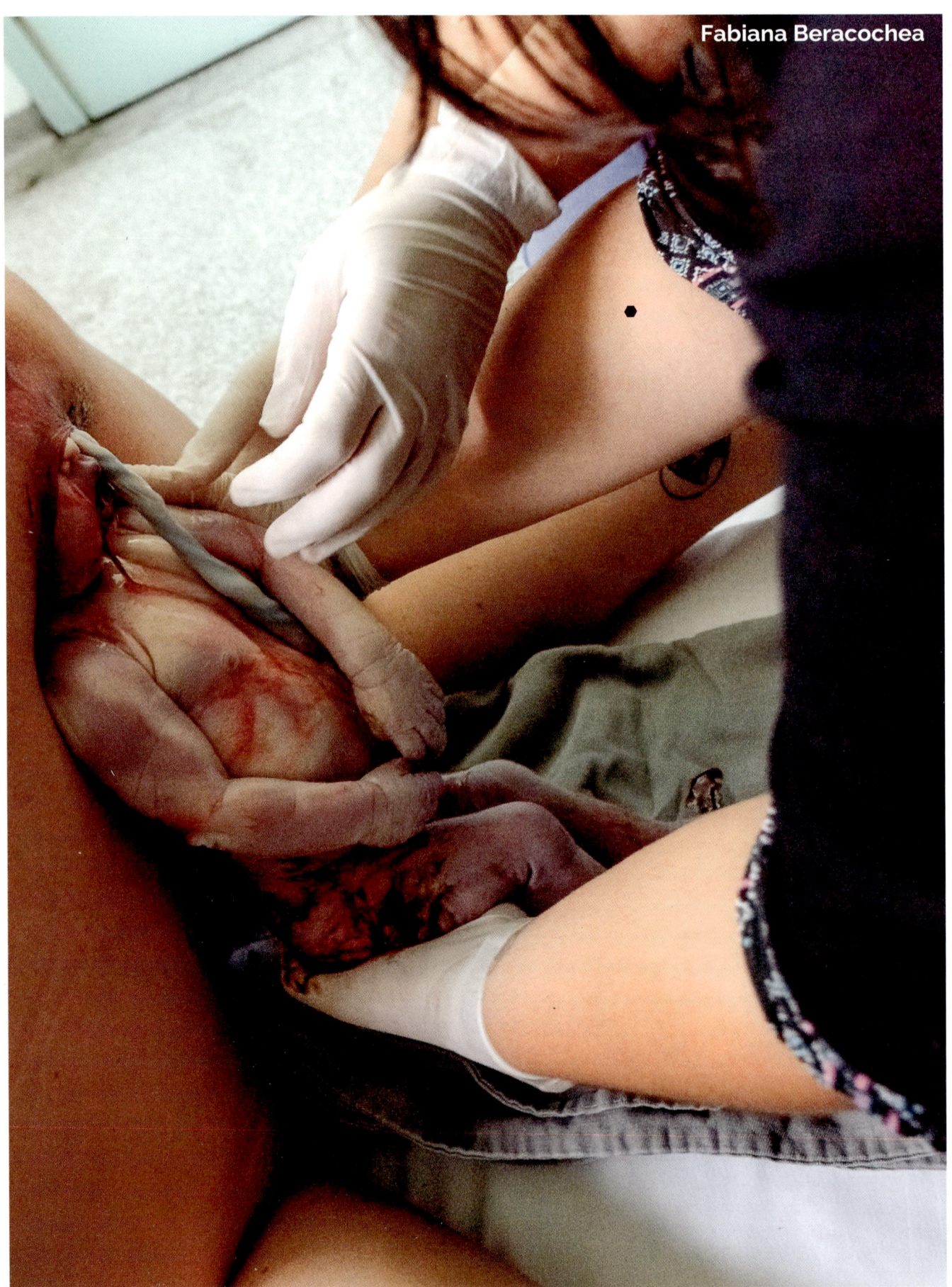

Fabiana Beracochea